MATRIX METALLOPROTEINASE INHIBITORS IN CANCER THERAPY

CANCER DRUG DISCOVERY AND DEVELOPMENT

Beverly A. Teicher, Series Editor

Matrix Metalloproteinase Inhibitors in Cancer Therapy

Edited by

Neil J. Clendeninn, MD, PhD

Corporate V.P., Clinical Affairs
Agouron Pharmaceuticals Inc., San Diego, CA

and

Krzysztof Appelt, PhD

Department of Research Pharmacology,
Agouron Pharmaceuticals Inc., San Diego, CA

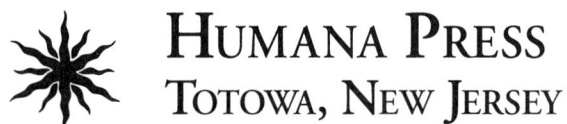

Humana Press
Totowa, New Jersey

© 2001 Humana Press Inc.
999 Riverview Drive, Suite 208
Totowa, New Jersey 07512

For additional copies, pricing for bulk purchases, and/or information about other Humana titles, contact Humana at the above address or at any of the following numbers: Tel.: 973-256-1699; Fax: 973-256-8341; E-mail: humana@humanapr.com or visit our Website: http://humanapress.com

Due diligence has been taken by the publishers, editors, and authors of this book to assure the accuracy of the information published and to describe generally accepted practices. The contributors herein have carefully checked to ensure that the drug selections and dosages set forth in this text are accurate and in accord with the standards accepted at the time of publication. Notwithstanding, as new research, changes in government regulations, and knowledge from clinical experience relating to drug therapy and drug reactions constantly occurs, the reader is advised to check the product information provided by the manufacturer of each drug for any change in dosages or for additional warnings and contraindications. This is of utmost importance when the recommended drug herein is a new or infrequently used drug. It is the responsibility of the treating physician to determine dosages and treatment strategies for individual patients. Further it is the responsibility of the health care provider to ascertain the Food and Drug Administration status of each drug or device used in their clinical practice. The publisher, editors, and authors are not responsible for errors or omissions or for any consequences from the application of the information presented in this book and make no warranty, express or implied, with respect to the contents in this publication.

This publication is printed on acid-free paper. ∞
ANSI Z39.48-1984 (American National Standards Institute) Permanence of Paper for Printed Library Materials.

Cover design by Patricia F. Cleary.

Photocopy Authorization Policy:
Authorization to photocopy items for internal or personal use, or the internal or personal use of specific clients, is granted by Humana Press Inc., provided that the base fee of US $10.00 per copy, plus US $00.25 per page, is paid directly to the Copyright Clearance Center at 222 Rosewood Drive, Danvers, MA 01923. For those organizations that have been granted a photocopy license from the CCC, a separate system of payment has been arranged and is acceptable to Humana Press Inc. The fee code for users of the Transactional Reporting Service is: [0-89603-668-5/01 $10.00 + $00.25].

Printed in the United States of America.   10 9 8 7 6 5 4 3 2 1

Library of Congress Cataloging-in-Publication Data

Matrix metalloproteinase inhibitors in cancer therapy / edited by Neil J. Clendeninn and Krzysztof Appelt.
      p. ; cm.—(Cancer drug discovery and development)
   Includes bibliographical references and index.
   ISBN 0-89603-668-5 (alk. paper)
   1. Metalloproteinases—Inhibitors—Therapeutic use. 2. Extracellular matrix proteins. 3. Cancer—Chemotherapy. I. Clendeninn, Neil J. II. Appelt, Krzysztof. III. Series.
   [DNLM: 1. Metalloproteinases—antagonists & inhibitors. 2.
   Neoplasms—drug therapy. QU 136 M4338 2000]
   RC271.M43 M38 2000
   616.99'4061—dc21
                                                         99-089543

PREFACE

Remodeling of the extracellular matrix is a well-ordered biological process necessary for many functions, including tissue growth and regeneration, angiogenesis, collagen turnover, and cellular migration. Perturbation of the remodeling process is a hallmark of several diseases and pathological stages, such as tumor growth, invasion and metastasis, rheumatoid- and osteoarthritis, and a variety of pathologies that include neovascularization. Although several pathways for the degradation of extracellular matrices have been identified, the most universal yet-discovered utilizes enzymes known as matrix metalloproteinases (MMPs). MMPs are a family of highly homologous, zinc- and calcium-dependent endopeptidases that cleave most, if not all, components of the extracellular matrix.

More than 20 members of the family of human MMPs have been identified. The enzymes share a high degree of structural homology, but differ significantly in substrate specificity. Collagenases 1, 2, and 3 (MMPs 1, 8, and 13 or fibroblast, neutrophil, and osteoblast collagenases, respectively) efficiently degrade triple helical collagens I, II, and III at neutral pH. Gelatinases A and B (MMPs 2 and 9) degrade basement membrane collagen type IV, gelatin, and other proteoglycan components of the extracellular matrix. Highly related stromelysins 1 and 2 (MMPs 3 and 10) and the smallest member of the family, matrilysin (MMP 7), degrade various collagens, as well as fibronectin, laminin, and other proteoglycan components. In addition, the activity of various MMPs is required for activation of particular proteolytic cascades or for degradation of serpins, natural inhibitors of serine proteases.

Matrix metalloproteinases are expressed by many cell types in response to cytokines and growth factors, and in most cases are secreted as proenzymes. Enzyme activation in the extracellular environment requires coordinated activity of various serine proteases and an autoactivation step critical for optimal activity on natural substrates. In addition, the activation and activity of MMPs are further controlled by coordinated expressions of natural MMP inhibitors, the "tissue inhibitors of metalloproteinases" (TIMPs). In a variety of pathological processes, the balance of TIMP and MMP expression is perturbed, leading to locally increased proteolytic activity of MMPs and uncontrolled degradation of the extracellular matrix.

Expression of MMPs by tumors and surrounding stromal components has been studied extensively by *in situ* hybridization techniques, immunofluorescence, and enzyme zymography. The emerging pattern of MMP expression is complicated, and there is some controversy over which MMPs are most commonly associated with growing and invasive tumors.

Matrix Metalloproteinase Inhibitors in Cancer Therapy covers the entire field, from the biology of MMPs through current clinical studies. In the first half of the book several authors discuss the molecular mechanisms of the enzymes, substrates, and natural inhibitors, as well as the design strategy for MMP inhibitors. The remainder of the book is devoted to many of the individual pharmaceutical companies and their particular research on MMP inhibitors. Each company will approach this by discussing their own design strategy, providing the in vitro activity, animal model work, and if available, toxicology and human clinical trial safety and efficacy of their respective MMP inhibitors.

All of this represents a work in progress. We each recognize that our knowledge within this field is being expanded rapidly through new discoveries and analysis of current information. It is hoped that *Matrix Metalloproteinase Inhibitors in Cancer Therapy* not only provides a background for students, scientists, and clinicians, but will also help continue our efforts aimed at our understanding of the biologic process of extracellular matrix remodeling and its implications for human disease.

Neil J. Clendeninn, MD, PhD
Krzysztof Appelt, PhD

CONTENTS

CONTRIBUTORS

KRZYSZTOF APPELT, PhD • *Department of Research Pharmacology, Agouron Pharmaceuticals Inc., San Diego, CA*

R. BANNISTER, PhD • *Chiroscience R & D Ltd., Cambridge, UK*

A.D. BAXTER, PhD • *Chiroscience R & D Ltd., Cambridge, UK*

STEVE BENDER, PhD • *Department of Research Pharmacology, Agouron Pharmaceuticals, Inc., San Diego, CA*

R. BHOGAL, PhD • *Chiroscience R & D Ltd., Cambridge, UK*

J.B. BIRD, PhD • *Chiroscience R & D Ltd., Cambridge, UK*

HANS BRANDSTETTER, PhD • *Structural Research, Max-Planck-Institute for Biochemistry, Martinsried, Germany*

PETER D. BROWN, DPhil • *British Biotech Pharmaceuticals Ltd., Oxford, UK*

GEORGE CLEMENS, PhD • *Pharmaceutical Division, Bayer Corporation, West Haven, CT*

NEIL J. CLENDENINN, MD, PhD • *Agouron Pharmaceuticals Inc., San Diego, CA*

MARY COLLIER, BS • *Department of Research Pharmacology, Agouron Pharmaceuticals Inc., San Diego, CA*

LISA M. COUSSENS, PhD • *Cancer Research Institute, Department of Pathology, UCSF, San Francisco, CA*

ALAN H. DAVIDSON, MA, PhD • *British Biotech Pharmaceuticals Ltd., Oxford, UK*

ALAN H. DRUMMOND, PhD • *British Biotech Pharmaceuticals Ltd., Oxford, UK*

DYLAN R. EDWARDS, PhD • *School of Biological Sciences, University of East Anglia, Norwich, Norfolk, UK*

RICHARD A. ENGH, PhD • *Chemical Research, Roche Diagnostics GmbH, Mannheim, Germany*

BARBARA FINGLETON, PhD • *Department of Cell Biology, Vanderbilt University Medical Center, Nashville, TN*

ANDREW GEARING, PhD • *British Biotech Pharmaceuticals Ltd., Oxford, UK*

DAGMAR GLITZ, PhD • *Biological Research, Roche Diagnostics GmbH, Penzberg, Germany*

ERICH GRAF V. ROEDERN, PhD • *Max-Planck-Institute for Biochemistry, Bioorganic Chemistry, Martinsried, Germany*

FRANK GRAMS, PhD • *Molecular Design, F. Hoffman-La Roche Ltd., Basel, Switzerland*

J. HENSHILWOOD, PhD • *Chiroscience R & D Ltd., Cambridge, UK*

BARBARA HIBNER, PhD • *Pharmaceutical Division, Bayer Corporation, West Haven, CT*

RACHEL HUMPHREY, MD • *Pharmaceutical Division, Bayer Corporation, West Haven, CT*

ROBERT C. JACKSON, PhD • *Chiroscience R&D Ltd., Cambridge, UK*

HAROLD KLUENDER, PhD • *Pharmaceutical Division, Bayer Corporation, West Haven, CT*

HANS-WILLI KRELL, PhD • *Biological Research, Roche Diagnostics GmbH, Penzberg, Germany*

VALERIA LIVI, PhD • *Novuspharma SpA, Monza, Italy*

D.T. MANALLACK, PhD • *Chiroscience R & D Ltd., Cambridge, UK*

LYNN M. MATRISIAN, PhD • *Department of Cell Biology, Vanderbilt University Medical Center, Nashville, TN*

ERNESTO MENTA, PhD • *Novuspharma SpA, Monza, Italy*

LORI-ANN MINASI, PhD • *Scientific Communication, Pharmaceutical Division, Bayer Corporation, West Haven, CT*

J. MONTANA, PhD • *Chiroscience R & D Ltd., Cambridge, UK*

LUIS MORODER, PhD • *Bioorganic Chemistry, Max-Planck-Institute for Biochemistry, Martinsried, Germany*

J. CONSTANZE D. MÜLLER, PhD • *Bioorganic Chemistry, Max-Planck-Institute for Biochemistry, Martinsried, Germany*

HIDEAKI NAGASE, PhD • *The Kennedy Institute of Rheumatology, London, UK*

MICHAEL R. NEISMAN, PhD • *Agouron Pharmaceuticals Inc., San Diego, CA.*

ANTHONY NERI, PhD • *Department of Research Pharmacology, Agouron Pharmaceuticals Inc., San Diego, CA*

D.A. OWEN, PhD • *Chiroscience R & D Ltd., Cambridge, UK*

YAZDI PITHAVALA, PhD • *Department of Research Pharmacology, Agouron Pharmaceuticals Inc., San Diego, CA*

DAVID R. SHALINSKY, PhD • *Department of Research Pharmacology, Agouron Pharmaceuticals Inc., San Diego, CA*

BHASKER SHETTY, PhD • *Department of Research Pharmacology, Agouron Pharmaceuticals Inc., San Diego, CA*

MARK D. STERNLICHT, PhD • *Department of Anatomy, UCSF,*
  San Francisco, CA

THIENNU H. VU, MD, PhD • *Department of Anatomy, UCSF, San*
  Francisco, CA

R.W. WATSON, PhD • *Chiroscience R & D Ltd., Cambridge, UK*

STEPHANIE WEBBER, PhD • *Department of Research Pharmacology,*
  Agouron Pharmaceuticals Inc., San Diego, CA

ZENA WERB, PhD • *Department of Anatomy, UCSF, San Francisco, CA*

MARK WHITTAKER, DPhil • *British Biotech Pharmaceuticals Ltd.,*
  Oxford, UK

SCOTT WILHELM, PhD • *Pharmaceutical Division, Bayer Corporation,*
  West Haven, CT

GERD ZIMMERMANN, PhD • *Chemical Research, Roche Diagnostics*
  Boehringer Mannheim GmbH, Mannheim, Germany

MATRIX METALLOPROTEINASE
INHIBITORS IN CANCER THERAPY

1 Biology and Regulation of the Matrix Metalloproteinases

Mark D. Sternlicht, PhD,
Lisa M. Coussens, PhD,
Thiennu H. Vu, MD, PhD,
and Zena Werb, PhD

1. INTRODUCTION

Matrix metalloproteinases (MMPs) are the predominant family of enzymes that degrade extracellular matrix and cell surface molecules. Like the proteins they modify, the MMPs and their endogenous inhibitors, the tissue inhibitors of metalloproteinases (TIMPs), play a critical role in diverse physiologic and pathologic processes, including embryonic development, tissue morphogenesis, wound re-

From: *Cancer Drug Discovery and Development:*
Matrix Metalloproteinase Inhibitors in Cancer Therapy
Edited by: Neil J. Clendeninn and Krzysztof Appelt © Humana Press Inc., Totowa, NJ

pair, arthritis, and cancer *(1–3)*. Indeed, several MMPs were first cloned from cancer cell lines, and most human MMPs have been detected in one tumor cell line or another *(1,4)*. In actual carcinomas however, the MMPs are usually expressed by the adjacent and intervening stromal cells rather than by the malignant cells themselves *(1,4)*. Nevertheless, the overexpression of MMPs usually correlates with more aggressive tumor behavior and a poor prognosis. Moreover, cancer cells can be made even more aggressive in vitro and in vivo by MMP overexpression or TIMP down-regulation, or they can be made less aggressive by MMP down-regulation, TIMP overexpression, or the addition of exogenous MMP inhibitors. Thus several MMPs have been shown to act as key agonists during tumor invasion, metastasis, and angiogenesis *(1,4)*. In addition, some MMPs may contribute to initial tumor development *(5–9)*, thus raising the possible clinical utility of inhibiting select MMPs during early as well as late stages of cancer progression.

The MMPs constitute a multigene family of enzymes within the metalloproteinase class and "metzincin" superfamily of endopeptidases *(10)*. As a class, metalloproteinases are distinguished from "serine," "cysteine," and "aspartic" proteinases by their essential catalytic group and their sensitivity to the class-specific inhibitor 1,10-phenanthroline *(10)*. Metzincins, in turn, are distinguished from other metalloproteinases by a conserved structural topology, a consensus motif containing three histidines that bind zinc at the catalytic site, and a conserved methionine-containing "Met-turn" motif that sits below the active site zinc (Fig. 1) *(11)*. The signature three-histidine zinc-binding motif of the metzincins is **HEBXHXBGBXHZ**, where bold amino acids are invariant, B is a bulky hydrophobic residue, X is a variable residue, and Z is a family-specific residue.* Likewise, the "Met-turn" contains a number of family-specific residues *(11)*. In the case of the MMPs, the zinc-binding motif is usually **HEF/LGHS/ALGLXHS**,

---

*Metzincins are separated into four distinct families based on, among other things, the identity of the ultimate residue of the zinc-binding motif: i.e., Z is Asp in the "ADAMs/adamalysins," Glu in the "astacins," Pro in the "serralysins," and Ser in all but a few MMPs *(11)*. The adamalysins (reprolysins) are soluble snake venom proteins and the ADAMs are transmembrane cell surface proteins that contain both a disintegrin and metalloproteinase domain *(12)*. The ADAMs can potentially mediate proteolysis, cell adhesion, cell-cell fusion, and cellular signaling via their various domains, and thus they are likely to be important mediators of several physiologic processes *(13)*. The astacins include bone morphogenetic protein-1 which is the type I procollagen C-proteinase, mammalian tolloid which may activate certain growth factors, and meprins A and B which are thought to process peptide hormones and possibly extracellular matrix molecules as well *(14)*. Serralysins are large bacterial enzymes, some of which play an important part in the virulence and pathogenicity of certain bacteria *(15)*. Some of these metzincins as well as some nonmetzincin metalloproteinases warrant consideration during the design of MMP inhibitors due to their potential susceptibility to such inhibitors as well as their possible value as targets for inhibition.

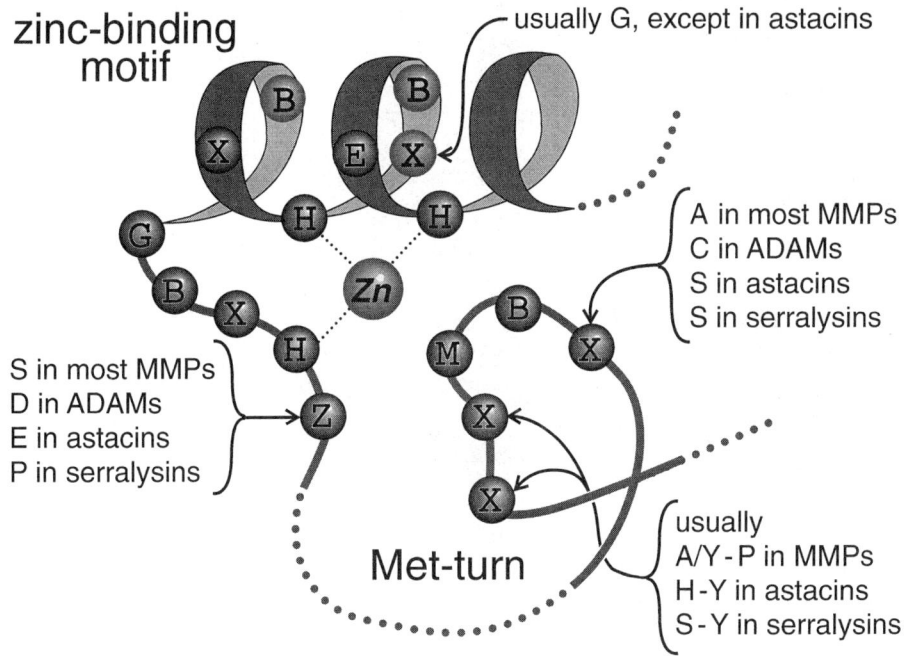

Fig. 1. Structural model of the conserved zinc-binding region of the metzincins. In addition to the standard single-letter amino acid designations, **B** represents a bulky hydrophobic residue, and **Z** is a family-specific residue (see footnote on p. 2). Modified from *(11)*.

and the "Met-turn" is usually AL**M**YP (Fig. 2). As their name implies, the matrix metalloproteinases possess overlapping substrate specificities against virtually all extracellular matrix molecules (Table 1). Other features that distinguish the MMPs are: 1) a strict requirement that zinc be bound at their catalytic site; 2) a dependence on calcium for their structural integrity and activity; 3) their inhibition by chelating agents, α2-macroglobulin and TIMPs; 4) an N-terminal signal sequence that directs their synthesis to the endoplasmic reticulum so that most MMPs are secreted while others are expressed as transmembrane proteins; 5) a propeptide domain situated N-terminal to the catalytic domain that maintains the enzyme as an inactive zymogen until it is removed by limited proteolysis; and 6) their in vitro activation by diverse reagents, including organomercurials (e.g., 4-aminophenylmercuric acetate, APMA), detergents, chaotropes, oxidants, heavy metals, disulfide compounds, and sulfhydryl-alkylating agents *(10,11,16)*.

To date, 20 distinct vertebrate MMPs and 18 human homologs have been identified* (Table 1) together with a number of nonvertebrate MMPs (embryonic

*MMP numbers 4–6 were dropped from the numbering system used to identify sequentially discovered MMPs when it was determined that MMPs 2 and 5 were identical and MMPs 4 and 6 were not true MMPs.

Collagenases

Hu MMP-1	Y N L H R V A A	H E L G H S L G L S H S	T D I G A L M Y P S Y
Por MMP-1	Y N L Y R V A A	H E L G H S L G L S H S	T D I G A L M Y L N Y
Bov MMP-1	Y N L Y R V A A	H E F G H S L G L A H S	T D I G A L M Y P S Y
Rab MMP-1	Y N L Y R V A A	H E L G H S L G L S H S	T D I G A L M Y P N Y
Bfr MMP-1	Y N L Y R V A A	H E L G H S L G L S H S	T D I G A L M Y P T Y
Hu MMP-8	Y N L F L V A A	H E F G H S L G L A H S	S D P G A L M Y P N Y
Hu MMP-13	Y N L F L V A A	H E F G H S L G L D H S	K D P G A L M F P I Y
Mus MMP-13	Y N L F I V A A	H E L G H S L G L D H S	K D P G A L M F P I Y
Rat MMP-13	Y N L F I V A A	H E L G H S L G L D H S	K D P G A L M F P I Y
Rab MMP-13	Y N L F L V A A	H E F G H S L G L D H S	K D P G A L M F P I Y
Nwt MMP-13	Y N L F I V A A	H E F G H A L G L D H S	R D P G S L M Y P V Y
Xe MMP-13	Y N L F V V A A	H E F G H A L G L D H S	R D P G S L M F P V Y
Xe MMP-18	Y N L F L V A A	H E F G H S L G L S H S	T D Q G A L M Y P T Y

Gelatinases

Hu MMP-2	Y S L F L V A A	H E F G H A M G L E H S	Q D P G A L M A P I Y
Mus MMP-2	Y S L F L V A A	H E F G H A M G L E H S	Q D P G A L M A P I Y
Rat MMP-2	Y S L F L V A A	H E F G H A M G L E H S	Q D P G A L M A P I Y
Rab MMP-2	Y S L F L V A A	H E F G H A M G L E H S	Q D P G A L M A P I Y
Ch MMP-2	Y S L F L V A A	H E F G H A M G L E H S	E D P G A L M A P I Y
Hu MMP-9	Y S L F L V A A	H E F G H A L G L D H S	S V P E A L M A P M Y
Rab MMP-9	Y S L F L V A A	H E F G H A L G L D H S	S V P E R L M A P M Y
Bov MMP-9	Y S L F L V A A	H E F G H A L G L D H T	S V P E A L M A P M Y
Mus MMP-9	Y S L F L V A A	H E F G H A L G L D H S	S V P E A L M A P L Y

Stromelysins and Matrilysin

Hu MMP-3	T N L F L V A A	H E I G H S L G L F H S	A N T E A L M Y P L Y
Rab MMP-3	T N L F L V A A	H E L G H S L G L F H S	A N P E A L M Y P V Y
Rat MMP-3	T N L F L V A A	H E L G H S L G L F H S	A N A E A L M Y P V Y
Mus MMP-3	T N L F L V A A	H E L G H S L G L Y H S	A K A E A L M Y P V Y
Hu MMP-7	I N F L Y A A T	H E L G H S L G M G H S	S D P N A V M Y P T Y
Mus MMP-7	V N F L F A A T	H E F G H S L G L Q H S	N N P K S V M Y P T Y
Hu MMP-10	T N L F L V A A	H E L G H S L G L F H S	A N T E A L M Y P L Y
Rat MMP-10	T N L F L V A A	H E L G H S L G L F H S	N N K E S L M Y P V Y
Hu MMP-11	T D L L Q V A A	H E F G H V L G L Q H T	T A A K A L M S A F Y
Mus MMP-11	T D L L Q V A A	H E F G H V L G L Q H T	T A A K A L M S P F Y
Xe MMP-11	T D L L Q V A A	H E F G H M L G L Q H S	S I S K S L M S P F Y

Membrane-type MMPs

Hu MMP-14	N D I F L V A V	H E L G H A L G L E H S	S D P S A I M A P F Y
Mus MMP-14	N D I F L V A V	H E L G H A L G L E H S	N D P S D I M S P F Y
Rat MMP-14	N D I F L V A V	H E L G H A L G L E H S	N D P S A I M A P F Y
Rab MMP-14	N D I F L V A V	H E L G H A L G L E H S	N D P S A I M A P F Y
Hu MMP-15	N N L F L V A V	H E L G H A L G L E H S	S N P N A I M A P F Y
Hu MMP-16	N D L F L V A V	H E L G H A L G L E H S	N D P T A I M A P F Y
Ch MMP-16	N D L F L V A V	H E L G H A L G L E H S	N D P T A I M A P F Y
Hu MMP-17	M D L F L V A V	H E F G H A I G L S H V	A A A H S I M R P Y Y

Other MMPs

Hu MMP-12	T N L F L T A V	H E I G H S L G L G H S	S D P K A V M F P T Y
Mus MMP-12	T N L F L V A V	H E L G H S L G L Q H S	N N P K S I M Y P T Y
Hu MMP-19	V N L R I I A A	H E V G H A L G L G H S	R Y S Q A L M A P V Y
Hu MMP-20	F N L F T V A A	H E F G H A L G L A H S	T D P S A L M Y P T Y
Por MMP-20	F N L F T V A A	H E F G H A L G L A H S	T D P S A L M Y P T Y
Hu MMP-21	T D L V H V A A	H E I G H A L G L M H S	Q H G R A L M H L N A
Hu MMP-22	T D L V H V A A	H E I G H A L G L M H S	Q H G R A L M H L N A
Xe MMP-x	I S L L K V A A	H E I G H V L G L S H I	H R V G S I M Q P N Y
Ur MMP-y	T N L F Q V A A	H E F G H S L G L Y H S	T V R S A L M Y P - Y
Sb MMP-z	F D L E S V A V	H E I G H L L G L G H S	S D L R A I M Y P S I

Fig. 2. Primary structure of the zinc-binding region of the MMPs. Highly conserved amino acid residues are shaded and the zinc-binding and "Met-turn" motifs are underlined. The aligned region corresponds to residues 210–240 of human MMPs 1 and 3. Abbreviations: Hu, human; Por, porcine; Bov, bovine; Mus, mouse; Rab, Rabbit; Ch, Chicken; Xe, frog (*Xenopus*); Bfr, bullfrog (*Rana*); Nwt, newt; Ur, sea urchin; Sb, soybean. Data are from (*16–21*) and corresponding GenBank entries.

sea urchin hatching enzyme (envelysin) *[17]*, *C. elegans* MMPs C31, H19, and Y19 *[22]*, soybean leaf metalloendopeptidase-1 *[18]*, and gamete lytic enzyme from green alga *[23]*). A comparison of the amino acid sequences of 30 MMPs from 8 species has revealed 30–99% overall sequence identity and 49–99% sequence similarity among the examined MMPs *(16)*. Some recently identified MMPs, however, exhibit lower levels of homology, such as a transiently expressed *Xenopus* MMP (MMP-x) that is most closely related to stromelysin-3 at only 20% identity *(20)*. Although subdividing the MMPs according to such homology considerations may prove useful, traditional MMP names and groupings have been based on substrate specificities and protein domain considerations. Thus MMPs are conventionally classified as "collagenases," "gelatinases," "stromelysins," "membrane-type MMPs," and "other MMPs." An alternative domain-based classification scheme is shown in Figure 3.

All MMPs possess an N-terminal signal sequence or "Pre" domain, a propeptide "Pro" domain that maintains enzyme latency until it is removed during enzyme activation, and a conserved catalytic domain. With the exception of matrilysin and two putative MMPs (MMPs 21 and 22), all other MMPs contain a hemopexin/vitronectin-like domain and a hinge domain that links the catalytic and hemopexin-like domains. The hemopexin-like domain mediates enzyme-TIMP interactions for the gelatinases, but appears to be involved in both inhibitor and substrate binding for the collagenases. The hinge region varies in length and composition among the different MMPs and may also play a role in defining substrate specificity. A cysteine-rich domain with homology to the collagen-binding region of fibronectin is present within the catalytic domain of gelatinases A and B, and is required for collagen binding and cleavage *(24)*. Finally, the membrane-type MMPs (MT-MMPs) possess a transmembrane domain and a short C-terminal cytoplasmic tail.

All MMPs are initially synthesized as inactive proenzymes or zymogens. Crystallographic studies have confirmed that ProMMP latency is maintained by coordination of the active site zinc by an unpaired cysteine sulfhydryl group within a highly conserved sequence motif (usually **P**R**CGVPD**) at the carboxy end of the propeptide domain *(25)*. Thus, whether MMP activation is initiated by normal proteolytic removal of the propeptide domain or by ectopic perturbants, ultimate activation requires interruption of this cysteine-zinc interaction, allowing water to replace the blocking cysteine *(26)*. In addition, once this "cysteine switch" is opened, further autocatalytic processing of the propeptide results in final cleavage at a highly conserved site.

Although most MMPs are secreted as latent zymogens, stromelysin-3 and all MT-MMPs contain an **RXK/RR** recognition motif in their propeptide domain that enables them to be activated intracellularly by calcium-dependent transmembrane serine proteinases of the subtilisin family such as furin *(27)*. Indeed, insertion of the recognition sequence from stromelysin-3 into procollagnease-1

Table 1
The MMP Multigene Family[a]

Common name	Other names	Substrates
Collagenases		
Collagenase-1	MMP-1, Interstitial Collagenase, Fibroblast Collagenase, EC 3.4.24.7	Collagens I, II, III, VII, X, Gelatins, Entactin, Link Protein, Aggrecan, Tenascin, L-Selectin, IGF-Binding Proteins, ProMMPs 2 & 9
Collagenase-2	MMP-8, Neutrophil Collagenase, EC 3.4.24.34	Collagens I, II, III, Gelatins, Aggrecan
Collagenase-3	MMP-13	Collagens I, II, III, Gelatins, Aggrecan
Collagenase-4	MMP-18	Collagen I, Gelatins
Gelatinases		
Gelatinase A	MMP-2, 72 kDa Gelatinase, 72 kDa Type IV Collagenase, EC 3.4.24.24	Gelatins, Collagens I, IV, V, VII, X, Elastin, Fibronectin, Laminin, Link Protein, Aggrecan, Galectin-3, IGF-Binding proteins, Vitronectin, Fibulin-2, FGF Receptor-1, ProMMPs 9 & 13
Gelatinase B	MMP-9, 92 kDa Gelatinase, 92 kDa type IV Collagenase, EC 3.4.24.35	Gelatin, Collagens IV, V, XI, Elastin, Link Protein, Vitronectin, Aggrecan, Galectin-3, Plasminogen, ProMMP-2
Stromelysins 1 & 2		
Stromelysin-1	MMP-3, Transin-1, Procollagenase Activating Protein, Proteoglycanase, EC 3.4.24.17	Proteoglycans, Laminin, Fibronectin, Gelatins, Collagens III, IV, V, IX, X, XI, Link Protein, Fibrin, Entactin, SPARC, Tenascin, Vitronectin, ProMMPs 1, 8, 9 & 13, α1-Antichymotrypsin, PAI-2, Antithrombin III, α2-Macroglobulin, α1-PI, L-Selectin, E-Cadherin, HB-EGF
Stromelysin-2	MMP-10, Transin-2, EC 3.4.24.22	Proteoglycans, Laminin, Gelatins, Elastin, Collagens III, IV, V, IX, Fibronectin, Link Protein, ProMMP-1

Membrane-type MMPs

MT1-MMP	MMP-14, MT-MMP-1, Membrane-type MMP-1	Collagens I, II, III, Gelatins, Fibronectin, Laminin, Vitronectin, Proteoglycans, ProMMPs 2 & 13, α1-PI, α2-Macroglobulin
MT2-MMP	MMP-15, MT-MMP-2	Pro-MMP-2
MT3-MMP	MMP-16, MT-MMP-3	Pro-MMP-2, Collagen III, Fibronectin
MT4-MMP	MMP-17, MT-MMP-4	Unknown

Other MMPs

Matrilysin	MMP-7, Matrin, PUMP-1, Small Uterine Metalloproteinase, EC 3.4.24.23	Proteoglycans, Laminin, Gelatins, Collagen IV, Entactin, Fibronectin, Link Protein, Vitronectin, Elastin, Tenascin, Fibulins, ProMMPs 1, 2 & 9
Stromelysin-3	MMP-11	Laminin, Fibronectin, Aggrecan, α1-PI, α2-Macroglobulin
Metalloelastase	MMP-12, Macrophage Elastase, EC 3.4.24.65	Elastin, Fibrinogen, Fibronectin, Laminin, Proteoglycans, Entactin, Collagen IV, IgGs, Myelin Basic Protein, Plasminogen, α1-PI
Enamelysin	MMP-20	Amelogenin
	MMP-19	Unknown
	MMP-21	Unknown
	MMP-22	Unknown

[a] Abbreviations: EC, Enzyme Commission; IGF, insulin-like growth factor; FGF, fibroblast growth factor; PAI-2, plasminogen activator inhibitor type-2; α1-PI, α1-proteinase inhibitor (α1-antitrypsin); HB-EGF, heparin-binding epidermal growth factor-like growth factor. Data are from (1,16, 19,34,45–58).

Minimal Domain MMPs *(Matrilysin)*

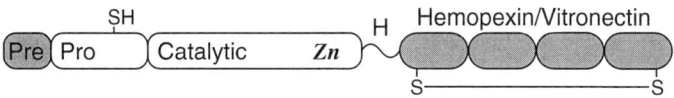

Hemopexin/Vitronectin Domain MMPs

A Simple *(Collagenases, Stromelysins 1 & 2, Metalloelastase, MMP-19, Enamelysin)*

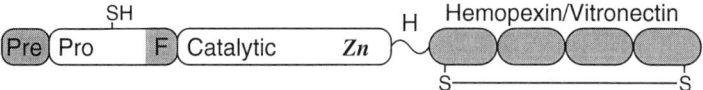

B Furin-activated *(Stromelysin-3)*

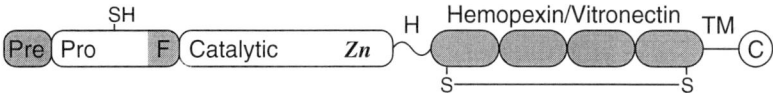

C Transmembrane Furin-activated *(MT-MMPs)*

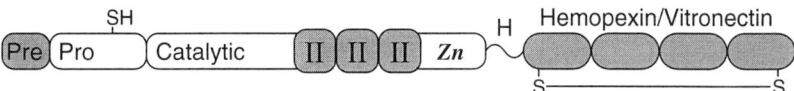

D Gelatin-binding *(Gelatinases A & B)*

Fig. 3. Domain structure of the MMPs. Pre, signal sequence; Pro, propeptide with a free zinc-ligating thiol group; F, furin-like enzyme-recognition motif; Zn, zinc-binding site; II, collagen-binding fibronectin type II inserts; H, hinge region; TM, transmembrane domain; C, cytoplasmic tail. The hemopexin/vitronectin-like C-terminal domain contains four repeats, the first and fourth being connected by a disulfide bridge. Modified from *(1)*.

results in intracellular activation of the latter proenzyme. The two most recently discovered MMPs (MMP-21 and MMP-22) also contain a furin-like enzyme recognition sequence between their propeptide and catalytic domains, indicating that they too are likely targets of furin/PACE/kex-2-like proprotein convertases *(21)*. However, MMPs 21 and 22 are unique in that they lack the conserved cysteine that is otherwise responsible for maintaining enzyme latency. All other MMPs lack the furin-like enzyme recognition motif and are thus activated outside the cell. Extracellular serine proteinases such as plasmin, urokinase-type plasminogen activator (uPA), elastase and trypsin can cleave peptide bonds within the prodomains of collagenase-1, stromelysin-1 and gelatinase B, and thus initiate further autocatalytic activation of these MMPs. Gelatinase A, on the other hand, appears to be refractory to serine proteinase activation. It can, however, be activated by a multistep pericellular pathway involving MT1-, MT2-, or MT3-MMP, with MT1-MMP being the most efficient activator of gelatinase A. First, MT1-MMP is activated intracellularly by a furin-like enzyme in the trans-Golgi network, or it is activated at the cell surface by plasmin. Active cell surface MT1-MMP, in turn, acts as a receptor for TIMP-2, and this binary complex acts as a further receptor for progelatinase A, which binds to TIMP-2 via its C-terminal hemopexin-like domain *(28)*. Finally, another MT1-MMP molecule that is not inhibited by TIMP-2 cleaves and activates the tethered progelatinase A. Recent data indicate that gelatinase A can also be activated by furin prior to its secretion at an RQPR site in its propeptide domain *(29)*. In addition, other activated MMPs can activate still other proMMPs, or they can inactivate endogenous serine proteinase inhibitors (Table 1). Other potential means of localizing MMPs to the cell surface include the binding of gelatinase A by $\alpha v \beta 3$ integrin *(30)*, and the presence of cell surface receptors for MMP-activating enzymes such as uPA, plasmin(ogen), and elastase. Such cell surface-localized proteolysis may confer enhanced proenzyme activation, protection against inhibitors, concentration of required molecules, and spatial limits on the extent of proteolysis *(1)*.

Another obvious means of regulating MMPs is at the level of transcription. For example, the collagenase-1, stromelysin-1, and gelatinase B genes can be up- or down-regulated by 12-O-tetradecanoylphorbol-13-acetate (TPA) *(31)*, EGF, basic FGF, TGFβ *(32)*, TNFα *(33)*, leukotriene D4 *(34)*, p53 *(35)*, integrin-derived signals *(36)*, alterations in cell shape *(37)*, and extracellular matrix proteins such as osteonectin/SPARC *(38)*. Collagenase-1 expression is also induced by extracellular matrix metalloproteinase inducer (EMMPRIN, tumor cell-derived collagenase stimulatory factor)*(39)*, and MT1-MMP expression is induced by various growth factors *(40)* and concanavalin A *(41)*. Many of these factors first induce the expression of *c-fos* and *c-jun* proto-oncogene products, which in turn recognize an activator protein-1 (AP-1) site (or TPA-responsive element) within the MMP gene promoter. Other motifs found in MMP promoter regions include PEA-3 sequences (which bind *ets* gene family products), AP-2 sites, GC box/SP-1-binding sites, CA-rich sequences, and TGF-β inhibitory elements *(42)*. In addition, polymorphisms have been identified within the human collagenase-1 and stromelysin-1 gene promoters that alter gene transcription and appear to play a role in malignant and atherosclerotic disease progression, respectively *(43,44)*. Thus MMPs can be strictly controlled at the level of transciption, as well as at the protein level via enzyme activators and inhibitors.

2. COLLAGENASES

Four MMP collagenases have been identified: collagenase-1 (MMP-1), collagenase-2 (MMP-8), collagenase-3 (MMP-13), and *Xenopus* collagenase-4 (MMP-18). These MMPs readily cleave the triple-helical domain of native fibrillar collagens I, II, and III. Gelatinase A can also cleave native type I collagen, but with a lower efficiency than the collagenases *(59)*, and the lysosomal cysteine proteinase cathepsin K found primarily in osteoclasts and chondroclasts can cleave within the helical domain of type II collagen *(60)*. Soluble MT1- and MT3-MMPs also exhibit collagenolytic activity *(49,61)*. Cleavage of each collagen α-chain occurs at a specific Gly-Ile/Leu peptide bond located three-quarters of the distance from the N- to C-terminus, resulting in the generation of characteristic 3/4- and 1/4-length collagen fragments *(47)*. Following cleavage, the helical collagen fragments spontaneously denature, and in so doing they become susceptible to further degradation by gelatinolytic enzymes. In addition to cleaving fibrillar collagens at a single site, collagenases can also degrade a number of other matrix molecules with variable efficiency (Table 1).

Insight into the functions of the various collagenase domains has come from examining the activities and affinities of various deletion mutants and chimeric constructs. For example, C-terminally truncated collagenase-1 can still cleave gelatin, casein, and peptide substrates, and can still be inhibited by TIMPs, but it can no longer cleave native triple-helical collagens, indicating that the hinge and hemopexin-like domains are required for triple helicase activity *(62,63)*. Chimeric enzymes containing the catalytic domain of collagenase-1 linked to the C-terminal domain of stromelysin-1 or -2, and a chimeric enzyme containing the stromelysin-1 catalytic domain linked to the collagenase C-terminal domain all lack triple helicase activity, but retain their caseinase and gelatinase activities, indicating that the triple helicase activity of collagenase-1 derives from both ends of the enzyme *(62,63)*. Furthermore, gelatin cleavage product fingerprints from the various chimeras indicate that the cleavage specificity of a given MMP is conferred by the zinc-binding region within its catalytic domain *(63)*. Active-site specificity mapping with synthetic substrates has also shown that collagenase-1 is an esterase that prefers lipophilic sequences *(64)*. The specificity of the collagenases may derive from three collagenase-specific residues that flank the three-histidine zinc-binding motif: a Tyr 8 residues upstream of the first His residue, and Asp and Gly residues that sit 3 and 5 residues downstream of the third His residue, respectively (Fig. 2) *(63)*. It is also worth noting that although collagenases are thought to be activated in vivo by serine proteinases such as plasmin, the latter enzyme can also cleave the collagenase C-terminal domain, an event that would, given the importance of this domain, abolish collagenolytic activity *(45)*.

As a group, the collagenases are highly homologous to one another, yet interesting differences do exist. All collagenases, other than the somewhat shorter bullfrog collagenase-1, have 447–452 amino acid latent forms with predicted molecular weights of 51–52 kDa, and 368–369 amino acid active forms with predicted weights of 42 kDa *(16,47,65)*. Their apparent molecular weights, however, depend on the presence or absence of Asn-linked glycosylation

(66,67). Thus, collagenase-1 and collagenase-2 each have 42 kDa active forms, but collagenase-1 has two latent forms of 52 and 57 kDa, whereas collagenase-2 has a 75 kDa latent form that is readily proteolyzed during extraction to a 58 kDa form that retains its latency. Collagenase-3 has latent and active forms that are 60 and 48 kDa, respectively. Collagenase-1 is produced and immediately secreted from a variety of cell types of primarily mesenchymal origin in response to specific inducers *(67,68)*. Collagenase-2, in contrast, is primarily produced by neutrophils during their maturation in bone marrow, and it is then stored until the cells are stimulated to degranulate *(67,68)*. Collagenase-3 is found in bone, normal and pathologic cartilage, and various epithelial cancers, and it is the predominant collagenase in mice and rats, collagenase-1 being undetectable in these species *(68–71)*. Finally, *Xenopus* collagenase-4 is expressed only transiently during tadpole tail resorption, hindlimb morphogenesis and intestinal remodeling *(47)*. Subtle differences also exist in the enzymatic activities of the respective collagenases. Although each mammalian collagenase can degrade all of the fibrillar collagens, the preferred substrates for collagenases 1, 2, and 3 are collagens III, I, and II, respectively *(66,72,73)*. The specificity of collagenase-4 has only been characterized for type I collagen *(47)*.

X-ray crystal structures have been solved for truncated human collagenase-1, full-length porcine collagenase-1, the substrate analog-inhibited catalytic domains of human collagenases 1 and 2, and the C-terminal hemopexin-like domain of human collagenase-3 *(74)*. These data reveal a spherical catalytic domain with a zinc-containing active-site cleft. The catalytic domain is, in turn, attached via a flexible hinge domain to an ellipsoid disk-shaped C-terminal domain that is composed of four β-sheets arranged sequentially about a central funnel-like tunnel containing two calcium and two chloride ions, thus giving the C-terminal domain a "four-bladed β-propeller-like" appearance. The first and last "blades" of the propeller are covalently linked by a disulfide bridge between cysteines at the leading portion of blade I and the C-terminal end of blade IV. Beyond this, several subtle structural differences probably help define the binding and cleavage characteristics of the collagenases when compared with one another and with other MMPs.

Although mutant phenotypes have not been described for the collagenase genes, mice carrying a collagenase-resistant *COL1A1* transgene exhibit late embryonic lethality, and introduction of the same mutation into the endogenous *COL1A1* gene leads to impaired postpartum uterine involution and marked dermal lesions resembling human scleroderma *(75)*. These studies further suggest that collagen resorption can also be accomplished through proteolytic cleavage at a novel site within the nonhelical N-telopeptide domain of type I collagen. In another model, transgenic expression of human collagenase-1 in mouse skin led to hyperproliferative skin lesions and an increased sensitivity to chemical carcinogens *(8)*. Interestingly, a single nucleotide polymorphism has been identified within the human collagenase-1 gene promoter that creates a functional Ets binding site, and the proportion of tested tumor cell lines that were homozygous for this polymorphism was significantly greater than the proportion of individuals within a control population, suggesting that enhanced gene transcription due to the presence of this polymorphism may contribute to cancer progression (43). Collagenase-3 expression is induced in chronically inflamed oral mucosal epithelium, indicating that it may contribute to the matrix degradation seen during chronic periodontitis (76).

3. GELATINASES

Gelatinases A and B (MMPs 2 and 9) are distinguished from other MMPs by three head-to-tail repeats within the catalytic domain that resemble the type II repeats of the gelatin-binding region of fibronectin (77–81). These fibronectin-like repeats are encoded by three extra exons (82,83), and play an important role in the particular ability of the gelatinases to degrade denatured collagens. Indeed, deletion of these repeats from gelatinase A abolishes its ability to bind collagen and lowers its gelatinolytic activity over 90%; however these deletions have little or no effect on the membrane-mediated activation of gelatinase A, on its TIMP-1 or TIMP-2-binding capacity, or on its ability to cleave small peptide substrates (84). Furthermore, gelatinase A, gelatinase B, and fibronectin compete with one another for binding to collagen, whereas collagenase-1 and stromelysin-1, which bind collagen via their C-terminal domains, do not compete (24). In addition to this collagen-binding domain, gelatinase B has an extended proline-rich hinge region of unknown significance that shows homology to the $\alpha 2(V)$ chain of collagen V (81). Progelatinase A is 72 kDa, which is comparable to its predicted size of 71 kDa, whereas human and mouse progelatinase B have predicted molecular weights of 76 and 79 kDa, but apparent molecular weights of 92 and 105 kDa due to N- and O-linked glycosylation, as well as to 16 additional residues in the murine collagen V-like hinge domain (77,81). Activated gelatinase A is 62 kDa, and slow autolytic cleavages eventually yield an active C-terminally truncated form of 42 kDa and several inactive breakdown products (77). Gelatinase B has active forms of 82 to 65 kDa, the smaller forms being the result of progressive proteolytic and autolytic processing of its N- and C-termini (77,85,86).

Gelatinases A and B have similar, but not identical, substrate specificities (Table 1), but differ in terms of their transcriptional regulation, extracellular activation, and inhibition (77,83). For example, macrophages, neutrophils, and keratinocytes express gelatinase B but not gelatinase A, whereas melanoma cells and fibroblasts exhibit the opposite pattern of expression (81). In addition, constitutive gelatinase A expression in HT-1080 fibrosarcoma cells is unaffected by TPA, whereas the otherwise low expression of gelatinase B is strongly induced (83). Although tumor cell lines of diverse origin can produce gelatinase

A and gelatinase B, their mRNA in epithelial cancers is generally limited to stromal fibroblasts for gelatinase A, and monocytes, neutrophils, and endothelial cells for gelatinase B *(1)*. Gelatinase B is also expressed by cytotrophoblasts during implantation, and by chondroclasts and osteoclasts during bone development. Mice that contain a gelatinase B promoter-driven lacZ reporter transgene have also been used to examine gelatinase B gene expression and have shown substantial promoter activity within developing bone and neural tissues as well as in migrating epithelia during wound repair *(87)*. Gelatinase B-null mice exhibit delayed growth plate vascularization and endochondral ossification, and a subtle shortening of their long bones *(88)*. These mice also exhibit abnormal implantation sites, suggesting other possible roles for gelatinase B (unpublished data).

Both the latent and active forms of gelatinase A and gelatinase B are bound and inhibited by TIMPs 1-3, however TIMP-1 binds more strongly to gelatinase B, TIMP-2 binds gelatinase A more strongly, and TIMP-3 inhibits either enzyme equally well *(1)*. This binding results from strong interactions between the C-terminal regions of both the enzyme and inhibitor, and inhibition results from interactions between the N-terminal domain of the inhibitor and the catalytic domain of the activated enzyme *(77)*. Because progelatinase-TIMP complexes that form upon mixing individually purified enzyme and inhibitor tend to dissociate more readily than do cell-derived enzyme-inhibitor complexes, the latter complexes are thought to cotranslationally fold together within the cell prior to their cosecretion *(77)*.

Exposure of MMPs to organomercurial agents and other perturbants generally initiates self-processing of their prodomains. However, unlike gelatinase A, gelatinase B cannot remove the final 13 residues of its own prodomain including the blocking cysteine residue *(85)*. The peptide bond separating the pro and catalytic domains of gelatinase B can, however, be cleaved by collagenase-1, stromelysin-1, matrilysin, and trypsin *(85)*. Other enzymes that activate gelatinase B in vitro include plasmin, cathepsin G, tissue kallikrein, and gelatinase A *(77,86)*. Gelatinase A itself, however, cannot be activated directly by any serine proteinase tested thus far, although neutrophil elastase cleaves within the hemopexin-like domain of APMA-treated gelatinase A yielding a 40 kDa product with fourfold greater gelatinolytic activity *(89)*. In the absence of gelatin, however, at least two sites within the fibronectin-like gelatin-binding domain of gelatinase A are cleaved by neutrophil elastase, thus inactivating the enzyme. Another serine proteinase, thrombin, can induce the activation of gelatinase A in endothelial cells *(90)*. This thrombin-mediated induction requires the presence of the cells themselves, and is inhibited by thrombin inhibitors, TIMP-2 and a C-terminal fragment of gelatinase A. Studies showing that progelatinase A binds to cell membranes via its C-terminal domain, and that it can be activated by cell membrane fractions *(84,91,92)* presaged the discovery of the

MT-MMPs, and the demonstration that they could indeed bind progelatinase A to the cell surface via TIMP-2 and, then, induce its activation *(28,93)*. Gelatinase A may also interact with other cell surface proteins, such as integrin αvβ3 *(30)*. A 190 kDa cell surface binding protein for gelatinase B has been identified as the α2(IV) chain of type IV collagen *(94)*. Gelatinase B also binds to the cell surface hyaluronan receptor CD44, and its binding appears to play an important role in CD44-mediated tumor cell invasion *(95)*.

Both gelatinases are active at neutral pH and each prefers to cleave peptide bonds between small Gly or Ala residues and aliphatic or hydrophobic residues *(77)*. Gelatinase A and gelatinase B share a number of common substrates which they both degrade in an apparently similar manner. These are gelatins, elastin, fibrillar collagen V, and basement membrane collagen IV, the latter being cleaved at a single unknown site to yield 1/4- and 3/4-length fragments *(77)*. Both enzymes also cleave cartilage link protein and aggrecan, but with differences in their respective activities *(96,97)*. In addition, gelatinase A can remove cell surface fibroblast growth factor (FGF) receptor 1 *(50)*, and gelatinase A, but not gelatinase B, can cleave triple-helical type I collagen to yield 3/4- and 1/4-length fragments at about 1/10 the K_{cat}/K_M of collagenase-1 *(59)*. These subtle differences in the substrate specificities of the two enzymes are most likely due to minor differences in their active sites.

4. STROMELYSINS 1 AND 2

Stromelysins 1 and 2 can degrade several structural substrates, activate other MMPs, and inactivate several serine proteinase inhibitors. They are distinguished from other MMPs by their close sequence similarity to one another, their extended hinge domains, and their similar substrate specificities. Stromelysin-1 (MMP-3) was first isolated by biochemical means *(98,99)*. It is secreted as a 56 kDa inactive zymogen that is processed to yield 45–48 and 28 kDa active forms with identical N-termini and indistinguishable activities and specificities (although the 28 kDa C-terminally truncated form no longer binds to type I collagen, indicating the importance of the C-terminal hemopexin-like domain in this regard) *(98,100)*. Single Asn glycosylation sites are present in its catalytic and C-terminal domains. Accordingly, about 20% of stromelysin-1 from fibroblasts is secreted as a 59 kDa glycoprotein, the remainder being unglycosylated *(98)*. Stromelysin-2 (MMP-10) was later discovered by molecular cloning *(101)*. It also has a 57 kDa latent form, and active forms of 45–47 and 28 kDa *(98)*. Both stromelysins share considerable sequence homology with one another, and they are further distinguished by a 9-residue insert in their hinge domain that is absent from most other MMPs.

Crystallographic studies indicate that the Cys-75 residue in the prodomain of stromelysin-1 ligates the active site zinc and thus maintains enzyme latency

(98). Like most other secreted MMPs, stromelysin-1 and stromelysin-2 are activated extracellularly. Their activation can be accomplished using perturbants such as APMA or serine proteinases such as plasmin, plasma kallikrein, neutrophil elastase, chymases, tryptase, chymotrypsin, or trypsin *(98).* Once activated, stromelysin-1 can hydrolyze numerous structural proteins, activate procollagenases 1–3 and progelatinase B, and inactivate a number of serpins (Table 1). In addition, stromelysin-1 can digest the telopeptides of collagens I and II *(98).* Activity against collagen III and elastin is weak, however, and activation of procollagenase-1 requires prior removal of a more proximal portion of its prodomain by another enzyme *(98).* Still, the activation of procollagenases by stromelysin-1 leaves the N-terminal Phe that is required for expression of their full enzymatic activity. Stromelysin-1 can cause the cleavage of cell surface E-cadherin *(102),* it can release soluble L-selectin from leukocytes *(54),* and it releases active heparin-binding EGF-like growth factor from cell surfaces by cleaving at a single site just outside the cell membrane *(58).* Cleavage-site and synthetic substrate analyses indicate that stromelysin-1 readily cleaves between P1 and P1′ residues when a hydrophobic residue is in the P1′ position, whereas there seem to be no strict requirements for the P1 residue *(98).* Stromelysin-1 is most active against aggrecan, gelatin, and Azocoll at pH 5.3–5.5, but it remains 30–50% active at pH 7.5–8.0 *(98).* The enzymatic activity of stromelysin-2 against various substrates is generally weaker than that of stromelysin-1.

Stromelysin-1 knockout mice exhibit hypomorphic virgin and pregnant mammary glands, altered involution and delayed closure of excisional wounds (unpublished observations). Mice that express an autoactivating stromelysin-1 transgene targeted to mammary epithelium display a gain-of-function with precocious virgin glandular development, unscheduled apoptosis during midpregnancy, formation of a reactive stroma, and the development of premalignant and malignant mammary gland lesions *(5,103).* Moreover, stromelysin-1 can trigger epithelial-to-mesenchymal phenotypic conversion of cultured mammary epithelial cells and induces otherwise noninvasive and nontumorigenic cells to form highly infiltrative tumors in immunocompromised mice *(5,102).* These data indicate that in addition to its traditional proinvasive activity *(104),* stromelysin-1 can promote the development of early premalignant lesions and can foster late phenotypic changes associated with more aggressive tumor behavior. Although stromelysin-1 is present in cartilage in rheumatoid arthritis and osteoarthritis, stromelysin-1 knockout mice are just as susceptible as wild-type mice to collagen-induced arthritis, and both types of mice exhibit cleavage of the Asn^{341}-Phe^{342} peptide bond of the cartilage proteoglycan aggrecan *(105).* Thus additional "aggrecanases" are likely to play a role in arthritic cartilage destruction. Finally, stromelysin-1 has also been implicated in coronary atherosclerosis. Interestingly, a common polymorphism (6A) in the stromelysin-1 gene promoter leads to reduced gene expression, and those atherosclerosis patients who are homozygous for 6A exhibit more rapid disease progression *(44)*.

5. MATRILYSIN

Matrilysin (MMP-7), which was first identified and purified from involuting rat uterus *(106,107)* and later cloned from a human tumor cDNA library *(101,108)*, differs from other MMPs in several regards. With the exception of two recently discovered putative MMPs, matrilysin is the only other MMP that is synthesized without a hemopexin-like C-terminal domain, and thus it is comparably small in size; having 28 and 19 kDa latent and active forms, respectively *(109,110)*. Nevertheless, matrilysin can cleave a wide array of extracellular matrix substrates and it can activate procollagenase-1 and progelatinases A and B (Table 1). Indeed, it cleaves aggrecan, versican, link protein, and entactin more readily than other MMPs, including stromelysin-1 *(96,111)*. Cleavage-site analyses further indicate that matrilysin prefers a large hydrophobic side chain at the P1' position.

Unlike other MMPs which are primarily expressed by stromal cells, matrilysin expression is restricted to glandular epithelium and is secreted apically. Matrilysin has been implicated in early tumor development *(7,112)* and late-stage invasion *(113)*, however unlike other MMPs which are expressed by the stromal cells that surround and infiltrate epithelial tumors, only matrilysin and possibly collagenase-3 are expressed by the tumor cells themselves *(1)*. However, reports of matrilysin expression in osteosarcomas and in fibroblasts surrounding breast carcinomas indicate that its expression may not be limited to epithelial cells *(1)*. Although matrilysin null mice have no apparent phenotype, when mice carrying the Apc^{Min} mutation are rendered deficient in matrilysin, they develop fewer and smaller intestinal adenomas than usual, suggesting that matrilysin may contribute to early tumor formation *(7)*. Interestingly, matrilysin immunolocalizes to the apical rather than basal surface of premalignant cells, suggesting that it may promote tumor development by degrading molecules other than those of the extracellular matrix *(7)*. Matrilysin is normally located apically in Paneth cells of the normal epithelium, again suggesting the existence of apical nonmatrix substrates *(114,115)*. Mice that overexpress a matrilysin transgene driven by the mouse mammary tumor virus (MMTV) promoter exhibit precocious mammary gland differentiation, preneoplastic mammary gland lesions, and male infertility *(114,116)*. In addition, mammary tumorigenesis in transgenic mice that express an MMTV-driven *neu* oncogene was accelerated when these MMTV-*neu* mice were crossed with the matrilysin overexpressing MMTV-matrilysin transgenic mice, again suggesting a role for matrilysin in promoting early tumor formation *(9,116)*. Matrilysin has

also been implicated in the rupture of atherosclerotic plaques where it is expressed by lipid-laden macrophages at potential rupture sites and colocalizes
with deposits of versican, a proteoglycan substrate *(117)*.

6. MEMBRANE-TYPE MMPS

The discovery of the membrane-type MMPs (MT-MMPs) represented a significant breakthrough in our understanding of the mechanisms that underlie the
pericellular activation of some MMPs. Using degenerate PCR primers, Sato et
al. *(118)* cloned the first of these integral plasma membrane enzymes (MT1-
MMP; MMP-14). Since then, three more MT-MMPs have been cloned: MT2-,
MT3-, and MT4-MMP (MMPs 15–17) *(93,119,120)*. In addition to their signal,
pro, catalytic, hinge, and hemopexin-like domains, the MT-MMPs have a
10–12-residue insert with a potential furin-like enzyme recognition motif
(RRK/RR) situated between their pro and catalytic domains that is similar to the
insert seen in stromelysin-3, an 8-residue insert of unknown significance in the
mid-proximal portion of the catalytic domain (this insert is absent in MT4-
MMP), and a final 75–105-residue insert containing a transmembrane domain
of about 24 residues and a short cytoplasmic C-terminal tail. MT1-MMP is synthesized as a 63 kDa latent enzyme that is processed to a 60 kDa active form.*
Such processing may be catalyzed by furin-like proprotein convertases in the
Golgi apparatus, although unprocessed 63 kDa MT1-MMP has also been detected at the cell surface *(118)*. Recombinant and transmembrane domain-
deleted MT1-MMP can indeed be activated by furin *(121,122)*. However,
MT1-MMP remains activatable despite the use of a furin inhibitor or the substitution of its RRKR residues with ARAA by site-directed mutagenesis *(123)*.
Pro-MT1-MMP can also be activated at the cell surface by extracellular plasmin, but not by any other extracellular trypsin-like serine proteinase *(124)*. Thus
MT-MMP activation may occur both within the cell and at the cell surface.

Once activated, MT1-MMP binds TIMP-2, and this complex can then bind
and activate ProMMP-2 or -13 (Fig. 4) *(28,45,124,125)*. Indeed, there appears
to be strict coexpression of the MT1-MMP and TIMP-2 genes duing development, suggesting a common gene regulatory pathway *(126)*. Because a hydrox-
aminic acid-derived MMP inhibitor blocks TIMP-2 binding, it was realized that
the MT1-MMP active site is involved in TIMP-2 binding *(127)*. Thus another
separate MT1-MMP molecule without bound TIMP-2 activates the ProMMP
that is bound via TIMP-2 to an otherwise inhibited MT1-MMP *(127)*. MT1-
MMP and TIMP-2 can also be secreted as a bimolecular complex that can then
interact with progelatinase A *(125)*. This secretion probably results from cleavage that occurs at a juxtamembrane site when the MT-MMP is undergoing

---

*Latent MT2-, MT3-, and MT4-MMP have apparent molecular weights of 72, 64,
and 70 kDa, respectively *(93,119,120)*.

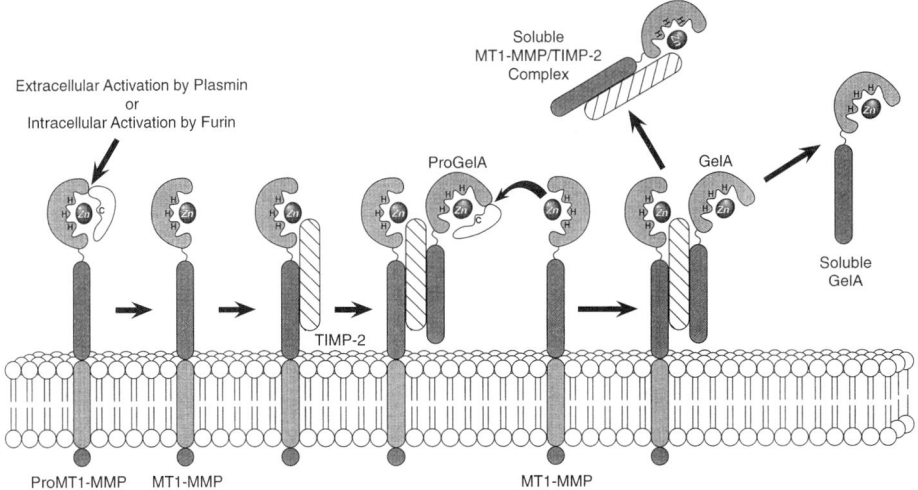

Fig. 4. Cell-surface activation of progelatinase A by MT1-MMP. ProMT1-MMP is activated at the cell surface by plasmin or in the trans-Golgi network by a furin-like enzyme during its passage to the cell surface. Activated MT1-MMP interacts with TIMP-2 and then progelatinase A binds to the TIMP-2 to form a trimolecular complex. Because TIMP-2 blocks the MT1-MMP active site, another uninhibited MT1-MMP removes the proGelatinase A propeptide thus yielding free active gelatinase A. The bimolecular MT1-MMP/TIMP-2 complex can also be shed from the cell surface by an unknown enzyme that cleaves MT1-MMP outside its transmembrane domain.

transport to the cell surface or once it is present at the cell surface, and this cleavage may be carried out by another nearby MT-MMP. On the other hand, a soluble form of MT3-MMP that can cleave type III collagen and fibronectin is the product of alternative mRNA splicing rather than proteolytic shedding *(61)*. By artificially deleting the MT1-MMP transmembrane domain or by replacing it with the IL-2 receptor α chain transmembrane domain, it has been shown that the MT1-MMP transmembrane domain is required for the recruitment of MT1-MMP to sites of active extracellular matrix degradation (invadopodia) *(128)*.

Membrane-associated MT1-, MT2-, and MT3-MMP can each activate progelatinase A *(93,118)*, and MT1-MMP can also activate procollagenase-3 *(45,129)*. Secreted MT1-MMP and an MT1-MMP deletion mutant lacking the transmembrane domain can also cleave gelatin, cartilage proteoglycan, fibronectin, vitronectin, laminin-1, α1-proteinase inhibitor, and α2-macroglobulin *(49,122,125)*. Furthermore, soluble MT1-MMP can cleave collagens I, II, and III at specific Gly-Ile/Leu bonds to yield the same characteristic 3/4- and 1/4-length fragments as do the collagenases, even though MT1-MMP lacks the conserved Tyr, Asp, and Gly residues that flank the zinc-binding motif of the collagenases and which are thought to confer specificity for fibrillar collagens *(49)*. Because

MT1-MMP is sensitive to inhibition by TIMP-2 and TIMP-3, but not TIMP-1, it can still function as a proenzyme activator and broad-spectrum proteinase even in the presence of high levels of TIMP-1 *(130)*. The proteolytic activities of MT4-MMP remain to be characterized; however, it is worth noting that MT4-MMP has a Val rather than Ser residue following the final His residue of the three-histidine zinc-binding motif, a feature that sets it apart from all other metzincins.

Each MT-MMP shows a unique pattern of expression by Northern blot analysis. MT1-MMP is expressed in numerous normal tissues, but is unde-tectable in brain and leukocytes *(93,119)*. MT2-MMP expression is also unde-tectable in brain and leukocytes, but is stronger than MT1-MMP expression in liver, heart and skeletal muscle, and is weak or absent in ovary, prostate, thy-mus, and spleen *(119)*. On the other hand, MT3-MMP mRNA is detectable in brain, as well as in placenta, lung, and heart *(93)*, and MT4-MMP expression is strongest in brain, leukocytes, colon, ovary, and testis *(120)*. MT1-MMP ex-pression is up-regulated in invasive tumors as compared to adjacent normal tis-sues *(118)*, and although its transcripts are most often seen in adjacent stromal cells by *in situ* hybridization *(131)*, carcinoma cells themselves may also over-express this enzyme *(132)*. MT1-MMP knockout mice have several develop-mental problems, fail to thrive and die a few days after birth (K. Holmbeck and H. Birkedal-Hansen, personal communication).

7. STROMELYSIN-3

Stromelysin-3 (MMP-11) was initially identified from a subtracted breast cancer cDNA library and found to be specifically expressed by stromal cells surrounding invasive tumors *(133)*. Stromelysin-3 has a latent form of about 60 kDa, active forms of 45-47 kDa, and an active 28 kDa C-terminally trun-cated form *(27,134)*. Unlike stromelysins-1 and -2 from various species which show 76% sequence identity and 86% similarity to one another, stromelysin-3 shares only 39% identity and 56% similarity with the other stromelysins, and only 36% identity and 55% similarity with all other MMPs *(16)*. Furthermore, whereas most other secreted MMPs are activated extracellularly, processed stromelysin-3 can be found within cells, and both latent and active stromelysin-3 are rapidly detected in cell-conditioned medium, yet their relative amounts re-main stable over time, suggesting intracellular rather than extracellular activation *(27)*. Like the MT-MMPs, stromelysin-3 has a 10-residue insert at the end of its prodomain that harbors an RxK/RR furin-like enzyme recognition motif, and the Golgi-associated enzyme furin activates stromelysin-3 prior to its secretion by cleaving the bond between the final Arg of the insert and the sub-sequent Phe residue *(27)*. Although most furin-processed proteins contain only an RxK/RR site, the stromelysin-3 sequence (RNRQKR) contains an added Arg residue that potentiates its furin-catalyzed activation *(27)*. Indeed, substitution of the upstream Arg decreases stromelysin-3 processing some 90%, and mutation of the Lys or other Arg residues abolishes processing altogether. Processing is also blocked by a furin-specific inhibitor, α1-antitrypsin Pittsburg. A cell line that lacks functional furin can activate stromelysin-3 only when these cells are cotransfected with furin in addition to stromelysin-3, thus indicating the obligate nature of this activation mechanism.

Once activated, stromelysin-3 exhibits relatively weak proteolytic activity against α1-proteinase inhibitor and several structural proteins with a substrate specificity like that of stromelysins-1 and -2 (Table 1). Despite its weak activity against these particular substrates in vitro, stromelysin-3 apparently plays an important role in cancer progression. It represents an independent prognostic factor for disease-free survival in certain breast cancers, and even though it is normally expressed by adjacent stromal cells of mesenchymal origin rather than the malignant epithelial cells themselves, it is apparently induced in certain advanced cancers when the epithelial tumor cells undergo epithelial-to-mesenchymal conversion *(135)*. Moreover, stromelysin-3 knockout mice develop fewer and smaller chemically-induced tumors than wild-type mice, and whereas wild-type fibroblasts foster the tumorigenicity of human MCF7 breast cancer cells in nude mice, stromelysin-3-deficient fibroblasts do not *(6)*. Further evidence indicates that this apparent tumor promoting activity of stromelysin-3 derives from its ability to release and/or activate growth factors that are sequestered in the extracellular matrix *(6)*.

8. METALLOELASTASE

It has long been recognized that stimulated mouse macrophages secrete a metallo-enzyme with elastinolytic activity *(136)*. Since then, a 22 kDa murine macrophage metalloelastase (MMP-12) has been purified *(137)* and its murine and human genes cloned *(138,139)*. The molecular mass of the proenzyme is 53–54 kDa, and the mature 22 kDa active form apparently derives from both standard propeptide removal (which yields a 45 kDa active intermediate) and atypical C-terminal processing *(138)*. In addition to elastin, macrophage metalloelastase can cleave a wide array of other proteins (Table 1). Although macrophage metalloelastase is about 30% as active as the serine proteinase neutrophil elastase at degrading elastin, it can also inactivate the major inhibitor of neutrophil elastase, α1-proteinase inhibitor *(55)*. The peptide substrate specificities and inhibitor sensitivities of mouse metalloelastase have also been described *(56)*. Metalloelastase is required for tissue invasion by macrophages *(140)*. It also plays a role in pulmonary emphysema and is indeed required for tobacco smoke-induced emphysema in mice *(55,141,142)*. Metalloelastase has also been implicated in vascular aneurysm formation *(55,142)*, and it can generate the angiogenesis inhibitor angiostatin by cleaving plasminogen *(143)*.

9. ENAMELYSIN

The enamelysin (MMP-20) cDNA was initially isolated from a porcine enamel organ cDNA library *(144)*. The human cDNA was subsequently cloned *(145)* and an orthologous bovine cDNA has also been obtained (P.K. DenBesten, personal communication). The predicted protein has 483 amino acids, a molecular weight of 54 kDa, and a characteristic MMP domain structure, but it lacks distinctive features of the collagenase, gelatinase, stromelysin, and MT-MMP subgroups. It also diverges from all other MMPs in terms of three otherwise invariant amino acids found in the hemopexin-like domain. Enamelysin mRNA transcripts of 2.5 and 4.3 kb have only been detected in the enamel organ. During tooth enamel formation, ameloblast cells of this organ secrete an organic matrix made up mostly of amelogenin that is continuously turned over as biomineralization proceeds. Gelatin zymograms done on acid extracts of developing porcine enamel matrix show two major metalloproteinases at 50–65 kDa that may or may not represent enamelysin *(144)*. Multiple 21–25 kDa enzymes that probably do represent truncated forms of enamelysin have been purified from neutral extracts of bovine enamel matrix *(146)*. These have poor enzymatic activity against gelatin, but readily cleave casein and isoforms of amelogenin, the ameloblast-derived protein that forms the organic matrix of tooth enamel (P.K. DenBesten, personal communication). Furthermore, recombinant human enamelysin can hydrolyze amelogenin and is fully inhibited by TIMP-2 *(145)*. Taken together, these data strongly suggest that enamelysin may be a key player in the processing of enamel matrix.

10. MMP-19

Human MMP-19 cDNAs have been cloned from a liver cDNA library *(19)*, from a cDNA library obtained from the inflamed synovium of a rheumatoid arthritis patient *(147)*, and by performing 5'-RACE on an expressed sequence tag with MMP sequence homology *(148)*.* The predicted protein has 508 amino acids, a molecular weight of 57.4 kDa, two potential N-glycosylation sites, and characteristic pre, pro, catalytic, and hemopexin-like MMP domains. MMP-19, however, lacks specific features that would otherwise distinguish it as a collagenase, gelatinase, or membrane-type MMP. Furthermore, the hinge region of MMP-19 contains a 16-residue acidic insert rather than the 9-residue hydrophobic insert typical of the stromelysins. MMP-19 also has a unique threonine-rich C-terminal region and the highly conserved MMP propeptide sequence PRCGVPD reads PRCGLED in MMP-19. Its mRNA is expressed in a

---

*Because the GenBank sequences submitted as human MMPs 18 *(148)* and 19 *(19)* are identical to one another, but diverge considerably from the *Xenopus* MMP-18 sequence, they have been designated MMP-19.

variety of human tissues, particularly placenta, lung, pancreas, ovary, spleen, and intestine. In addition, MMP-19 has been detected on the surface of activated peripheral blood mononuclear cells *(147)*.

Recombinant MMP-19 can hydrolyze fluorogenic MMP substrates only after trypsin activation, and this activity is abolished by TIMP-2 and EDTA *(19)*. Peptide substrate mapping further indicates that its enzymatic activity is most like that of the stromelysins and not at all similar to that of the collagenases. MMP-19 has weak but definite gelatinolytic activity *(147)*, however the specific substrates of MMP-19 remain unknown. Still, when one considers that its cDNA was cloned from an arthritic synovium cDNA library, that it is present on the surface of activated inflammatory cells, and that it is recognized by autoantibodies present in the sera of about one in four rheumatoid arthritis patients *(147)*, it is apparent that MMP-19 may play a role in arthritic joint destruction.

11. OTHER MMPS

The closely linked and most likely duplicated MMP-21 and MMP-22 genes were recently discovered while screening for possible tumor suppressor genes within a chromosomal region (1p36.3) that is frequently deleted in a number of different cancers *(21)*. The predicted open reading frames of both MMPs are highly similar and only exhibit silent degenerate base changes or changes that encode a similar amino acid. Both MMPs are unique in that neither has the conserved propeptide cysteine residue that is required for proenzyme latency. Like the MT-MMPs, stromelysin-3 and many ADAMs, MMPs 21, and 22 have a furin-like enzyme recognition sequence (RRRR) between their propeptide and catalytic domains, suggesting that not only is the propeptide domain unable to maintain enzyme latency, but it is also probably removed by intracellular furin-like enzymes. However, the catalytic domains of MMPs 21 and 22 are followed not by hinge and hemopexin-like domains, but by a cysteine-rich domain similar to the cysteine-rich domains of ADAM metalloproteinases, a proline-rich domain, an interleukin-1 type II receptor-like domain, and putative transmembrane and cytoplasmic domains. The MMP-21 and MMP-22 genes also express alternatively spliced mRNAs that encode additional stretches of amino acids just before and after the zinc-binding region of the catalytic domain. MMP-21/22 transcripts have been detected in human placenta, ovary, testis, prostate, pancreas, and heart, however the function of these MMPs remains entirely unknown. Another recently cloned human cDNA that has been called MMP-23 also maps to 1p36 and shares 98% identity with the MMP-21/22 sequences *(149)*, indicating that it may very well represent a cDNA from the MMP-21 or 22 gene. The latter investigators failed to detect proteolytic activity after expressing their cDNA in bacteria, but obtained weak activity against one of three synthetic peptide substrates examined when they used a chimeric enzyme containing the MMP-19 propeptide domain and their newly cloned catalytic domain. The recombinant chimeric enzyme also lacked gelatinolytic activity. Another cDNA has been submitted to GenBank (accession number AJ010262) as mouse MMP-21 or membrane-type MMP-5 (MT5-MMP), however its otherwise unpublished sequence lacks similarity to the human MMP-21 sequence.

A novel *Xenopus* MMP cDNA (MMP-x) was recently cloned and found to be transiently expressed in gastrula and neurula stage embryos *(20)*. MMP-x and *Xenopus* collagenase-4 represent the only vertebrate MMPs for which mammalian homologs have not been found. MMP-x is only distantly related to other MMPs, with stromelysin-3 being most closely related at only 20% sequence identity. It has a signal peptide, suggesting that it is secreted, and a predicted molecular weight of 70 kDa. Unlike other MMPs, MMP-x has a 37-amino acid vitronectin-like insert in its propeptide domain, and it lacks a proline-rich hinge region between its catalytic and C-terminal domains. Like stromelysin-3, MMP-x has an RRKR furin-like enzyme recognition motif at the distal end of its pro domain, suggesting that it, too, may be secreted as an active enzyme.

12. TISSUE INHIBITORS OF METALLOPROTEINASES

Just as the MMPs are instrumental in normal and pathologic matrix remodeling, so too are their natural endogenous inhibitors, the TIMPs. To date, four members of the TIMP multigene family (TIMPs 1–4) have been cloned in humans and other species *(1,150,151)*. They exhibit 37–51% overall sequence identity, with TIMPs 2, 3, and 4 being more similar to one another than to TIMP-1. Features that distinguish the TIMPs are:

1. Their extracellular secretion mediated by a transient 23–29-residue N-terminal signal sequence;
2. Their ability to bind latent and active MMPs with 1:1 stoichiometry;
3. Their ability to inhibit the autocatalytic activation of latent MMPs and the proteolytic function of activated MMPs;
4. Their ability to bind and inhibit subsequent MMPs after enzyme-inhibitor dissociation and dis-inhibition of the initial target occurs;
5. Their conserved gene structure;
6. Their 12 required and similarly separated Cys residues that form 6 disulfide bonds and a conserved 6-loop structure (Fig. 5);
7. Their inactivation by reducing agents; and
8. Their highly conserved N-terminal domain (loops 1–3) that is both necessary and sufficient for MMP inhibition *(150,152,153)*. Differences between individual family members exist in terms of their C-terminal domains (loops 4–6 and a free tail), their preferred MMP targets, their overall gene sizes, their gene regulation, and their tissue-specific patterns of expression *(152,153)*.

Human TIMP-1 is a 184-residue, 28.5 kDa glycoprotein with heterogeneous N-linked glycosylation at two sites *(153)*. On the other hand, TIMP-2 is an unglycosylated, 194-residue, 21 kDa protein with an extended and negatively charged C-terminus *(153)*. TIMP-3 is a 188-residue, 27 kDa glycoprotein with a single N-glycosylation site near its C-terminus *(152)*, and TIMP-4 is an apparently unglycosylated, 195-residue, 22 kDa protein *(150)*. TIMP-1 was found to be identical to the already cloned erythroid-potentiating activity (EPA), indicating that it also has growth promoting activity that may be independent of its MMP inhibitory activity *(154)*. Like TIMP-1, TIMP-2 may also have growth factor-like activity *(153)*.

The TIMPs specifically and reversibly inhibit the MMPs, but they are not known to inhibit any other metalloproteinases *(153)*. The C-terminal domains of TIMPs 1 and 2 interact strongly with the C-terminal domains of gelatinases B and A, respectively, resulting in preferential binding of TIMP-1 to gelatinase B and of TIMP-2 to gelatinase A *(153)*. Because C-terminally truncated "tiny TIMPs" containing only the first three loops of TIMPs 1 or 2 can still inhibit MMPs, it is clear that a portion of the N-terminal domain of the TIMPs binds to the MMP active site *(152,155)*. Nuclear magnetic resonance (NMR) chemical shift analyses further indicate that much of one face of the TIMP-2 N-terminal domain binds to the stromelysin-1 catalytic domain *(156)*, and X-ray crystallography has revealed that the disulphide-linked Cys^1-Thr^2-Cys^3-Val^4 and Ser^{68}-Val^{69} segments of TIMP-1 bind opposite sides of the active site zinc of stromelysin-1, that the Cys^1 residue coordinates the zinc ion from directly above, and that the Thr^2 residue occupies the large S1′ specificity pocket of stromelysin-1 *(157)*. Altogether, four separate segments from the TIMP-1 N-terminal domain and two short segments from the C-terminal domain contact the stromelysin-1 catalytic domain. Still, single-site mutations at several conserved sites within the N-terminal domain of TIMP-1 have had little effect on its ability to bind and inhibit matrilysin, although single-residue replacements in the anchored region between Cys-3 and Cys-13 do diminish its affinity for matrilysin *(158)*. Most of this anchored region, however, does not bind the active site, but helps maintain overall TIMP conformation *(153,157)*. Synthetic TIMP-1 peptides that can inhibit collagenase-1 and which compete with TIMP-1 for binding to collagenase-1 tend to surround the second "disulfide knot" between loops 3 and 4 (Fig. 5) *(155)*. Furthermore, two neutralizing TIMP-1 antibodies recognize epitopes in this same region of loop 3, whereas nonblocking antibodies recognize portions of loops 1, 4, and 6 *(155)*. Analysis of single-residue mutations in and around the collagenase-1 active site suggests that TIMP-1 binding requires a properly folded, but not necessarily functional, active site *(159)*. Taken together, these findings suggest that both the N- and C-terminal domains of the TIMPs contribute to their binding properties, whereas TIMP inhibitory activity derives from the N-terminal domain alone, and in particular from the region surrounding the first disulfide knot.

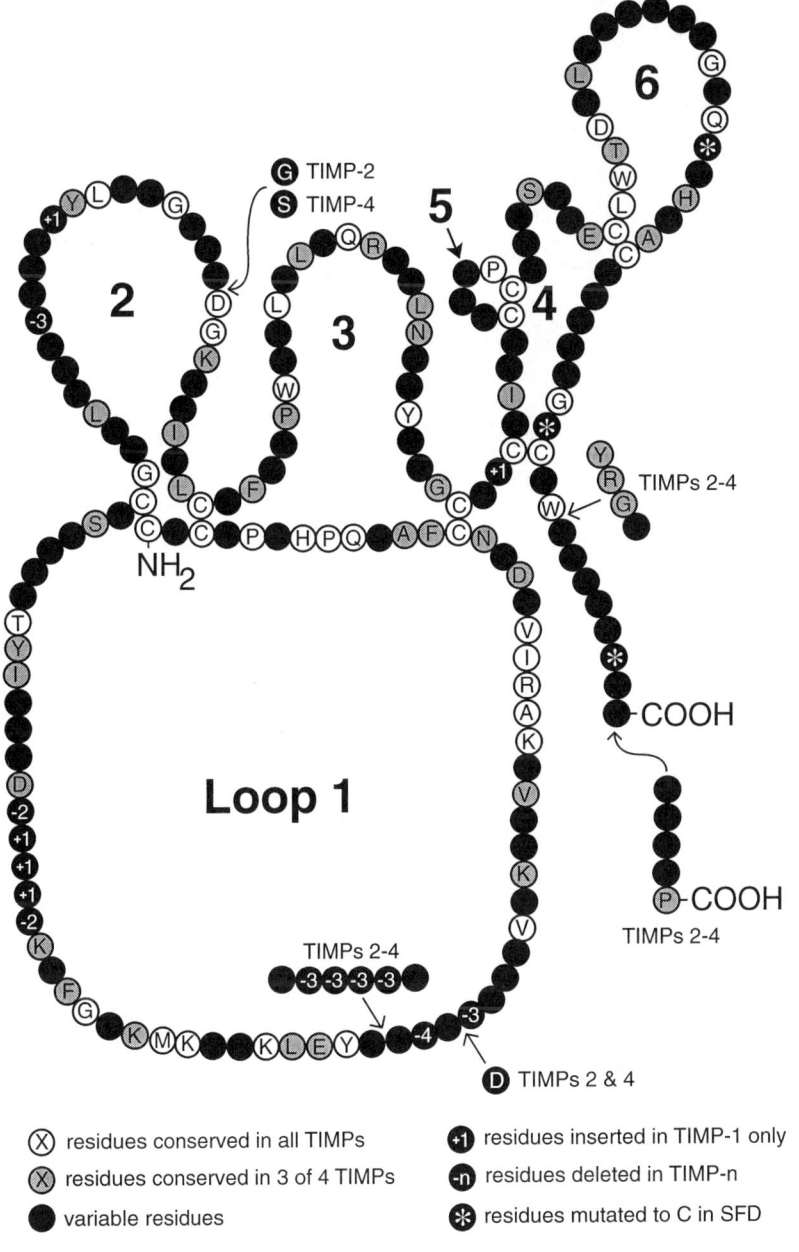

Fig. 5. Structural model of human TIMPs 1-4. The composite model is based on a structural model of human TIMP-1 *(155)* and the aligned amino acid sequences of the other human TIMPs. Unshaded residues are common to all human TIMPs, and shaded residues are common to any three of the four cloned TIMPs. Gaps and insertions in the aligned primary sequences are also indicated, as are the three mutated residues in TIMP-3 that have been linked to Sorsby's fundus dystrophy (SFD).

TIMP-1 is primarily expressed in adult bone and ovary and in tissues undergoing remodeling or inflammation *(160)*. TIMP-1 mRNA levels are usually greater in tumors than in adjacent normal tissues, whereas TIMP-2 mRNA levels tend to be similar in tumors and matched normal tissues *(161,162)*. Furthermore, TIMP-2 expression is down-regulated by TGF-β1 and is unaffected by serum and phorbol esters, whereas TIMP-1 expression is increased by each of these treatments *(161,162)*. Both TIMP-1 and TIMP-3 are induced by mitogenic stimuli (indeed, TIMP-3 was cloned as mitogen-inducible gene 5), however unlike other TIMPs, TIMP-3 is specifically up-regulated during G1 cell-cycle progression *(163)*. TIMP-3 is expressed in a variety of developing tissues, most notably uterine decidua during implantation, and cartilage, muscle, various epithelia, and placental trophoblasts during late gestation *(152)*. TIMP-3 is also expressed in a variety of adult tissues, and in certain cancers and diseases of the eye *(164–166)*. The importance of TIMP-3 in the eye is suggested by its increased expression in simplex retinitis pigmentosa *(166)*, by its immunolocalization to Bruch's membrane and drusen *(167)*, and by the presence of TIMP-3 mutations in patients with Sorsby's fundus dystrophy (SFD), an autosomal dominant disorder characterized by progressive degeneration of the central retina with relatively early onset *(168,169)*. Specifically, three point mutations that introduce an additional Cys residue into the C-terminal domain of TIMP-3 have been found in the affected members of three SFD families (Fig. 5). These mutations may result in intra- or inter-molecular disulfide bonds and may thus disrupt the conserved disulfide bonds that are required for proper protein folding and MMP inhibitory activity. Interestingly, TIMP-3 is the only known endogenous inhibitor that can inhibit TNFα convertase (TACE) and possibly other ADAMs family members as well *(170)*. In addition, methylation-associated inactivation of the TIMP-3 gene promoter is often seen in human cancers and may contribute to their progression *(171)*. Finally, TIMP-4 is distinguished by its abundant expression in adult heart tissue, and its relatively low expression in certain other adult tissues *(150,151)*. It is also expressed in stromal fibroblasts of normal and benign but not malignant breast tissue.

13. CONCLUDING REMARKS

Extracellular matrix-degrading enzymes such as the MMPs give malignant cancers their defining ability to invade and metastasize *(1)*. Indeed, without these enzymes, cancer cells could not cross the extracellular matrix barriers that otherwise contain their spread, and they would instead remain effectively benign. By this rationale, therapeutic strategies are being developed to thwart the activities of the responsible proinvasive enzymes. In addition, an MMP-generated fragment of α1-proteinase inhibitor fosters tumor growth by mechanisms that may involve the modulation of NK cell activity *(172)*. Recent data also suggest that some MMPs contribute to the initial development of preneoplastic and premalignant lesions and can trigger cellular phenotypic changes associated with more aggressive tumor behavior. The involvement of MMPs in these added processes may thus expand the ultimate clinical utility of selective MMP inhibitors, as may their involvement in other disease processes such as atherosclerosis, emphysema, and arthritis. Conversely, some MMPs, such as metalloelastase, matrilysin, and gelatinase B which can cleave plasminogen to generate the angiogenesis inhibitor angiostatin, may actually *defy* tumor progression *(3,173)*. These data also point out that MMPs do more than just degrade extracellular matix barriers and scaffolds. Rather, MMPs can affect cellular signaling and can potentially compromise genomic stability *(174–176)*. By remodeling extracellular matrices, which are by no means passive, MMPs alter matrix-derived signals and cause the release of bioactive matrix fragments. MMPs can also cleave a growing list of cell-surface proteins such as E-cadherin, a known contributor to cell-cell signaling and cancer progression. Moreover, they can potentially cause the release or inactivation of growth and angiogenesis factors, inhibitors, binding proteins, and receptors. Thus MMPs can alter cell-matrix, cell-cell and paracrine signals that, in turn, control such basic processes as cell growth, morphogenesis, differentiation, migration, tissue repair, and cell death. Thus the importance of MMPs in normal physiologic processes and the potential for untoward effects must be considered when designing and undertaking interventions that target these enzymes.

ACKNOWLEDGMENTS

This work was supported by grants from the National Cancer Institute (CA57621 and CA72006), the National Heart, Lung and Blood Institute (HL03880), and the U.S. Army Medical Research and Materiel Command (DAMD17-97-1-7246).

REFERENCES

1. Coussens, L. M. and Werb, Z. (1996) Matrix metalloproteinases and the development of cancer. *Chem. Biol.* 3, 895–904.
2. Woessner, J. F. (1998) in *Matrix Metalloproteinases* (Parks, W. C. and Mecham, R. P., eds.), Academic Press, San Diego, pp. 1–14.
3. Shapiro, S. D. (1998) Matrix metalloproteinase degradation of extracellular matrix: biological consequences. *Curr. Opin. Cell Biol.* 10, 602–608.
4. Giambernardi, T. A., Grant, G. M., Taylor, G. P., Hay, R. J., Maher, V. M., McCormick, J. J., and Klebe, R. J. (1998) Overview of matrix metalloproteinase expression in cultured human cells. *Matrix Biol.* 16, 483–496.
5. Sternlicht, M. D., Lochter, A., Sympson, C. J., Huey, B., Rougier, J. P., Gray, J. W., Pinkel, D., Bissell, M. J. and Werb, Z. (1999) The stromal proteinase MMP-3/stromelysin-1 promotes mammary carcinogenesis. *Cell* 98, 137–146.
6. Masson, R., Lefebvre, O., Noël, A., Fahime, M. E., Chenard, M. P., Wendling, C., et al. (1998) In vivo evidence that the stromelysin-3 metalloproteinase contributes in a paracrine manner to epithelial cell malignancy. *J. Cell Biol.* 140, 1535–1541.

7. Wilson, C. L., Heppner, K. J., Labosky, P. A., Hogan, B. L. and Matrisian, L. M. (1997) Intestinal tumorigenesis is suppressed in mice lacking the metalloproteinase matrilysin. *Proc. Natl. Acad. Sci. (USA)* 94, 1402–1407.

8. D'Armiento, J., DiColandrea, T., Dalal, S. S., Okada, Y., Huang, M. T., Conney, A. H. and Chada, K. (1995) Collagenase expression in transgenic mouse skin causes hyperkeratosis and acanthosis and increases susceptibility to tumorigenesis. *Mol. Cell. Biol.* 15, 5732–5739.

9. Rudolph-Owen, L. A., Chan, R., Muller, W. J. and Matrisian, L. M. (1998) The matrix metalloproteinase matrilysin influences early-stage mammary tumorigenesis. *Cancer Res.* 58, 5500–5506.

10. Rawlings, N. D. and Barrett, A. J. (1995) Evolutionary families of metallopeptidases. *Methods Enzymol.* 248, 183–228.

11. Stöcker, W., Grams, F., Baumann, U., Reinemer, P., Gomis-Rüth, F. X., McKay, D. B. and Bode, W. (1995) The metzincins—topological and sequential relations between the astacins, adamalysins, serralysins, and matrixins (collagenases) define a superfamily of zinc-peptidases. *Protein Sci.* 4, 823–840.

12. Wolfsberg, T. G. and White, J. M. (1996) ADAMs in fertilization and development. *Dev. Biol.* 180, 389–401.

13. Black, R. A. and White, J. M. (1998) ADAMs: focus on the protease domain. *Curr. Opin. Cell Biol.* 10, 654–659.

14. Sternlicht, M. D. and Werb, Z. (1999) ECM proteinases, in *Guidebook to the Extracellular Matrix and Adhesion Proteins* (Kreis, T. and Vale, R., eds.), Oxford University Press, New York, pp. 503–603.

15. Maeda, H. and Morihara, K. (1995) Serralysin and related bacterial proteinases. *Methods Enzymol.* 248, 395–413.

16. Sang, Q. A. and Douglas, D. A. (1996) Computational sequence analysis of matrix metalloproteinases. *J. Protein Chem.* 15, 137–160.

17. Lepage, T. and Gache, C. (1990) Early expression of a collagenase-like hatching enzyme gene in the sea urchin embryo. *EMBO J.* 9, 3003–3012.

18. McGeehan, G., Burkhart, W., Anderegg, R., Becherer, J. D., Gillikin, J. W. and Graham, J. S. (1992) Sequencing and characterization of the soybean leaf metalloproteinase: structural and functional similarity to the matrix metalloproteinase family. *Plant Physiol.* 99, 1179–1183.

19. Pendás, A. M., Knäuper, V., Puente, X. S., Llano, E., Mattei, M. G., Apte, S., Murphy, G. and López-Otín, C. (1997) Identification and characterization of a novel human matrix metalloproteinase with unique structural characteristics, chromosomal location, and tissue distribution. *J. Biol. Chem.* 272, 4281–4286.

20. Yang, M., Murray, M. T. and Kurkinen, M. (1997) A novel matrix metalloproteinase gene (XMMP) encoding vitronectin-like motifs is transiently expressed in Xenopus laevis early embryo development. *J. Biol. Chem.* 272, 13527–13533.

21. Gururajan, R., Grenet, J., Lahti, J. M. and Kidd, V. J. (1998) Isolation and characterization of two novel metalloproteinase genes linked to the CdC2L locus on human chromosome 1p36.3. *Genomics* 52, 101–106.

22. Wada, K., Sato, H., Kinoh, H., Kajita, M., Yamamoto, H. and Seiki, M. (1998) Cloning of three Caenorhabditis elegans genes potentially encoding novel matrix metalloproteinases. *Gene* 211, 57–62.

23. Kinoshita, T., Fukuzawa, H., Shimada, T., Saito, T. and Matsuda, Y. (1992) Primary structure and expression of a gamete lytic enzyme in Chlamydomonas reinhardtii: similarity of functional domains to matrix metalloproteases. *Proc. Natl. Acad. Sci. (USA)* 89, 4693–4697.

24. Allan, J. A., Docherty, A. J., Barker, P. J., Huskisson, N. S., Reynolds, J. J. and Murphy, G. (1995) Binding of gelatinases A and B to type-I collagen and other matrix components. *Biochem. J.* 309, 299–306.

25. Birkedal-Hansen, H. (1995) Proteolytic remodeling of the extracellular matrix. *Curr. Opin. Cell Biol.* 7, 728–735.

26. Van Wart, H. E. and Birkedal-Hansen, H. (1990) The cysteine switch: a principle of regulation of metalloproteinase activity with potential applicability to the entire matrix metalloproteinase gene family. *Proc. Natl. Acad. Sci. (USA)* 87, 5578–5582.

27. Pei, D. and Weiss, S. J. (1995) Furin-dependent intracellular activation of the human stromelysin-3 zymogen. *Nature* 375, 244–247.

28. Strongin, A. Y., Collier, I., Bannikov, G., Marmer, B. L., Grant, G. A. and Goldberg, G. I. (1995) Mechanism of cell surface activation of 72-kDa type IV collagenase. Isolation of the activated form of the membrane metalloprotease. *J. Biol. Chem.* 270, 5331–5338.

29. Cao, J., Rehemtulla, A., Conner, C., Drews, M., Bahou, W. and Zucker, S. (1999) Furin directly processes pro-gelatinase A within the secretory pathway of cells. *Proc. American Association for Cancer Research* 40, 520 (#3432).

30. Brooks, P. C., Strömblad, S., Sanders, L. C., von Schalscha, T. L., Aimes, R. T., Stetler-Stevenson, W. G., Quigley, J. P. and Cheresh, D. A. (1996) Localization of matrix metalloproteinase MMP-2 to the surface of invasive cells by interaction with integrin alpha v beta 3. *Cell* 85, 683–693.

31. Angel, P., Baumann, I., Stein, B., Delius, H., Rahmsdorf, H. J. and Herrlich, P. (1987) 12-O-tetradecanoyl-phorbol-13-acetate induction of the human collagenase gene is mediated by an inducible enhancer element located in the 5'-flanking region. *Mol. Cell. Biol.* 7, 2256–2266.

32. Edwards, D. R., Murphy, G., Reynolds, J. J., Whitham, S. E., Docherty, A. J., Angel, P. and Heath, J. K. (1987) Transforming growth factor beta modulates the expression of collagenase and metalloproteinase inhibitor. *EMBO J.* 6, 1899–1904.

33. Brenner, D. A., O'Hara, M., Angel, P., Chojkier, M. and Karin, M. (1989) Prolonged activation of jun and collagenase genes by tumour necrosis factor-alpha. *Nature* 337, 661–663.

34. Rajah, R., Nunn, S. E., Herrick, D. J., Grunstein, M. M. and Cohen, P. (1996) Leukotriene D4 induces MMP-1, which functions as an IGFBP protease in human airway smooth muscle cells. *Am. J. Physiol.* 271, L1014–L1022.

35. Bian, J. and Sun, Y. (1997) Transcriptional activation by p53 of the human type IV collagenase (gelatinase A or matrix metalloproteinase 2) promoter. *Mol. Cell. Biol.* 17, 6330–6338.

36. Tremble, P., Damsky, C. H. and Werb, Z. (1995) Components of the nuclear signaling cascade that regulate collagenase gene expression in response to integrin-derived signals. *J. Cell Biol.* 129, 1707–1720.

37. Kheradmand, F., Werner, E., Tremble, P., Symons, M. and Werb, Z. (1998) Role of Rac1 and oxygen radicals in collagenase-1 expression induced by cell shape change. *Science* 280, 898–902.

38. Tremble, P. M., Lane, T. F., Sage, E. H and Werb, Z. (1993) SPARC, a secreted protein associated with morphogenesis and tissue remodeling, induces expression of metalloproteinases in fibroblasts through a novel extracellular matrix-dependent pathway. *J. Cell Biol.* 121, 1433–1444.

39. Biswas, C., Zhang, Y., DeCastro, R., Guo, H., Nakamura, T., Kataoka, H. and Nabeshima, K. (1995) The human tumor cell-derived collagenase stimulatory factor (renamed EMMPRIN) is a member of the immunoglobulin superfamily. *Cancer Res.* 55, 434–439.

40. Lohi, J., Lehti, K., Westermarck, J., Kähäri, V. M. and Keski-Oja, J. (1996) Regulation of membrane-type matrix metalloproteinase-1 expression by growth factors and phorbol 12-myristate 13-acetate. *Eur. J. Biochem.* 239, 239–247.

41. Yu, M., Sato, H., Seiki, M., Spiegel, S. and Thompson, E. W. (1998) Elevated cyclic AMP suppresses ConA-induced MT1-MMP expression in MDA-MB-231 human breast cancer cells. *Clin. Exp. Metastasis* 16, 185–191.

42. Gaire, M., Magbanua, Z., McDonnell, S., McNeil, L., Lovett, D. H. and Matrisian, L. M. (1994) Structure and expression of the human gene for the matrix metalloproteinase matrilysin. *J. Biol. Chem.* 269, 2032–2040.

43. Rutter, J. L., Mitchell, T. I., Butticè, G., Meyers, J., Gusella, J. F., Ozelius, L. J. and Brinckerhoff, C. E. (1998) A single nucleotide polymorphism in the matrix metalloproteinase-1 promoter creates an Ets binding site and augments transcription. *Cancer Res.* 58, 5321–5325.

44. Ye, S., Eriksson, P., Hamsten, A., Kurkinen, M., Humphries, S. E. and Henney, A. M. (1996) Progression of coronary atherosclerosis is associated with a common genetic variant of the human stromelysin-1 promoter which results in reduced gene expression. *J. Biol. Chem.* 271, 13055–13060.

45. Knäuper, V., Will, H., López-Otin, C., Smith, B., Atkinson, S. J., Stanton, H., Hembry, R. M. and Murphy, G. (1996) Cellular mechanisms for human procollagenase-3 (MMP-13) activation. Evidence that MT1-MMP (MMP-14) and gelatinase a (MMP-2) are able to generate active enzyme. *J. Biol. Chem.* 271, 17124–17131.

46. Fosang, A. J., Last, K. and Maciewicz, R. A. (1996) Aggrecan is degraded by matrix metalloproteinases in human arthritis. Evidence that matrix metalloproteinase and aggrecanase activities can be independent. *J. Clin. Invest.* 98, 2292–2299.

47. Stolow, M. A., Bauzon, D. D., Li, J., Sedgwick, T., Liang, V. C., Sang, Q. A. and Shi, Y. B. (1996) Identification and characterization of a novel collagenase in Xenopus laevis: possible roles during frog development. *Mol. Biol. Cell* **7**, 1471–1483.

48. Imai, K., Shikata, H. and Okada, Y. (1995) Degradation of vitronectin by matrix metalloproteinases-1, -2, -3, -7 and -9. *Febs Lett.* 369, 249–251.

49. Ohuchi, E., Imai, K., Fujii, Y., Sato, H., Seiki, M. and Okada, Y. (1997) Membrane type 1 matrix metalloproteinase digests interstitial collagens and other extracellular matrix macromolecules. *J. Biol. Chem.* 272, 2446–2451.

50. Levi, E., Fridman, R., Miao, H. Q., Ma, Y. S., Yayon, A. and Vlodavsky, I. (1996) Matrix metalloproteinase 2 releases active soluble ectodomain of fibroblast growth factor receptor 1. *Proc. Natl. Acad. Sci. (USA)* 93, 7069–7074.

51. Sasaki, T., Mann, K., Murphy, G., Chu, M. L. and Timpl, R. (1996) Different susceptibilities of fibulin-1 and fibulin-2 to cleavage by matrix metalloproteinases and other tissue proteases. *Eur. J. Biochem.* 240, 427–434.

52. Mayer, U., Mann, K., Timpl, R. and Murphy, G. (1993) Sites of nidogen cleavage by proteases involved in tissue homeostasis and remodelling. *Eur. J. Biochem.* 217, 877–884.

53. Ochieng, J., Fridman, R., Nangia-Makker, P., Kleiner, D. E., Liotta, L. A., Stetler-Stevenson, W. G. and Raz, A. (1994) Galectin-3 is a novel substrate for human matrix metalloproteinases-2 and -9. *Biochemistry* 33, 14109–14114.

54. Preece, G., Murphy, G. and Ager, A. (1996) Metalloproteinase-mediated regulation of L-selectin levels on leucocytes. *J. Biol. Chem.* 271, 11634–11640.

55. Gronski, T. J., Jr., Martin, R. L., Kobayashi, D. K., Walsh, B. C., Holman, M. C., Huber, M., Van Wart, H. E. and Shapiro, S. D. (1997) Hydrolysis of a broad spectrum of extracellular matrix proteins by human macrophage elastase. *J. Biol. Chem.* 272, 12189–12194.

56. Banda, M. J., Clark, E. J. and Werb, Z. (1985) Macrophage elastase: regulatory consequences of the proteolysis of non-elastin tissue substrates, in *Mononuclear Phagocytes: Characteristics, Physiology and Function.* (van Furth, R., ed.), Martinus Nijhoff, The Hague, pp. 295–301.

57. Giannelli, G., Falk-Marzillier, J., Schiraldi, O., Stetler-Stevenson, W. G. and Quaranta, V. (1997) Induction of cell migration by matrix metalloprotease-2 cleavage of laminin-5. *Science* 277, 225–228.

58. Suzuki, M., Raab, G., Moses, M. A., Fernandez, C. A. and Klagsbrun, M. (1997) Matrix metalloproteinase-3 releases active heparin-binding EGF-like growth factor by cleavage at a specific juxtamembrane site. *J. Biol. Chem.* 272, 31730–31737.

59. Aimes, R. T. and Quigley, J. P. (1995) Matrix metalloproteinase-2 is an interstitial collagenase. Inhibitor-free enzyme catalyzes the cleavage of collagen fibrils and soluble native type I collagen generating the specific 3/4- and 1/4-length fragments. *J. Biol. Chem.* 270, 5872–5876.

60. Kafienah, W., Bromme, D., Buttle, D. J., Croucher, L. J. and Hollander, A. P. (1998) Human cathepsin K cleaves native type I and II collagens at the N-terminal end of the triple helix. *Biochem. J.* 331, 727–732.
61. Matsumoto, S., Katoh, M., Saito, S., Watanabe, T. and Masuho, Y. (1997) Identification of soluble type of membrane-type matrix metalloproteinase-3 formed by alternatively spliced mRNA. *Biochim. Biophys. Acta* 1354, 159–170.
62. Murphy, G., Allan, J. A., Willenbrock, F., Cockett, M. I., O'Connell, J. P. and Docherty, A. J. (1992) The role of the C-terminal domain in collagenase and stromelysin specificity. *J. Biol. Chem.* 267, 9612–9618.
63. Sanchez-Lopez, R., Alexander, C. M., Behrendtsen, O., Breathnach, R. and Werb, Z. (1993) Role of zinc-binding- and hemopexin domain-encoded sequences in the substrate specificity of collagenase and stromelysin-2 as revealed by chimeric proteins. *J. Biol. Chem.* 268, 7238–7247.
64. Weingarten, H., Martin, R. and Feder, J. (1985) Synthetic substrates of vertebrate collagenase. *Biochemistry* 24, 6730–6734.
65. Oofusa, K., Yomori, S. and Yoshizato, K. (1994) Regionally and hormonally regulated expression of genes of collagen and collagenase in the anuran larval skin. *Int. J. Dev. Biol.* 38, 345–350.
66. Knäuper, V., López-Otin, C., Smith, B., Knight, G. and Murphy, G. (1996) Biochemical characterization of human collagenase-3. *J. Biol. Chem.* 271, 1544-1550.
67. Dioszegi, M., Cannon, P. and Van Wart, H. E. (1995) Vertebrate collagenases. *Methods Enzymol.* 248, 413–431.
68. Jeffrey, J. J. (1998) Interstitial collagenases, in *Matrix Metalloproteinases* (Parks, W. C. and Mecham, R. P., eds.), Academic Press, San Diego, pp. 15–42.
69. Freije, J. M., Díez-Itza, I., Balbín, M., Sánchez, L. M., Blasco, R., Tolivia, J. and López-Otín, C. (1994) Molecular cloning and expression of collagenase-3, a novel human matrix metalloproteinase produced by breast carcinomas. *J. Biol. Chem.* 269, 16766–16773.
70. Reboul, P., Pelletier, J. P., Tardif, G., Cloutier, J. M. and Martel-Pelletier, J. (1996) The new collagenase, collagenase-3, is expressed and synthesized by human chondrocytes but not by synoviocytes. A role in osteoarthritis. *J. Clin. Invest.* 97, 2011–2019.
71. Mitchell, P. G., Magna, H. A., Reeves, L. M., Lopresti-Morrow, L. L., Yocum, S. A., Rosner, P. J., Geoghegan, K. F. and Hambor, J. E. (1996) Cloning, expression, and type II collagenolytic activity of matrix metalloproteinase-13 from human osteoarthritic cartilage. *J. Clin. Invest.* 97, 761–768.
72. Hasty, K. A., Jeffrey, J. J., Hibbs, M. S. and Welgus, H. G. (1987) The collagen substrate specificity of human neutrophil collagenase. *J. Biol. Chem.* 262, 10048–10052.
73. Welgus, H. G., Jeffrey, J. J. and Eisen, A. Z. (1981) The collagen substrate specificity of human skin fibroblast collagenase. *J. Biol. Chem.* 256, 9511–9515.
74. Gomis-Rüth, F. X., Gohlke, U., Betz, M., Knäuper, V., Murphy, G., López-Otín, C. and Bode, W. (1996) The helping hand of collagenase-3 (MMP-13): 2.7 A crystal structure of its C-terminal haemopexin-like domain. *J. Mol. Biol.* 264, 556–566.
75. Liu, X., Wu, H., Byrne, M., Jeffrey, J., Krane, S. and Jaenisch, R. (1995) A targeted mutation at the known collagenase cleavage site in mouse type I collagen impairs tissue remodeling. *J. Cell Biol.* 130, 227–237.
76. Uitto, V. J., Airola, K., Vaalamo, M., Johansson, N., Putnins, E. E., Firth, J. D., Salonen, J., López-Otín, C., Saarialho-Kere, U. and Kähäri, V. M. (1998) Collagenase-3 (matrix metalloproteinase-13) expression is induced in oral mucosal epithelium during chronic inflammation. *Am. J. Pathol.* 152, 1489–1499.
77. Murphy, G. and Crabbe, T. (1995) Gelatinases A and B. *Methods Enzymol.* 248, 470–484.
78. Yu, A. E., Murphy, A. N. and Stetler-Stevenson, W. G. (1998) 72-kDa gelatinase (gelatinase A): structure, activation, regulation, and substrate specificity, in *Matrix Metalloproteinases* (Parks, W. C. and Mecham, R. P., eds.), Academic Press, San Diego, pp. 85–113.

79. Vu, T. H. and Werb, Z. (1998) Gelatinase B: structure, regulation, and function, in *Matrix Metalloproteinases* (Parks, W. C. and Mecham, R. P., eds.), Academic Press, San Diego, CA, pp. 115–148.

80. Collier, I. E., Wilhelm, S. M., Eisen, A. Z., Marmer, B. L., Grant, G. A., Seltzer, J. L., Kronberger, A., He, C. S., Bauer, E. A. and Goldberg, G. I. (1988) H-ras oncogene-transformed human bronchial epithelial cells (TBE-1) secrete a single metalloprotease capable of degrading basement membrane collagen. *J. Biol. Chem.* 263, 6579–6587.

81. Wilhelm, S. M., Collier, I. E., Marmer, B. L., Eisen, A. Z., Grant, G. A. and Goldberg, G. I. (1989) SV40-transformed human lung fibroblasts secrete a 92-kDa type IV collagenase which is identical to that secreted by normal human macrophages (published erratum appears in J Biol Chem 1990 Dec 25;265(36):22570). *J. Biol. Chem.* 264, 17213–17221.

82. Huhtala, P., Chow, L. T. and Tryggvason, K. (1990) Structure of the human type IV collagenase gene. *J. Biol. Chem.* 265, 11077–11082.

83. Huhtala, P., Tuuttila, A., Chow, L. T., Lohi, J., Keski-Oja, J. and Tryggvason, K. (1991) Complete structure of the human gene for 92-kDa type IV collagenase. Divergent regulation of expression for the 92- and 72-kilodalton enzyme genes in HT-1080 cells. *J. Biol. Chem.* 266, 16485–16490.

84. Murphy, G., Nguyen, Q., Cockett, M. I., Atkinson, S. J., Allan, J. A., Knight, C. G., Willenbrock, F. and Docherty, A. J. (1994) Assessment of the role of the fibronectin-like domain of gelatinase A by analysis of a deletion mutant. *J. Biol. Chem.* 269, 6632–6636.

85. Sang, Q. X., Birkedal-Hansen, H. and Van Wart, H. E. (1995) Proteolytic and non-proteolytic activation of human neutrophil progelatinase B. *Biochim. Biophys. Acta* 1251, 99–108.

86. Fridman, R., Toth, M., Peña, D. and Mobashery, S. (1995) Activation of progelatinase B (MMP-9) by gelatinase A (MMP-2). *Cancer Res.* 55, 2548–2555.

87. Mohan, R., Rinehart, W. B., Bargagna-Mohan, P. and Fini, M. E. (1998) Gelatinase B/lacZ transgenic mice, a model for mapping gelatinase B expression during developmental and injury related tissue remodeling. *J. Biol. Chem.* 273, 25903–25914.

88. Vu, T. H., Shipley, J. M., Bergers, G., Berger, J. E., Helms, J. A., Hanahan, D., Shapiro, S. D., Senior, R. M. and Werb, Z. (1998) MMP-9/gelatinase B is a key regulator of growth plate angiogenesis and apoptosis of hypertrophic chondrocytes. *Cell* 93, 411–422.

89. Rice, A. and Banda, M. J. (1995) Neutrophil elastase processing of gelatinase A is mediated by extracellular matrix. *Biochemistry* 34, 9249–9256.

90. Zucker, S., Conner, C., DiMassmo, B. I., Ende, H., Drews, M., Seiki, M. and Bahou, W. F. (1995) Thrombin induces the activation of progelatinase A in vascular endothelial cells. Physiologic regulation of angiogenesis. *J. Biol. Chem.* 270, 23730–23738.

91. Murphy, G., Willenbrock, F., Ward, R. V., Cockett, M. I., Eaton, D. and Docherty, A. J. (1992) The C-terminal domain of 72 kDa gelatinase A is not required for catalysis, but is essential for membrane activation and modulates interactions with tissue inhibitors of metalloproteinases [published erratum appears in Biochem. J. 1992 Jun 15;284(Pt 3):935]. *Biochem. J.* 283, 637–641.

92. Strongin, A. Y., Marmer, B. L., Grant, G. A. and Goldberg, G. I. (1993) Plasma membrane-dependent activation of the 72-kDa type IV collagenase is prevented by complex formation with TIMP-2. *J. Biol. Chem.* 268, 14033–14039.

93. Takino, T., Sato, H., Shinagawa, A. and Seiki, M. (1995) Identification of the second membrane-type matrix metalloproteinase (MT-MMP-2) gene from a human placenta cDNA library. MT-MMPs form a unique membrane-type subclass in the MMP family. *J. Biol. Chem.* 270, 23013–23020.

94. Olson, M. W., Toth, M., Gervasi, D. C., Sado, Y., Ninomiya, Y. and Fridman, R. (1998) High affinity binding of latent matrix metalloproteinase-9 to the alpha2(IV) chain of collagen IV. *J. Biol. Chem.* 273, 10672–10681.

95. Yu, Q. and Stamenkovic, I. (1999) Localization of matrix metalloproteinase 9 to the cell surface provides a mechanism for CD44-mediated tumor invasion. *Genes Dev.* 13, 35–48.
96. Nguyen, Q., Murphy, G., Hughes, C. E., Mort, J. S. and Roughley, P. J. (1993) Matrix metalloproteinases cleave at two distinct sites on human cartilage link protein. *Biochem. J.* 295, 595–598.
97. Lark, M. W., Williams, H., Hoernner, L. A., Weidner, J., Ayala, J. M., Harper, C. F., Christen, A., Olszewski, J., Konteatis, Z., Webber, R. and et al. (1995) Quantification of a matrix metalloproteinase-generated aggrecan G1 fragment using monospecific anti-peptide serum. *Biochem. J.* 307, 245–252.
98. Nagase, H. (1995) Human stromelysins 1 and 2. *Methods Enzymol.* 248, 449–470.
99. Chin, J. R., Murphy, G. and Werb, Z. (1985) Stromelysin, a connective tissue-degrading metalloendopeptidase secreted by stimulated rabbit synovial fibroblasts in parallel with collagenase. Biosynthesis, isolation, characterization, and substrates. *J. Biol. Chem.* 260, 12367–12376.
100. Nagase, H. (1998) Stromelysins 1 and 2, in *Matrix Metalloproteinases* (Parks, W. C. and Mecham, R. P., eds.), Academic Press, San Diego, pp. 43–84.
101. Muller, D., Quantin, B., Gesnel, M. C., Millon-Collard, R., Abecassis, J. and Breathnach, R. (1988) The collagenase gene family in humans consists of at least four members. *Biochem. J.* 253, 187–192.
102. Lochter, A., Galosy, S., Muschler, J., Freedman, N., Werb, Z. and Bissell, M. J. (1997) Matrix metalloproteinase stromelysin-1 triggers a cascade of molecular alterations that leads to stable epithelial-to-mesenchymal conversion and a premalignant phenotype in mammary epithelial cells. *J. Cell Biol.* 139, 1861–1872.
103. Sympson, C. J., Talhouk, R. S., Bissell, M. J. and Werb, Z. (1995) The role of metalloproteinases and their inhibitors in regulating mammary epithelial morphology and function in vivo. *Persp. Drug Discovery Design* 2, 401–411.
104. Lochter, A., Srebrow, A., Sympson, C. J., Terracio, N., Werb, Z. and Bissell, M. J. (1997) Misregulation of stromelysin-1 expression in mouse mammary tumor cells accompanies acquisition of stromelysin-1-dependent invasive properties. *J. Biol. Chem.* 272, 5007–5015.
105. Mudgett, J. S., Hutchinson, N. I., Chartrain, N. A., Forsyth, A. J., McDonnell, J., Singer, I. I., Bayne, E. K., Flanagan, J., Kawka, D., Shen, C. F., Stevens, K., Chen, H., Trumbauer, M. and Visco, D. M. (1998) Susceptibility of stromelysin 1-deficient mice to collagen-induced arthritis and cartilage destruction. *Arthritis Rheum.* 41, 110–121.
106. Sellers, A. and Woessner, J. F., Jr. (1980) The extraction of a neutral metalloproteinase from the involuting rat uterus, and its action on cartilage proteoglycan. *Biochem. J.* 189, 521–531.
107. Woessner, J. F., Jr. and Taplin, C. J. (1988) Purification and properties of a small latent matrix metalloproteinase of the rat uterus. *J. Biol. Chem.* 263, 16918–16925.
108. Quantin, B., Murphy, G. and Breathnach, R. (1989) Pump-1 cDNA codes for a protein with characteristics similar to those of classical collagenase family members. *Biochemistry* 28, 5327–5334.
109. Wilson, C. L. and Matrisian, L. M. (1998) Matrilysin, in *Matrix Metalloproteinases* (Parks, W. C. and Mecham, R. P., eds.), Academic Press, San Diego, pp. 149–184.
110. Woessner, J. F., Jr. (1995) Matrilysin. *Methods Enzymol.* 248, 485–495.
111. Sires, U. I., Griffin, G. L., Broekelmann, T. J., Mecham, R. P., Murphy, G., Chung, A. E., Welgus, H. G. and Senior, R. M. (1993) Degradation of entactin by matrix metalloproteinases. Susceptibility to matrilysin and identification of cleavage sites. *J. Biol. Chem.* 268, 2069–2074.
112. Witty, J. P., McDonnell, S., Newell, K. J., Cannon, P., Navre, M., Tressler, R. J. and Matrisian, L. M. (1994) Modulation of matrilysin levels in colon carcinoma cell lines affects tumorigenicity in vivo. *Cancer Res.* 54, 4805–4812.
113. Powell, W. C., Knox, J. D., Navre, M., Grogan, T. M., Kittelson, J., Nagle, R. B. and Bowden, G. T. (1993) Expression of the metalloproteinase matrilysin in DU-145 cells in-

creases their invasive potential in severe combined immunodeficient mice. *Cancer Res.* 53, 417–422.

114. Rudolph-Owen, L. A. and Matrisian, L. M. (1998) Matrix metalloproteinases in remodeling of the normal and neoplastic mammary gland. *J. Mammary Gland Biol. Neoplasia* 3, 177–189.

115. Saarialho-Kere, U. K., Crouch, E. C. and Parks, W. C. (1995) Matrix metalloproteinase matrilysin is constitutively expressed in adult human exocrine epithelium. *J. Invest. Dermatol.* 105, 190–196.

116. Rudolph-Owen, L. A., Cannon, P. and Matrisian, L. M. (1998) Overexpression of the matrix metalloproteinase matrilysin results in premature mammary gland differentiation and male infertility. *Mol. Biol. Cell* 9, 421–435.

117. Halpert, I., Sires, U. I., Roby, J. D., Potter-Perigo, S., Wight, T. N., Shapiro, S. D., Welgus, H. G., Wickline, S. A. and Parks, W. C. (1996) Matrilysin is expressed by lipid-laden macrophages at sites of potential rupture in atherosclerotic lesions and localizes to areas of versican deposition, a proteoglycan substrate for the enzyme. *Proc. Natl. Acad. Sci. (USA)* 93, 9748–9753.

118. Sato, H., Takino, T., Okada, Y., Cao, J., Shinagawa, A., Yamamoto, E. and Seiki, M. (1994) A matrix metalloproteinase expressed on the surface of invasive tumour cells. *Nature* 370, 61–65.

119. Will, H. and Hinzmann, B. (1995) cDNA sequence and mRNA tissue distribution of a novel human matrix metalloproteinase with a potential transmembrane segment. *Eur. J. Biochem.* 231, 602–608.

120. Puente, X. S., Pendás, A. M., Llano, E., Velasco, G. and López-Otín, C. (1996) Molecular cloning of a novel membrane-type matrix metalloproteinase from a human breast carcinoma. *Cancer Res.* 56, 944–949.

121. Sato, H., Kinoshita, T., Takino, T., Nakayama, K. and Seiki, M. (1996) Activation of a recombinant membrane type 1-matrix metalloproteinase (MT1-MMP) by furin and its interaction with tissue inhibitor of metalloproteinases (TIMP)-2. *FEBS Lett.* 393, 101–104.

122. Pei, D. and Weiss, S. J. (1996) Transmembrane-deletion mutants of the membrane-type matrix metalloproteinase-1 process progelatinase A and express intrinsic matrix-degrading activity. *J. Biol. Chem.* 271, 9135–9140.

123. Cao, J., Rehemtulla, A., Bahou, W. and Zucker, S. (1996) Membrane type matrix metalloproteinase 1 activates pro-gelatinase A without furin cleavage of the N-terminal domain. *J. Biol. Chem.* 271, 30174–30180.

124. Okumura, Y., Sato, H., Seiki, M. and Kido, H. (1997) Proteolytic activation of the precursor of membrane type 1 matrix metalloproteinase by human plasmin. A possible cell surface activator. *FEBS Lett.* 402, 181–184.

125. Imai, K., Ohuchi, E., Aoki, T., Nomura, H., Fujii, Y., Sato, H., Seiki, M. and Okada, Y. (1996) Membrane-type matrix metalloproteinase 1 is a gelatinolytic enzyme and is secreted in a complex with tissue inhibitor of metalloproteinases 2. *Cancer Res.* 56, 2707–2710.

126. Apte, S. S., Fukai, N., Beier, D. R. and Olsen, B. R. (1997) The matrix metalloproteinase-14 (MMP-14) gene is structurally distinct from other MMP genes and is co-expressed with the TIMP-2 gene during mouse embryogenesis. *J. Biol. Chem.* 272, 25511–25517.

127. Zucker, S., Drews, M., Conner, C., Foda, H. D., DeClerck, Y. A., Langley, K. E., Bahou, W. F., Docherty, A. J. and Cao, J. (1998) Tissue inhibitor of metalloproteinase-2 (TIMP-2) binds to the catalytic domain of the cell surface receptor, membrane type 1-matrix metalloproteinase 1 (MT1-MMP). *J. Biol. Chem.* 273, 1216–1222.

128. Nakahara, H., Howard, L., Thompson, E. W., Sato, H., Seiki, M., Yeh, Y. and Chen, W. T. (1997) Transmembrane/cytoplasmic domain-mediated membrane type 1-matrix metalloprotease docking to invadopodia is required for cell invasion. *Proc. Natl. Acad. Sci. (USA)* 94, 7959–7964.

129. Cowell, S., Knäuper, V., Stewart, M. L., D'Ortho, M. P., Stanton, H., Hembry, R. M., López-Otín, C., Reynolds, J. J. and Murphy, G. (1998) Induction of matrix metalloproteinase activation cascades based on membrane-type 1 matrix metalloproteinase: associated activation of gelatinase A, gelatinase B and collagenase 3. *Biochem. J.* 331, 453–458.

130. Atkinson, S. J., Crabbe, T., Cowell, S., Ward, R. V., Butler, M. J., Sato, H., Seiki, M., Reynolds, J. J. and Murphy, G. (1995) Intermolecular autolytic cleavage can contribute to the activation of progelatinase A by cell membranes. *J. Biol. Chem.* 270, 30479–30485.

131. Okada, A., Bellocq, J. P., Rouyer, N., Chenard, M. P., Rio, M. C., Chambon, P. and Basset, P. (1995) Membrane-type matrix metalloproteinase (MT-MMP) gene is expressed in stromal cells of human colon, breast, and head and neck carcinomas. *Proc. Natl. Acad. Sci. (USA)* 92, 2730–2734.

132. Ohtani, H., Motohashi, H., Sato, H., Seiki, M. and Nagura, H. (1996) Dual over-expression pattern of membrane-type metalloproteinase-1 in cancer and stromal cells in human gastrointestinal carcinoma revealed by in situ hybridization and immunoelectron microscopy. *Int. J. Cancer* 68, 565–570.

133. Basset, P., Bellocq, J. P., Wolf, C., Stoll, I., Hutin, P., Limacher, J. M., Podhajcer, O. L., Chenard, M. P., Rio, M. C. and Chambon, P. (1990) A novel metalloproteinase gene specifically expressed in stromal cells of breast carcinomas. *Nature* 348, 699–704.

134. Murphy, G., Segain, J. P., O'Shea, M., Cockett, M., Ioannou, C., Lefebvre, O., Chambon, P. and Basset, P. (1993) The 28-kDa N-terminal domain of mouse stromelysin-3 has the general properties of a weak metalloproteinase. *J. Biol. Chem.* 268, 15435–15441.

135. Ahmad, A., Hanby, A., Dublin, E., Poulsom, R., Smith, P., Barnes, D., Rubens, R., Anglard, P. and Hart, I. (1998) Stromelysin 3: an independent prognostic factor for relapse-free survival in node-positive breast cancer and demonstration of novel breast carcinoma cell expression. *Am. J. Pathol.* 152, 721–728.

136. Werb, Z. and Gordon, S. (1975) Elastase secretion by stimulated macrophages. Characterization and regulation. *J. Exp. Med.* 142, 361–377.

137. Banda, M. J. and Werb, Z. (1981) Mouse macrophage elastase. Purification and characterization as a metalloproteinase. *Biochem. J.* 193, 589–605.

138. Shapiro, S. D., Griffin, G. L., Gilbert, D. J., Jenkins, N. A., Copeland, N. G., Welgus, H. G., Senior, R. M. and Ley, T. J. (1992) Molecular cloning, chromosomal localization, and bacterial expression of a murine macrophage metalloelastase. *J. Biol. Chem.* **267**, 4664–4671.

139. Shapiro, S. D., Kobayashi, D. K. and Ley, T. J. (1993) Cloning and characterization of a unique elastolytic metalloproteinase produced by human alveolar macrophages. *J. Biol. Chem.* 268, 23824–23829.

140. Shipley, J. M., Wesselschmidt, R. L., Kobayashi, D. K., Ley, T. J. and Shapiro, S. D. (1996) Metalloelastase is required for macrophage-mediated proteolysis and matrix invasion in mice. *Proc. Natl. Acad. Sci. (USA)* 93, 3942–3946.

141. Hautamaki, R. D., Kobayashi, D. K., Senior, R. M. and Shapiro, S. D. (1997) Requirement for macrophage elastase for cigarette smoke-induced emphysema in mice. *Science* 277, 2002–2004.

142. Shapiro, S. D. and Senior, R. M. (1998) Macrophage metalloelastase (MMP-12), in *Matrix Metalloproteinases* (Parks, W. C. and Mecham, R. P., eds.), Academic Press, San Diego, pp. 185–197.

143. Dong, Z., Kumar, R., Yang, X. and Fidler, I. J. (1997) Macrophage-derived metalloelastase is responsible for the generation of angiostatin in Lewis lung carcinoma. *Cell* 88, 801–810.

144. Bartlett, J. D., Simmer, J. P., Xue, J., Margolis, H. C. and Moreno, E. C. (1996) Molecular cloning and mRNA tissue distribution of a novel matrix metalloproteinase isolated from porcine enamel organ. *Gene* 183, 123–128.

145. Llano, E., Pendás, A. M., Knäuper, V., Sorsa, T., Salo, T., Salido, E., Murphy, G., Simmer, J. P., Bartlett, J. D. and López-Otín, C. (1997) Identification and structural and functional characterization of human enamelysin (MMP-20). *Biochemistry* 36, 15101–15108.

146. Punzi, J. S. and DenBesten, P. K. (1995) Multiple forms of a 21.5 kDa metalloproteinase in bovine enamel. *J. Dent. Res.* 74, 95.
147. Sedlacek, R., Mauch, S., Kolb, B., Schätzlein, C., Eibel, H., Peter, H. H., Schmitt, J. and Krawinkel, U. (1998) Matrix metalloproteinase MMP-19 (RASI-1) is expressed on the surface of activated peripheral blood mononuclear cells and is detected as an autoantigen in rheumatoid arthritis. *Immunobiology* 198, 408–423.
148. Cossins, J., Dudgeon, T. J., Catlin, G., Gearing, A. J. and Clements, J. M. (1996) Identification of MMP-18, a putative novel human matrix metalloproteinase. *Biochem. Biophys. Res. Commun.* 228, 494–498.
149. Valesco, G., Pendas, A. M., Fueyo, A., Knauper, V., Murphy, G. and Lopez-Otin, C. (1999) Cloning and characterization of human MMP-23, a new matrix metalloproteinase predominantly expressed in reproductive tissues and lacking conserved domains in other family members. *J. Biol. Chem.* 274, 4570–4576.
150. Greene, J., Wang, M., Liu, Y. E., Raymond, L. A., Rosen, C. and Shi, Y. E. (1996) Molecular cloning and characterization of human tissue inhibitor of metalloproteinase 4. *J. Biol. Chem.* 271, 30375–30380.
151. Leco, K. J., Apte, S. S., Taniguchi, G. T., Hawkes, S. P., Khokha, R., Schultz, G. A. and Edwards, D. R. (1997) Murine tissue inhibitor of metalloproteinases-4 (Timp-4): cDNA isolation and expression in adult mouse tissues. *FEBS Lett.* 401, 213–217.
152. Apte, S. S., Olsen, B. R. and Murphy, G. (1995) The gene structure of tissue inhibitor of metalloproteinases (TIMP)-3 and its inhibitory activities define the distinct TIMP gene family (published erratum appears in J. Biol. Chem. (1996) 271, 2874). *J. Biol. Chem.* 270, 14313–14318.
153. Murphy, G. and Willenbrock, F. (1995) Tissue inhibitors of matrix metalloendopeptidases. *Methods Enzymol.* 248, 496–510.
154. Docherty, A. J., Lyons, A., Smith, B. J., Wright, E. M., Stephens, P. E., Harris, T. J., Murphy, G. and Reynolds, J. J. (1985) Sequence of human tissue inhibitor of metalloproteinases and its identity to erythroid-potentiating activity. *Nature* 318, 66–69.
155. Bodden, M. K., Harber, G. J., Birkedal-Hansen, B., Windsor, L. J., Caterina, N. C., Engler, J. A. and Birkedal-Hansen, H. (1994) Functional domains of human TIMP-1 (tissue inhibitor of metalloproteinases). *J. Biol. Chem.* 269, 18943–18952.
156. Williamson, R. A., Carr, M. D., Frenkiel, T. A., Feeney, J. and Freedman, R. B. (1997) Mapping the binding site for matrix metalloproteinase on the N-terminal domain of the tissue inhibitor of metalloproteinases-2 by NMR chemical shift perturbation. *Biochemistry* 36, 13882–13889.
157. Gomis-Rüth, F. X., Maskos, K., Betz, M., Bergner, A., Huber, R., Suzuki, K., Yoshida, N., Nagase, H., Brew, K., Bourenkov, G. P., Bartunik, H. and Bode, W. (1997) Mechanism of inhibition of the human matrix metalloproteinase stromelysin-1 by TIMP-1. *Nature* 389, 77–81.
158. O'Shea, M., Willenbrock, F., Williamson, R. A., Cockett, M. I., Freedman, R. B., Reynolds, J. J., Docherty, A. J. and Murphy, G. (1992) Site-directed mutations that alter the inhibitory activity of the tissue inhibitor of metalloproteinases-1: importance of the N-terminal region between cysteine 3 and cysteine 13. *Biochemistry* 31, 10146–10152.
159. Windsor, L. J., Bodden, M. K., Birkedal-Hansen, B., Engler, J. A. and Birkedal-Hansen, H. (1994) Mutational analysis of residues in and around the active site of human fibroblast-type collagenase. *J. Biol. Chem.* 269, 26201–26207.
160. Logan, S. K., Garabedian, M. J., Campbell, C. E. and Werb, Z. (1996) Synergistic transcriptional activation of the tissue inhibitor of metalloproteinases-1 promoter via functional interaction of AP-1 and Ets-1 transcription factors. *J. Biol. Chem.* 271, 774–782.
161. Stetler-Stevenson, W. G., Brown, P. D., Onisto, M., Levy, A. T. and Liotta, L. A. (1990) Tissue inhibitor of metalloproteinases-2 (TIMP-2) mRNA expression in tumor cell lines and human tumor tissues. *J. Biol. Chem.* 265, 13933–13938.

162. Leco, K. J., Hayden, L. J., Sharma, R. R., Rocheleau, H., Greenberg, A. H. and Edwards, D. R. (1992) Differential regulation of TIMP-1 and TIMP-2 mRNA expression in normal and Ha-ras-transformed murine fibroblasts. *Gene* 117, 209–217.

163. Wick, M., Bürger, C., Brüsselbach, S., Lucibello, F. C. and Müller, R. (1994) A novel member of human tissue inhibitor of metalloproteinases (TIMP) gene family is regulated during G1 progression, mitogenic stimulation, differentiation, and senescence. *J. Biol. Chem.* 269, 18953–18960.

164. Wick, M., Härönen, R., Mumberg, D., Bürger, C., Olsen, B. R., Budarf, M. L., Apte, S. S. and Müller, R. (1995) Structure of the human TIMP-3 gene and its cell cycle-regulated promoter. *Biochem. J.* 311, 549–554.

165. Uría, J. A., Ferrando, A. A., Velasco, G., Freije, J. M. and López-Otín, C. (1994) Structure and expression in breast tumors of human TIMP-3, a new member of the metalloproteinase inhibitor family. *Cancer Res.* 54, 2091–2094.

166. Jones, S. E., Jomary, C. and Neal, M. J. (1994) Expression of TIMP3 mRNA is elevated in retinas affected by simplex retinitis pigmentosa. *FEBS Lett.* 352, 171–174.

167. Fariss, R. N., Apte, S. S., Olsen, B. R., Iwata, K. and Milam, A. H. (1997) Tissue inhibitor of metalloproteinases-3 is a component of Bruch's membrane of the eye. *Am. J. Pathol.* 150, 323–328.

168. Weber, B. H., Vogt, G., Pruett, R. C., Stöhr, H. and Felbor, U. (1994) Mutations in the tissue inhibitor of metalloproteinases-3 (TIMP3) in patients with Sorsby's fundus dystrophy. *Nature Genet.* 8, 352–356.

169. Felbor, U., Stöhr, H., Amann, T., Schönherr, U. and Weber, B. H. (1995) A novel Ser156Cys mutation in the tissue inhibitor of metalloproteinases-3 (TIMP3) in Sorsby's fundus dystrophy with unusual clinical features. *Hum. Mol. Genet.* 4, 2415–2416.

170. Amour, A., Slocombe, P. M., Webster, A., Butler, M., Knight, C. G., Smith, B. J., Stephens, P. E., Shelley, C., Hutton, M., Knauper, V., Docherty, A. J. and Murphy, G. (1998) TNF-alpha converting enzyme (TACE) is inhibited by TIMP-3. *FEBS Lett.* 435, 39–44.

171. Bachman, K. E., Herman, J. G., Corn, P. G., Merlo, A., Costello, J. F., Cavenee, W. K., Baylin, S. B. and Graff, J. R. (1999) Methylation-associated silencing of the tissue inhibitor of metalloproteinase-3 gene suggests a suppressor role in kidney, brain, and other human cancers. *Cancer Res.* 59, 798–802.

172. Kataoka, H., Uchino, H., Iwamura, T., Seiki, M., Nabeshima, K. and Koono, M. (1999) Enhanced tumor growth and invasiveness in vivo by a carboxyl-terminal fragment of α-proteinase inhibitor generated by matrix metalloproteinases: a possible modulatory role in natural killer cytotoxicity. *Am. J. Pathol.* 154, 457–468.

173. Patterson, B. C. and Sang, Q. A. (1997) Angiostatin-converting enzyme activities of human matrilysin (MMP-7) and gelatinase B/type IV collagenase (MMP-9). *J. Biol. Chem.* 272, 28823–28825.

174. Werb, Z. (1997) ECM and cell surface proteolysis: regulating cellular ecology. *Cell* 91, 439–442.

175. Lukashev, M. E. and Werb, Z. (1998) ECM signalling: orchestrating cell behaviour and misbehaviour. *Trends Cell Biol.* 8, 437–441.

176. Tlsty, T. D. (1998) Cell-adhesion-dependent influences on genomic instability and carcinogenesis. *Curr. Opin. Cell Biol.* 10, 647–653.

2 Substrate Specificity of MMPs

Hideaki Nagase, *PhD*

CONTENTS

INTRODUCTION
ACTIONS ON PROTEIN SUBSTRATES
PEPTIDE SUBSTRATE SPECIFICITY
CONCLUSIONS

1. INTRODUCTION

Matrix metalloproteinases (MMPs) are secreted or cell surface-bound zinc metalloendopeptidases that act on extracellular matrix (ECM) macromolecules. Thus, isolated MMPs have been tested against various components of ECM. Based on similarities in primary structure and the abilities to cleave ECM components, MMPs are grouped into collagenases, gelatinases, stromelysins, membrane-type MMP(MT-MMPs), and others which do not belong to those subgroups. Most MMPs consist of four typical domain structures: propeptide, catalytic, linker region, and a C-terminal hemopexin-like domains. The catalytic domain share structural similarity with interstitial collagenase (MMP-1). The propeptide domain has least similarities among MMPs, all but except MMP-23 *(1)* have the so-called cysteine switch sequence motif, PRCG[V/N]PD, whose cysteinyl residue ligates the catalytic zinc atom of the active site as the fourth ligand and maintain inactive proenzyme. Another conserved sequence is the zinc binding motif HEXGHXXGXXH, in which three histidines bind to Zn^{2+}. Three dimensional structures of the catalytic domains of MMPs [MMP-1 *(2–6)*, MMP-3 *(7–9)*, MMP-7 *(10)*, MMP-8 *(11,12)*, MMP-14 *(13)*] indicate that the polypeptide fold of the catalytic domains are essentially identical, although their substrate specificities are sufficiently different when peptide substrates were tested *(14)*. In addition, the action of MMPs on natural protein substrates is not only dectated by the subsite requirement of the

From: *Cancer Drug Discovery and Development:*
Matrix Metalloproteinase Inhibitors in Cancer Therapy
Edited by: Neil J. Clendeninn and Krzysztof Appelt © Humana Press Inc., Totowa, NJ

catalytic domains, but it is often influenced by the domains other than the catalytic domain. This chapter describes activities of MMPs on natural substrates and substrate specificity based on synthetic substrates.

2. ACTIONS ON PROTEIN SUBSTRATES

Earlier studies distinguished collagenases that degrade triple helical region of interstitial collagens *(15)* and gelatinases *(16,17)* that ready degrade denatured collagens (gelatins). A third metalloproteinase (MMP-3/stromylsin 1) was characterized for its ability to degrade various noncollagenous ECM components such as core protein of aggrecan, fibronectin, laminin, and type IV collagen *(18–20)*. Recent studies, however, have revealed that the actions of those enzymes are not restricted to those substrates but they can act on a large number of native protein substrates. Currently twenty-one vertebrate MMPs have been identified, and their potential substrates are listed in Table 1.

2.1. Collagenases

Collagenases are characterized for their abilities to cleave triple-helical regions of interstitial collagnes (types I, II, and III) at a site about three-fourths away from the N-terminus. Four MMPs belong to this subgroup: MMP-1 (interstitial collagenase/collagenase 1), MMP-8 (neutrophil collagenase/collogenase 2), MMP-13 (collagenase 3), and MMP-18 (collagenase 4). They consist of propeptide, catalytic domain, hinge region, and the C-terminal hemopexin-like domain, and they are about 50–55% identical in sequence. To express collagenolytic activity, they have to retain both the catalytic and hemopexin domains (the full-length enzyme), although the catalytic domain alone has proteolytic activity against other protein substrates and synthetic substrates. Those properties have been shown for MMP-1 *(21,22)*, MMP-8 *(23)*, and MMP-13 *(24)*. A similar principle probably applies to MMP-18. Nonetheless, it is not clear how the hemopexin domain help to cleave triple-helical collagens because the isolated hemopexin domains of MMP-8 and MMP-13 does not bind to collagen *(23,24)*, although the hemopexin domain of MMP-1 was reported to bind to type I collagen *(22)*. The hemopexin domain has two conserved cysteines that are disulfide bonded. Mutation of those cysteines to alanines *(25)* or reduction and alkylation destroys collagenolytic activity (K. Suzuki and H. Nagase, unpublished results). The three dimensional structures of collagenases *(2–6,11,12,26,27)* indicate that the active center has an extended substrate binding site about 5Å wide, but it is too narrow to accommodate a triple-helical structure of about 15 Å wide diameter *(28)*. This suggests that the binding of collagenases to collagen must partially unwind triple helix to allow cleavage of the individual α chains. Since heat-denatured collagens (gelatins) are poorer substrates at 37°C *(29)*, interaction of collagenase to interstitial collagen must induce conformational change in α chain of collagen that fits the substrate binding site of the catalytic domain, but the molecular basis of this mechanism is not known. The model of this triple helicase activity proposed by Gomis-Rüth et al. *(30)* suggests that the hemopexin domain folds over the catalytic site, sandwiching and trapping the triple-helical collagen molecule, and partially unwinding the triple helix. On the other hand, de Souza et al. *(31)* have hypothesized that the prolin-rich hinge region, which contains a repeated motif (Pro-Xaa-Yaa), might adopt a poly-proline II-like conformation. Their energy-minimized model of the complex of collagen triple helix and collagenase linker region proposes a "proline zipper-like" alignment between the linker and the two helix of the collagen, but experimental evidence for such interaction has not been provided.

Although all collagenases cleave interstitial collagens, each collagenase exhibit different preferences on collagen types. Table 2 lists the kinetic studies of three collagenases. Human MMP-1 degrade human collagens in the following preference: type III > type I >> type II. Whereas human type III collagen is most readily cleaved by MMP-1, guinea pig type III is a poorer substrate, suggesting that the action of MMP-1 on a particular collagen type may depend on species. Type II collagen is a poor substrate for MMP-1. However, MMP-13 digests type II collagen more readily than MMP-1 or MMP-8 (Table 2). Recently, Billinghurst et al. *(32)* reported that MMP-1, MMP-8, and MMP-13 initially cleave the Gly775-Leu776 bond of type II collagen then the Gly778-Gln779 bond of the C-terminal fragment. MMP-13 also digests aminotelopeptides of type I collagen and depolymenzes the crosslinked fibrillar collagen *(33)*. This action is primarily due to the catalytic domain of MMP-13 *(33,34)*. Digestion of types IV, IX, X, and XIV by MMP-13 does not require the hemopexin domain *(24)*. The best natural substrate of MMP-1 is α_2-macroglobulin ($\alpha_2 M$) with the association rate constant $k_2/K_i = 280 \times 10^4 \, M^{-1}s^{-1}$, which is approx 150-fold better substrate compared with human type I collagen ($k_{cat}/K_m = 1.8 \times 10^4 \, M^{-1}s^{-1}$) *(35)*.

As listed in Table 1, collagenases cleave a number of other ECM components and serum proteins.

2.2. Gelatinases

Gelatinase A (MMP-2) and gelatinase B (MMP-9) are in this subgroup, and both enzymes readily degrade heat-denatured collagens. These enzymes were once referred to as "type IV collagenases" because of their abilities to cleave type IV collagen, but their activity on type IV collagen is much weaker than that on type V collagen *(36,37)*. Senior et al. *(38)* reported that both gelatinases have elastolytic activity, and on a molar basis recombinant MMP-9 was 30% as active as human leukocyte elastase in solubilizing elastin and similar to that of macrophage metalloelastase (MMP-12) *(39)*. Both gelatinases possess three fibronectin type II-like repeats inserted in tandem just before the catalytic zinc

Table 1
Protein Substrates for the Matrix Metalloproteinases

Enzyme	MMP no.	Substrates
Collagenases		
Interstitial collagenase (collagenase 1)	MMP-1	Collagens I, II, III, VII, VIII[a], X, and XI[b], gelatin, Clq[c], entactin, tenascin, aggrecan, link protein[d], fibronectin[e], vitronectin[f], myelin basic protein[g], α₂-macroglobulin[h], ovostatin[h], α₁-proteinase inhibitor[i], α₁-antichymotrypsin[i], IL-1β[j], proTNF-α[k], IGFBP-3[l], casein[m], proMMP-2, proMMP-9
Neutrophil collagenase (collagenase 2)	MMP-8	Collagen I, II, and III, Clq[e], aggrecan, α₂M[r], ovostatin[g], α₁PI[h'], substrate P[i']
Collagenase 3	MMP-13	Collagen I[w], II[w], III[w], IV[w], IX[x'], X[x'] and XIV[x'], gelatin[z'], collagen telopeptides[y'], Clq[a'], fibronectin[x'], SPARC[x'], aggrecan[b''], α₂M[c'], casein[y']
Collagenase 4 (*Xenopus*)	MMP-18	Collagen I[g'], gelatin[g'']
Gelatinases		
Gelatinase A	MMP-2	Collagen I, III, IV, V, VII and X, gelatin, fibronectin, laminin, aggrecan, link protein[d], elastin, vitronectin[f], tenascin[p], SPARC[q], decorin[r], myelin basic protein[g], α₁PI[s], α₁-antichymotrypsin[s], IL-1β[j], proTNF-α[k], IGFBP-3[l], substance P[t]
Gelatinase B	MMP-9	Collagen IV, V, XI[k'], XIV[l'], elastin, aggrecan, link protein[d], decorin[r], laminin[n'], entactin, SPARC[q], myelin basic protein[m'], α₂M[n'], α₁PI[i'], IL-1β[j], proTNF-α[k], substrate P[i'], casein[o]
Stromelysins		
Stromelysin 1	MMP-3	Collagen III[u], IV, V[u], IX, X and XI, teropeptides (collagen I and II), gelatin, aggrecan, link protein[d], elastin, fibronectin, vitronectin[f], laminin, entactin[w], tenascin, SPARC[q], decorin[r], myelin basic protein[g], α₂-macroglobulin[h], ovostatin[h], α₁-PI[s], α₁-antichy-motrypsin[s], IL-1β[j], proTNF-α[k], IGFBP-3[l], substance P[x], T kininogen[z], casein[z], proMMP-1, proMMP-3[a'], proMMP-8, proMMP-9
Stromelysin 2	MMP-10	Collagen III[u], IV and V[u], gelatin, fibronectin, elastin, aggrecan, link protein[d], casein[p'], proMMP-1, proMMP-7[q], proMMP-8, proMMP-9[q']

MT-MMPs

MT1-MMP	MMP-14	proMMP-2, Collagen I[d''], II[d''], and III[d''], gelatin[e''], fibronectin[d''], vitronectin[d''], laminin[d''], entactin[e''], aggregan[f''], α_2M[r'], α_1Pl[f''], proTNF-α[r''], decorin[r'']
MT2-MMP	MMP-15	ProMMP-2[i''], laminin[f''], fibronectin[f''], tenascin[f''], entactin[f''], aggregan[f''], perlecan[f''], proTNF-α[f'']
MT3-MMP	MMP-16	ProMMP-2[k'']
MT4-MMP	MMP-17	Not known
MT5-MMP	MMP-24	Gelatin[e''], proMMP-2[l'']

Others

Matrilysin	MMP-7	Collagen IV, gelatin, aggrecan, link protein[d], elastin, fibronectin, vitronectin[f], laminin[b'], SPARC[q], enactin, docorin[r], myelin basic protein[g], tenascin, fibulin-1 and -2[h''], proTNF-α[k], casein[c'], α_1-Pl[d''], proMMP-1, proMMP-2, proMMP-9
Stromelysin 3	MMP-11	Collagen IV, gelatin[q], fibronectin, laminin, aggrecan, α_1Pl[r], α_2M[r']
Metalloelastase	MMP-12	Elastin, collagen IV[t], gelatin[s], fibronectin[t], vitronectin[t], laminin[t], entactin[t], aggrecan[t], myelin basic protein[s], α_2M[u''], α_1Pl[v''], proTNF-α[s]
Enamelysin	MMP-19	Gelatin[m''], large tenascin C[m''], aggrecan[m'']
XMMP (*Xenopus*)	MMP-20	Amelogenin[n'']
CMMP (Chicken)	MMP-21	Not known
	MMP-22	Caseine[o''], gelatin[o'']
	MMP-23	Autoproteolysis of proMMP-23[p''], Mca-peptide[p'']

[a]Sage et al. (106); [b]Gadher et al. (107); [c]Menzel and Smolen (108); [d]Nguyen et al. (109); [e]Fukai et al. (110); [f]Imai et al. (111); [g]Chandler et al. (112); [h]Enghild et al. (35); [i]Desrochers et al. (113); [j]Ito et al. (114); [k]Gearing et al. (115); [l]Fowlkes et al. (116); [m]Cawston and Taylor (117); [n]Siri et al. (118); [q]Sasaki et al. (119); [r]Imai et al. (120); [s]Mast et al. (121); [t]Nakagawa and Debuchi (122); [u]Nicholson et al. (50); [w]Mayer et al. (123); [x]Stein et al. (124); [y]Sakamoto et al. (125); [z]Chin et al. (19); [a']Nagase et al. (83); [b']Miyazaki et al. (126); [c']Quantin et al. (127); [d']Sires et al. (128); [e']Fletcher et al. (129); [f']Murphy et al. (130); [g']Kudo et al. (131); [h']Desrochers et al. (132); [i']Diekmann and Tschesche (133); [k']Hirose et al. (134); [l']Sires et al. (135); [m']Gijbels et al. (136); [n']Morodomi et al. (37); [o']Lyons et al. (137); [p']Sanchez-Lopez et al. (138); [q']Murphy et al. (70); [r']Pei et al. (72); [s']Chandler et al. (139); [t']Gronski et al. (39); [u']Banda and Werb (73); [v']Banda et al. (140); [w']Welgus et al. (141); [x']Knäuper et al. (24); [y']Lamaître et al. (34); [z']Welgus et al. (142); [a'']Eeckhout et al. (143); [b'']Fosang et al. (144); [c'']Nethery and O'Grady (145); [d'']Ohuchi et al.(67); [e'']Imai et al. (146); [f'']D'Ortho et al. (68); [g'']Stolow et al. (147); [h'']Sasaki et al. (148); [i'']Butler et al. (61); [k'']Takino et al. (62); [l'']Pei (63); [m'']Murphy et al. (149); [n'']Llano et al. (78); [o'']Yang and Kurkinen (80); [p'']Velsaco et al. (82); [q'']Nakamura et al. (57)

The list is after Sang and Douglas (105) unless otherwise noted.

Table 2
Kinetic Parameters of Collagenases (at 25°C, pH7.5)[a]

Enzyme	Substrate	K_m (μM)	k_{cat} ($s^{-1} \cdot 10^3$)	k_{cat}/K_m ($M^{-1} s^{-1} \times 10^{-3}$)	Ref.
MMP-1 (human)	Type I (human)	0.8	15	18	(150)
	Type I (calf)	0.8	9.5	12	(150)
	Type I (guinea pig)	0.9	6.0	7.0	(150)
	Type I (rat)	0.9	5.5	6.0	(150)
	Type II (human)	2.1	0.28	0.13	(150)
	Type II (calf)	1.6	0.75	0.47	(150)
	Type II (rat)	1.1	1.3	1.1	(150)
	Type III (human)	1.4	160	69	(150)
	Type III (guineas pig)	0.7	5.0	7.2	(150)
	α2-Macroglobulin (human)	0.17	483	2800	(35)
	Ovostatin (chicken)	0.32	0.17	1.8	(35)
MMP-8 (human)	Type I (human)	0.7	1.8	2.5	(151)
	Type II (human)	1.1	0.65	0.59	(151)
	Type III (human)	1.8	0.23	0.13	(151)
MMP-13 (human)	Type I (human)	ND	ND	ND	(152)
	Type II (human)	2	6.3	3.9	(152)
	Type III (human)	ND	ND	ND	(152)
MMP-13 (rat)	Type I (human)	1.1	3.8	3.4	(141)
	Type II (human)	0.9	3.9	4.3	(141)
	Type III (human)	1.7	5.6	3.2	(141)

[a]ND: not determined

binding site. Those repeats are responsible for binding of MMP-2 and MMP-9 to gelatin *(40,41)*, type I collagen *(42,43)*, collagen IV and laminin *(44)*. Deletion of the fibronectin-like domains from MMP-2 reduced the gelatinolytic activity and altered the digestion patterns of type IV collagen, although it did not influence the activity on a synthetic substrate *(45)*. MMP-2 and MMP-9 lacking the fibronectin domains did not exhibit elastase activity *(46)*. Matrilysin (MMP-7) and macrophage metalloelastase (MMP-12) lack fibronectin domain, but they possess elastolytic activities. Aimes and Quigley *(47)* reported that MMP-2 digests native type I collagen at the Gly775-Ile776/Leu776 bond and generates the ¾- and ¼-fragments characteristic of vertebrate collagenases. The k_{cat} and K_m values of MMP-2 against type I collagen were $4.4 \times 10^{-3} \ sec^{-1}$ and 8.5 μM, similar to those of MMP-1 *(47)*. Both gelatinases digests many other ECM components and soluble proteins. Cleavage of γ_2 chain of laminin 5 induces migration of normal breast epithelial cells *(48)*.

2.3. Stromelysins

Three MMPs are coined stromelysins, i.e., stromelysin 1 (MMP-3), stromelysin 2 (MMP-10), and stromelysin 3 (MMP-11). The enzymic activity and amino acid sequence of stromelysin 3 are significantly diverse from those of stromelysin 1 and 2. Thus, it is appropriate to place stromelysin 3 in the un-categorized subgroup.

MMP-3 and MMP-10 in humans are 79% identical in amino acid sequence and they are about 55% identical with MMP-1. However, neither of the enzymes are able to cleave triple-helical region of type I and II collagens. A weak activity was reported on type III collagen *(49,50)*. Both enzymes degrade a similar ECM component although the information of MMP-10 is limited (Table 1). In addition, the catalytic efficiency of MMP-10 is lower than that of MMP-3 *(50–52)*. Unlike collagenases, the catalytic domain of MMP-3 (28 kDa) and the full-length MMP-3 (45 kDa) have indistinguishable substrate specificities against protein substrates so far tested *(20)*. MMP-3 exhibits an acidic pH optimum activity around 5.5–6.0 for digestion of aggrecan and synthetic substrates, but it retains about 30–50% activity at pH 7.5 *(49,53)*. MMP-10 has optimal activity against Azocoll and synthetic substrates around pH 7.5–8.0 (K. Suzuki and H. Nagase, unpublished results). Both MMP-3 and MMP-10 participate in activation of proMMP-1, proMMP-7, proMMP-8, and proMMP-9 *(54–58)*. MMP-3 activates proMMP-13 *(59)*.

2.4. MT-MMPs

The first member of the MT-MMP subgroup was discovered by Sato et al. *(60)* and identified as the cell surface bound activation of proMMP-2. Currently five MT-MMPs have been identified and these enzymes have a single transmembrane and cytosolic domains after the hemopexin domains. In addition to

MT1-MMP, MT2-MMP *(61)*, MT3-MMP *(62)*, and MT5-MMP *(63)* were also shown to activate proMMP-2. Studies by Strogin et al., *(64)*, Butler et al., *(65)* and Kinoshita et al., *(66)* suggests that the cell surface activation of proMMP-2 by MT1-MMP requires the formation of a ternary complex, proMMP-2-TIMP-2-MT1-MMP on the cell surface which allows proMMP-2 to be correctly oriented and activated by free MT1-MMP. Such mechanism is considered to accumulate MMP-2 activity and locally express proteolytic activity. In addition to the ability activating proMMP-2, the soluble form of MT1-MMP was shown to digest interstitial collagen types I, II, and III into ¾- and ¼-fragments, but it is about 5–7-fold less efficient in cleaving type I collagen than MMP-1 *(67)*. Several other ECM components are also digested by MT1-MMP and MT2-MMP *(68)*. D'Ortho et al. *(68)* also reported that proTNF-α was processed by those two MT-MMPs. Localization of MT-MMPs restricts their actions on extracellular proteins near the cell surface.

2.5. Matrilysin

Matrilysin (MMP-7), consisting of a propeptide and a catalytic domain, is the smallest member of the family. MMP-7 digests a number of ECM components and nonmatrixin proteins, and its activity tends to be more proteolytic than that of MMP-3 *(51)*. Both human and rat MMP-7s have similar activities on protein substrate but a major difference is that the human enzyme digests elastin at a reasonable rate (190 μ*g/h/nmol* of enzyme) *(51)*, but little elastolytic activity is detected with the rat enzyme *(69)*.

2.6. Stromelysin 3

Only weak activity was reported to digest collagne IV, gelatin, fibronectin, laminin, and agrecan with mouse stromelysin 3 (MMP-11), but human MMP-11 expressed myeloma cells is unstable *(70)*. This instability of human enzyme is considered to be due Ala235 in place of the conserved Pro at this position immediately after the "Met-turn" that form a hydrophobic basis for the catalytic zinc atom in the metzincins *(71)*. Pei et al. *(72)* reported that MMP-11 cleaved α_1PI synthesized by breast cancer cell line MCF-7. It also cleaves $\alpha_2 M$ *(72)*.

2.7. Metalloelastase

Metalloelastase (MMP-12) was first purified from the conditioned medium of mouse macrophage and characterized as a metal-dependent elastase *(73)*. Recombinant human MMP-12 is approx 30% as active as human leukocyte elastase in solubilizing elastin *(39)*. The predicted molecular mass of the human MMP-12 is 54 kDa which contains the hemopexin domain. However, the enzyme readily undergoes N-terminal and C-terminal processing to the 22 kDa form which degrades insoluble elastin. Therefore, the C-terminal hemopexin domain does not appear to be an essential component for the elastolytic activity of MMP-12. In addition to elastin, the enzyme digests various other ECM components, α_1PI and processes proTNFα (Table 1).

2.8. Other MMPs

This group includes more recently discovered MMPs, i.e., MMP-19, MMP-20, MMP-21, MMP-22, and MMP-23. Thus, characterization of their enzymic actions on ECM components and other substrates is very limited.

MMP-19 was first identified by cDNA cloning and reported as MMP-18 by Cossins et al. *(74)*. Later, it is designated MMP-19 following collagenase 4 in *Xenopus* as MMP-18. The enzyme was also recognized as autoantigen by autoantibodies found in sera of patients with rheumatoid arthritis and systemic lupus erythematosus, and it was detected on the surface of activated peripheral blood monocytes, Th1 lymphocytes, and Jurkat T lymphocytes *(75)*. The recombinant enzyme hydrolyzes Mca-Pro-Leu-Ala-Nva-His-Ala-Dpa-NH$_2$ with $k_{cat}/K_m = 1.96 \times 10^4\ M^{-1}\ s^{-1}$ and Mca-Pro-Leu-Gly-Leu-Dpa-Ala-Arg-NH$_2$ with $k_{cat}/K_m = 1.3 \times 10^3\ M^{-1}\ s^{-1}$ *(76)*. It also digests gelatin, large tenascin C, and aggrecan *(149)*.

MMP-20 (enamelysin) is expressed by ameloblasts and odontoblasts immediately prior to the onset of dentin mineralization and continues to be expressed throughout the secretory stage of amelogenesis *(77)*. The recombinant MMP-20 digests amelogenis *(77,78)*, suggesting that the enzymes poly a role in enamel and dentin formation.

MMP-21 and MMP-22 were found in *Xenopus (79)* and chicken, respectively. MMP-21 (XMMP) mRNA is not detected in the blastula stage embryo, but expressed in gastrula stage and neurula stage embryos and down-regulated in pretailbud embryo *(79)*. However, the enzymic activity of MMP-21 was not reported. MMP-22 (CMMP) was found in chicken *(80)*. It is structurally related to collagenases, but it has a unique cysteine in the catalytic domain which is also found in MMP-19 and XMMP (MMP-21). Recombinant MMP-22 digests gelatin and casein *(80)*.

Two human MMP genes, originally designated as MMP-21 and MMP-22 *(81)*, were identified in two identical genomic regions in human chromosome 1p36.3, each of which contains a MMP gene in a tail-to-tail configuration *(1)*. This duplicated MMP gene, now designated as MMP-23 *(82)*, encodes an MMP with unique structural motifs. It lacks a recognizable signal sequence and has a short prodomain without a typical cysteine switch sequence. It also lacks a hemopexin domain. Instead, it has cysteine-rich, proline-rich, and IL-1 receptor like regions after the catalytic domain *(1,82)*. The recombinant catalytic domain of MMP-23 hydrolyzes Mca-Pro-Leu-Gly-Leu-Dpa-Ala-Arg-NH$_2$, but not gelatin *(82)*. TIMP-1 prevents the autolysis of the proenzyme *(82)*.

3. PEPTIDE SUBSTRATE SPECIFICITY

One of the goals of peptide-based specificity studies is to gain insights into the behavior of enzymes toward their natural substrates. However, peptide sequence specificities of MMPs do not necessarily match with protein specificities. This is due to conformational constraint of a potentially susceptible sequence in proteins. In addition, short peptides do not adopt a specific secondary structure and therefore they may be more readily accommodated in the substrate-binding groove of the enzyme. For example, MMP-3 cannot activate its proenzyme by cleaving the His-Phe bond of Asp-Val-Gly-His82#Phe83-Arg-Thr-Phe (# indicate the bond cleaved) in the junction of the propeptide and the catalytic domain in its native conformation, whereas this bond is readily cleaved by MMP-3 when an N-terminal part of the propeptide is removed by a proteinase *(83)*. Collagen sequence-based peptides are cleaved by most MMPs, but only a limited number of MMPs can cleave the triple-helical region of native collagens. On the other hand, although the Gly679-Leu680 in the bait region of $\alpha_2 M$ is cleaved by MMP-1 very rapidly, the oligopeptide containing the corresponding sequence is a poor substrate of MMP-1 *(84)*. Nonetheless, substrate specificity studies with peptides give us insights into the interaction of the substrate and the active site of the enzyme. The activity toward peptide is usually restricted to the catalytic domain. The truncation of the C-terminal hemopexin domain has little effect on peptide hydrolysis.

3.1. Substrate Binding Sites of MMPs

Three-dimensional structures of catalytic domains of MMPs revealed that their polypeptide folds are essentially superimposable and that all have a five stranded β-sheet, three α-helices, two zinc ions, and 1-3 calcium ions. The active site cleft is bordered by the 4th β-strand (strand IV), the 2nd α-helix, and a subsequent stretch of random coil. Based on the structure of MMP-8 catalytic domain with inhibitors Pro-Leu-Gly-NHOH that binds to the unprimed subsite (S site) of the enzyme *(11)* and 2-benzyl-3-mercaptopropanoyl-Ala-Gly-NH_2 that binds to the primed susbsite (S' site) *(85)*, Grams et al. *(85)* modeled the mode of interaction of a hexapeptide and the active site of MMP-8. In this model the peptide lies antiparallel to the edge strand IV by forming a number of hydrogen bonds. The N-terminal Pro at P_3 (the third residue on the left of the scissile bond) interacts with the hydrophobic cleft formed by side chains of His162, Ser151, and Phe164, whereas Leu at P_2 (the second residue on the right of the scissile bond) interacts with a shallow groove lined by His201, Ala206, and His207. The dominant interactions between the peptide and the enzyme are made by the phenyl side chain of the inhibitor and the large hydrophobic S_1' pocket (located to the right of the catalytic zinc) formed by side chains of His197, Val194, Tyr219, and the main chain segment of Pro217-Asn-Tyr219. The side chain of P_2' Ala points away from the enzyme and the C-terminal, P_3' Gly is located crossover segments Gly158-Leu160 and Pro217-Tyr219.

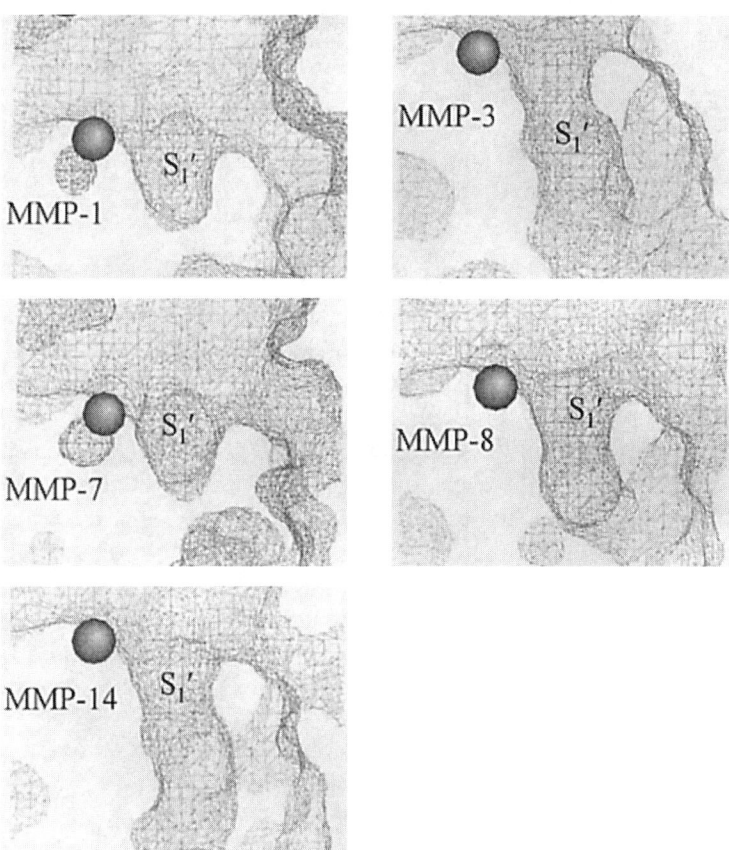

Fig. 1. Comparison of the S_1' pockets. Mesh representation of the molecular surface shows S_1' pocket of MMP-1, MMP-3, MMP-7, MMP-8, and MMP-14. Images are prepared from the Brookhaven Protein Data Bank entry 1hfc (MMP-1), 1hfs (MMP-3), 1mmp (MMP-7), 1 jan (MMP-8) and 1BQQ (MMP-14) using the program GRASP v1.2 *(104)*.

The most notable difference among MMP catalytic domains is the size of the S_1' specificity pocket (Fig. 1). Comparing between MMP-1 and MMP-8, the latter has the larger S_1' pocket. The main difference is due to the side chain of Arg195 in MMP-1 which delimits the S_1' pocket by projecting out toward the catalytic zinc, whereas Leu193 is found in the corresponding site in MMP-8. Leu193 enters the S_1' pocket but it orients away from the catalytic zinc. MMP-3 and MT1-MMP also have Leu at this position and form a very large, predominately hydrophobic S_1' pocket *(8,13)*. MMP-7 has Tyr193 in the corresponding position, which limits the size of S_1' pocket *(10)*, the enzyme prefers residues with aliphatic or aromatic side chain in the P_1' position *(86)*. Mutaiton of Tyr193 to Leu in MMP-7 altered the P_1' specificity making it similar to that of MMP-3, and reversal results were obtained with an MMP-3 (L197Y/V194A) mutant *(87)*. The S_1' pocket of MMP-2 and MMP-9 are thought to have a similar dimension as that of MMP-8 *(88)*.

Although the side chain of P_1' position is critical for substrate recognition, other subsites also influence substrate specificity of various MMPs *(see* Table 3).

3.2. Specificity Studies with Peptides

Initial peptide substrate studies were carried out with tadpole collagenase by Nagai and colleagues *(89,90)*. They were 6–8 amino acid residues based on collagenase cleavage site in α-chains of types I and III collagen. Weingarten and associates explored subsite preference of MMP-1 and MMP-2 *(91–94)* using a series of peptides, peptolides and peptide esters. Comprehensive sequence specificities of six MMPs were examined by Van Wart and associates *(86,95,96)* by measuring k_{cat}/K_m values of more than 45 oligopeptides covering the P_4 through P_4' subsites using the α1(I) collagen sequence Gly-Pro-Gln-Gly#Ile-Ala-Gly-Gln as the starting substrate *(see* Table 3). It is notable that the catalytic efficiency of MMPs depends on the length of the peptide substrate (Table 4). Little activity was detected with peptides less than three residues in either the P site (N-terminal side of the scissile bond) or the P′ site (the C-terminal side of the scissile bond) *(84,86,96)*. Niedzwiecki et al. *(97)* examined requirement of peptide length of the substrate for MMP-3 used more extended peptides, substance P analog, and reported that a peptide containing only three residue in the P site or two residue in the P′ site was not readily cleaved unless the N-terminal and the C-terminal ends are blocked (Table 5). Those results were somewhat different from those with collagen-based peptides but this may be due to extremely low activity of MMP-3 against Gly-Pro-Gln-Gly#Ile-Ala-Gly-Gln ($k_{cat}/K_m = 14.7\ M^{-1}\ s^{-1}$) *(14)* composed with a substance P analog ($k_{cat}/K_m = 1790\ M^{-1}\ s^{-1}$) *(97)*. These studies indicate that MMPs have an extended substrate binding site.

Comprehensive sequence specificity studies of six MMPs provided a number of important insights into differences and similarities in subsite requirement among those enzymes. As discussed earlier, the P_1' subsite plays a critical role. Little activity was detected with peptides with a charged group or proline at this position. Aliphatic side chains at P_1' position provide good substrates for all MMPs. Leu, Ile, and Met at this position are favored by all six enzymes. Aromatic groups are well tolerated by MMP-2, MMP-3, MMP-8, and MMP-9. This is due to relatively large hydrophobic S_1' pocket of these enzymes (Fig. 1). Ser is reasonably well tolerated by MMP-3, but a limited activity was detected with other MMPs.

Using dinitropheny-Arg-Pro-Leu-Ala#Leu-Trp-Arg-Ser-NH$_2$ peptide, Gronski et al. *(39)* examined the P_1' preference for macrophage metalloelastase

(MMP-12). Their studies indicated preference Leu>>Ala>Lys>Phe>Tyr> Trp>Arg>Ser. It is interesting that Ala-Lys and Ala-Arg bonds are cleaved by MMP-12.

A large enhancement in hydrolysis was observed with P_2' substitution. Crystal structures of MMPs with a peptide inhibitor indicate that the side chain of the P_2' position points away from the enzyme surface, but bulky aromatic side chains are much favored compared with Ala. Arg is well tolerated, but Hyp is a very poor substitution.

Substitution of the P_3' position has provided reasonably selective substrates for different MMPs. For example, Met is favored by MMP-3 and MMP-7, but the peptide with this substitution is about 10-fold less susceptible to MMP-2, MMP-8, and MMP-9. The P_4' substitution does not cause a large influence in specificity.

P_1 substitution for Gly has shown a marked influence in specificity. Ala in this position is most favored by MMP-1, MMP-3, MMP-7, and MMP-8. MMP-8 also well tolerates Glu at this position, but it only increases the rate of hydrolysis by MMP-3 about twofold. Interestingly, Pro at this position is reasonably tolerated for most cases. Bulky hydrophobic side chains are not favored by gelatinases (MMP-2 and MMP-9). Val substitution makes the peptide a poor substrate for most of the enzyme except MMP-3. For the P_2 position, however, aliphatic side chains (Leu, Met, Tyr) are favored by six MMPs. The best residue for the P_3 position for MMPs is Pro. This is also the case with substance P-based substrate for MMP-1 and MMP-3 *(97)*. When the MMP cleaved sites of naturally occurring protein substrate are aligned Pro is frequently found in P_3 position *(14)*.

3.3. Influence of Position 2
Side Chain of TIMP-1 on MMP Inhibition

The crystal structure of the complex formed between the catalytic domain of MMP-3 and TIMP-1 revealed the basic mode of interaction between MMPs and TIMPs and the inhibition mechanism of MMPs by TIMPs *(98)*. Six sequentially separate polypeptide segments of TIMP-1 interact with MMP-3 and the active site of MMP-3 is occupied by the N-terminal Cys1-Val4 and Ala65-Cys70 segments that are disulfide-bonded through Cys1 and Cys70. The α-amino group and peptide carbonyl group of Cys1 interacts with the catalytic Zn^{2+} of the metalloproteinase and the Cys1-Thr-Cys-Val4 segment bind to subsites S_1 to S_3' in a manner similar to a peptide substrate (P_1 to P_3'). The side chain of Thr2 extends into the large S_1' specificity pocket of MMP-3. Ser68 and Val69 occupy the part of S_2 and S_3 subsites, respectively, but they are arranged in a nearly opposite orientation to the P_3-P_2 segment of a peptide substrate.

Because the side chain of position 2 extends into the S_1' pocket, Meng et al. *(99)* generated fourteen variants of the N-terminal domain of TIMP-1 (N-

Table 3
Relative Substrate Specificities of Human MMPs[a,b]

Peptide sequence	Relative rate					
	MMP-1	MMP-8	MMP-2	MMP-9	MMP-3	MMP-7
Gly-Pro-Gln-Gly#Ile-Ala-Gly-Gln	100	100	100	100	100	100
Gly-Pro-Gln-Gly#Leu-Ala-Gly-Gln	130	180	88	80	110	300
Gly-Pro-Gln-Gly#Trp-Ala-Gly-Gln	<0.5	49	<5.0	<5.0	120	<5.0
Gly-Pro-Gln-Gly#Pro-Ala-Gly-Gln	<0.5	<0.5	<5.0	<5.0	<0.5	<5.0
Gly-Pro-Gln-Gly#Glu-Ala-Gly-Gln	<0.5	<0.5	<5.0	<5.0	<0.5	8.0
Gly-Pro-Gln-Gly#Tyr-Ala-Gly-Gln	50	390	50	96	150	21
Gly-Pro-Gln-Gly#Phe-Ala-Gly-Gln	20	46	55	24	140	24
Gly-Pro-Gln-Gly#Met-Ala-Gly-Gln	110	84	230	170	60	89
Gly-Pro-Gln-Gly#Val-Ala-Gly-Gln	9.1	9.0	30	25	53	17
Gly-Pro-Gln-Gly#Gln-Ala-Gly-Gln	28	10	34	20	38	<5.0
Gly-Pro-Gln-Gly#Ser-Ala-Gly-Gln	5.9	1.6	15	<5.0	45	5.5
Gly-Pro-Gln-Gly#Arg-Ala-Gly-Gln	<0.5	<0.5	<5.0	<5.0	<4.9	<5.0
Gly-Pro-Gln-Gly#Ile-Phe-Gly-Gln	360	510	380	390	130	140
Gly-Pro-Gln-Gly#Ile-Trp-Gly-Gln	840	930	310	240	280	330
Gly-Pro-Gln-Gly#Ile-Leu-Gly-Gln	430	400	400	240	280	250
Gly-Pro-Gln-Gly#Ile-Hyp-Gly-Gln	7.3	1.5	32	11	42	8.0
Gly-Pro-Gln-Gly#Ile-Arg-Gly-Gln	180	170	180	200	250	270
Gly-Pro-Gln-Gly#Ile-Glu-Gly-Gln	35	59	85	130	58	86
Gly-Pro-Gln-Gly#Ile-Ala-Val-Gln	100	57	26	49	170	170
Gly-Pro-Gln-Gly#Ile-Ala-Arg-Gln	55	34	35	45	490	220
Gly-Pro-Gln-Gly#Ile-Ala-Met-Gln	130	34	40	35	810	450
Gly-Pro-Gln-Gly#Ile-Ala-Ala-Gln	220	120	180	140	280	300
Gly-Pro-Gln-Gly#Ile-Ala-Ser-Gln	91	58	320	130	230	150
Gly-Pro-Gln-Gly#Ile-Ala-Gly-Ala	86	110	85	110	130	91

Gly-Pro-Gln-Gly#Ile-Ala-Gly-His	91	145	150	120	110	87
Gly-Pro-Gln-Gly#Ile-Ala-Gly-Thr	160	145	59	160	72	100
Gly-Pro-Gln-Met#Ile-Ala-Gly-Gln	200	140	22	12	110	150
Gly-Pro-Gln-Glu#Ile-Ala-Gly-Gln	28	330	15	29	190	170
Gly-Pro-Gln-Tyr#Ile-Ala-Gly-Gln	130	180	58	30	68	34
Gly-Pro-Gln-Ala#Ile-Ala-Gly-Gln	660	320	96	110	300	530
Gly-Pro-Gln-Pro#Ile-Ala-Gly-Gln	260	190	32	46	170	140
Gly-Pro-Gln-Gln#Ile-Ala-Gly-Gln	140	150	25	13	140	180
Gly-Pro-Gln-Phe#Ile-Ala-Gly-Gln	95	170	15	26	68	63
Gly-Pro-Gln-Leu#Ile-Ala-Gly-Gln	27	54	21	8.8	170	49
Gly-Pro-Gln-Val#Ile-Ala-Gly-Gln	5.5	7.9	<5.0	<5.0	32	<5.0
Gly-Pro-Gln-His#Ile-Ala-Gly-Gln	160	50	65	44	87	ND
Gly-Pro-Hyp-Gly#Ile-Ala-Gly-Gln	11	15	32	15	83	17
Gly-Pro-Asp-Gly#Ile-Ala-Gly-Gln	30	44	11	10	89	7.0
Gly-Pro-Val-Gly#Ile-Ala-Gly-Gln	32	30	130	110	160	57
Gly-Pro-Leu-Gly#Ile-Ala-Gly-Gln	150	260	330	290	190	420
Gly-Pro-Arg-Gly#Ile-Ala-Gly-Gln	17	32	160	83	96	13
Gly-Pro-Met-Gly#Ile-Ala-Gly-Gln	160	160	120	180	120	400
Gly-Pro-Tyr-Gly#Ile-Ala-Gly-Gln	200	110	200	150	230	240
Gly-Asn-Gln-Gly#Ile-Ala-Gly-Gln	17	45	60	<5.0	68	25
Gly-Ala-Gln-Gly#Ile-Ala-Gly-Gln	50	23	22	9.4	62	ND

[a]ND: Not determined.
[b]Data are from Refs. (14,86,95,96).

Table 4

Effect of N- and C-terminal Truncation on the Hydrolysis of Collagen Sequence-Based Substrate by MMPs at 30°C, pH 7.5[a]

Substrate	Relative rate					
P_4 P_3 P_2 P_1 P_1' P_2' P_3' P_4'	MMP-1	MMP-2	MMP-3	MMP-7	MMP-8	MMP-9
Gly-Pro-Gln-Gly#Ile-Ala-Gly-Gln	100	100	100	100	100	100
Ac-Pro-Gln-Gly#Ile-Ala-Gly-Gln	110	—	—	—	96	—
Pro-Gln-Gly#Ile-Ala-Gly-Gln	150	62	30	43	100	65
Gln-Gly#Ile-Ala-Gly-Gln	7.3	<5.0	26	8.3	<5.0	<5.0
Gly#Ile-Ala-Gly-Gln	<5.0	<5.0	<5.0	<5.0	<5.0	<5.0
Gly-Pro-Gln-Gly#Ile-Ala-Gly	68	60	64	99	54	93
Gly-Pro-Gln-Gly#Ile-Ala	13	<5.0	34	10	<5.0	<5.0
Gly-Pro-Gln-Gly#Ile	<5.0	<5.0	<5.0	<5.0	<5.0	<5.0

[a]The results are after Netzel-Arnett et al. (86,96) and Imper and Van Wart (84).

Table 5
Hydrolysis of Synthetic Peptides by MMP-3[a]

Substrate	K_{cat}/K_m $(s^{-1} M^{-1})$	Relative activity
P_6 P_5 P_4 P_3 P_2 P_1 P_1' P_2' P_3' P_4' P_5'		
Arg-Pro-Lys-Pro-Gln-Gln#Phe-Phe-Gly-Leu-Met-NH$_2$	1790 ± 140	100
Pro-Lys-Pro-Gln-Gln#Phe-Phe-Gly-Leu-Met-NH$_2$	800 ± 2	45
Lys-Pro-Gln-Gln#Phe-Phe-Gly-Leu-Met-NH$_2$	290 ± 84	16
Pro-Gln-Gln#Phe-Phe-Gly-Leu-Met-NH$_2$	<3	<0.1
Ac-Pro-Gln-Gln#Phe-Phe-Gly-Leu-Nle-NH$_2$	500 ± 200	28
Arg-Pro-Lys-Pro-Gln-Gln#Phe-Phe-Gly-Leu	1300 ± 91	73
Arg-Pro-Lys-Pro-Gln-Gln#Phe-Phe-Gly	790 ± 120	44
Arg-Pro-Lys-Pro-Gln-Gln#Phe-Phe	<3	<0.1
Arg-Pro-Lys-Pro-Gln-Gln#Phe-Phe-NH$_2$	1900 ± 380	106

[a]Data are from Niedzwiecki et al. *(97)*.

TIMP-1) at this position 2 and examined their affinity toward MMP-1, MMP-2, and MMP-3 (Table 6). The Gly mutant was the weakest inhibitor for all three MMPs. Negatively charged side chains at position 2 are unfavorable for all three MMPs. Nonpolar side chains of increasing size increase the affinity for MMP-2 and MMP-3, except Ile and Phe, but longer aliphatic chains reduced the affinity for MMP-1. A reasonably high affinity of Arg2 mutant with MMP-2 and MMP-3 was found although it was not an effective inhibitor of MMP-1. The unfavorable interaction of MMP-1 with the Arg2 mutant may be reflected by the structural feature of the S$_1'$ specificity pocket of MMP-1 where Arg195 and more cationic environment compared with those of MMP-2 and MMP-3.

The striking features of residue 2 of N-TIMP-1 are that mutation at this site significantly alters the affinity for three different MMPs and that this side chain apparently interacts with the S$_1'$ specificity pocket of MMPs differently from that of the P$_1'$ residue of a peptide substrate. As shown in Table 3, MMPs favor substrate with a large aliphatic or aromatic side chains at the P$_1'$ position. Peptides with Val, Ser, or a charged group at the P$_1'$ position are very poor substrates. However, the best inhibitor for MMP-1 was Val2 mutant, Leu2 mutant for MMP-2 and Ser2 mutant for MMP-3. Meng et al. *(99)* reported that there was a very poor correlation between -log K_i for TIMP mutants and log (k_{cat}/K_m) for peptide substrates with the sequence Gly-Pro-Gln-Gly#X-Ala-Gly-Gln, where the same amino acid was present at the P$_1'$ position (X) of the peptide and residue 2 of the N-TIMP-1 variant. This discrepancy is considered to be due to a greater loss of conformational entropy associated with peptide-MMP interaction a TIMP-MMP interaction. The orientation of residue 2 of TIMP-1 is probably influenced by the relatively rigid structure around the disulfide-bonded Cys1 with the catalytic Zn^{2+}.

Table 6
Inhibition Constants (K_i) of Position 2 Mutants of N-TIMP-1[a,b]

	K_i (nM)		
Amino Acid	MMP-1	MMP-2	MMP-3
Thr (wild-type)	3.0	1.1	1.9
ser	14.7	2.1	0.5
Gly	18×10^3[a]	103×10^3[a]	1380
Ala	2090	307	126
Val	1.6	4.5	3.0
Leu	93	1.0	3.2
Ile	262	5.6	20
Met	10.9	0.7	0.7
Phe	42	17	13
Asn	1970	16	44
Gln	870	12	29
Asp	8130	1250	1110
Glu	5730	433	468
Lys	1670	31	70
Arg	5010	12	28

[a] Estimated from the level of inhibition at a concentration of 8 μM.
[b] The results are from Meng et al. (99).

3.4. Zymogen Activiation and Substrate Specificity

Stromelysins (MMP-3 and MMP-10), MMP-2 and MMP-7 play a critical role in activation of procollagenases by cleaving the Gln80-Phe81 bond of proMMP-1 (54) and the Gly78-Phe79 bond of proMMP-8 (55). When procollagenases are treated with trypsin or an organomercurial, 4-aminophenylmercuric acetate (APMA), those bonds are not cleaved and only partial (10–25%) collagenolytic activity is detected. This was shown to be autoprocessing of procollagenase at bonds other than the above specific sites. Treatment of proMMP-1 with APMA results in generation of [Met78]MMP-1, [Val82] MMP-1, and [Leu83]MMP-1 (residues in brackets are the N-terminus), but not [Phe81]MMP-1, since Phe81 does not fit with the S_1' specificity pocket of MMP-1. Similarly [Met80]MMP-8 and [Leu83]MMP-8 with partial collagenolytic activity are generated by treatment with a mercurial compound (55). Reduced activity was also reported for MMP-3 when it retained several extra residues before the N-terminal Phe83 or when a few residues are trimmed from the N-terminus (100). This was also associated with changes in substrate specificity. The reduced activity of MMP-3 is due to an increase in K_m and a decrease in k_{cat} on a synthetic substrate *(100)*. It is not known how the differently processed N-termini of MMPs influences the enzyme activity and in some cases substrate specificity, but the crystal structures of the catalytic domains of [Phe79]MMP-8 and [Met80]MMP-8 indicated the structural differences between the two forms: In [Phe79]MMP-8, the ammonium group of Phe79 forms a salt bridge with the carboxylate side chain of Asp232 in the third helix of the catalytic domain *(101),* but without the Phe79 to N-terminal hexapeptide Met80-Leu-Thr-Pro-Gly-Asn85 of MMP-8 is disordered *(11)*. However, the geometry of the active site of the two forms are essentially identical. It is therefore postulated that disruption of the salt bridge may alter stabilization of the active site at the transition state or influence the substrate binding to the active site *(101)* but the experimental evidence to support these supposition is not currently available.

4. CONCLUSIONS

Substrate specificity studies of MMPs have been conducted with natural protein substrates as well as synthetic peptides. Those studies have demonstrated that many MMPs have a relatively broader substrate specificity on various ECM components and non-ECM proteins. Although degradation of interstitial collagens were originally thought to be only due to the action of the so-called collagenases, it is now known that at least six different MMPs, including gelatinase A (MMP-2) and MT1-MMP, have the collagenolytic activity. In addition, collagenases do have activities on various noncollagenous proteins. We have also learned that domains other than the catalytic domain play critical roles in expressing proteolytic activities on certain matrix components. Different propeptide processing results in active MMPs with different specific activities and substrate specificities in some cases. Although differently processed forms of MMPs are yet to be identified in the tissue, those points need to be considered in order to interpret biological and pathological implications of MMPs, since MMP activities may be altered by several fold. It should also be stressed that identification of MMP substrates in vivo is difficult. Biochemical studies using isolated macromolecules only suggest possibilities of substrates. For this purpose, antibodies that recognize specifically cleaved ECM components have been used *(32,102,103)*, and those studies have been informative.

Studies with a series of synthetic substrates have provided insights into the subsite requirements of MMPs and they were useful in designing active site-directed synthetic inhibitors of MMPs. Those studies have also indicated that the susceptibility of synthetic peptides modeled after the cleavage site of a natural substrate is often different from that of the native protein. More interestingly, recent mutagenesis studies of TIMP-1 indicated that the nature of the side chain of position 2 in TIMP-1 had a major influence on the affinity for MMPs, but it did not correlate with substrate specificity dictated by the P_1' side chain of substrates. The unique mode of interaction of TIMP with MMPs may provide the way to generate highly selective inhibitors of individual MMPs.

ACKNOWLEDGMENTS

I thank Dr. Deenlayal Dinakarpandian for preparation of mesh representation of S_1' pockets of MMPs. This work was supported by NIH grant AR 39189 and AR 40994.

REFERENCES

1. Gururajan, R., Grenet, J., Lahti, J. M., and Kidd, V. J. (1998) Isolation and characterization of two novel metalloproteinase genes linked to the Cdc2l locus on human chromosome 1p36.3. *Genomics* 52, 101–106.
2. Lovejoy, B., Cleasby, A., Hassell, A. M., Longley, K., Luther, M. A., Weigl, D., et al. (1994) Structure of the catalytic domain of fibroblast collagenase complexed with an inhibitor. *Science* 263, 375–377.
3. Borkakoti, N., Winkler, F. K., Williams, D. H., D'Arcy, A., Broadhurst, M. J., Brown, P. A., et al. (1994) Structure of the catalytic domain of human fibroblast collagenase complexed with an inhibitor. *Nat. Struct. Biol.* 1, 106–110.
4. Spurlino, J. C., Smallwood, A. M., Carlton, D. D., Banks, T. M., Vavra, K. J., Johnson, J. S., et al. (1994) 1.56 Å structure of mature truncated human fibroblast collagenase. *Proteins* 19, 98–109.
5. Moy, F. J., Chanda, P. K., Cosmi, S., Pisano, M. R., Urbano, C., Wilhelm, J., et al. (1998) High-resolution solution structure of the inhibitor-free catalytic fragment of human fibroblast collagenase determined by multidimensional NMR. *Biochemistry* 37, 1495–1504.
6. McCoy, M. A., Dellwo, M. J., Schneider, D. M., Banks, T. M., Falvo, J., Vavra, K. J., et al. (1997) Assignments and structure determination of the catalytic domain of human fibroblast collagenase using 3D double and triple resonance NMR spectroscopy. *J. Biomol. NMR* 9, 11–24.
7. Gooley, P. R., O'Connell, J. F., Marcy, A. I., Cuca, G. C., Salowe, S. P., Bush, B. L., et al. (1994) The NMR structure of the inhibited catalytic domain of human stromelysin-1. *Nat. Struct. Biol.* 1, 111–118.
8. Becker, J. W., Marcy, A. I., Rokosz, L. L., Axel, M. G., Burbaum, J. J., Fitzgerald, P. M., et al. (1995) Stromelysin-1: three-dimensional structure of the inhibited catalytic domain and of the C-truncated proenzyme. *Protein Sci.* 4, 1966–1976.
9. Dhanaraj, V., Ye, Q. Z., Johnson, L. L., Hupe, D. J., Ortwine, D. F., Dunbar, J. B., Jr., et al. (1996) X-ray structure of a hydroxamate inhibitor complex of stromelysin catalytic domain and its comparison with members of the zinc metalloproteinase superfamily. *Structure* 4, 375–386.
10. Browner, M. F., Smith, W. W., and Castelhano, A. L. (1995) Matrilysin-inhibitor complexes: common themes among metalloproteases. *Biochemistry* 34, 6602–6610.
11. Bode, W., Reinemer, P., Huber, R., Kleine, T., Schnierer, S., and Tschesche, H. (1994) The X-ray crystal structure of the catalytic domain of human neutrophil collagenase inhibited by a substrate analogue reveals the essentials for catalysis and specificity. *EMBO J.* 13, 1263–1269.
12. Stams, T., Spurlino, J. C., Smith, D. L., Wahl, R. C., Ho, T. F., Qoronfleh, M. W., et al. (1994) Structure of human neutrophil collagenase reveals large S1' specificity pocket. *Nat. Struct. Biol.* 1, 119–123.

13. Fernandez-Catalan, C., Bode, W., Huber, R., Turk, D., Calvete, J. J., Lichte, A., et al. (1998) Crystal structure of the complex formed by the membrane type 1-matrix metalloproteinase with the tissue inhibitor of metalloproteinases-2, the soluble progelatinase a receptor. *EMBO J.* 17, 5238–5248.

14. Nagase, H. and Fields, G. B. (1996) Human matrix metalloproteinase specificity studies using collagen sequence-based synthetic peptides. *Biopolymers* 40, 399–416.

15. Harris, E. D., Jr., and Krane, S. M. (1974) Collagenases. *N. Engl. J. Med.* 291, 557–563.

16. Harris, E. D., Jr., and Krane, S. M. (1972) An endopeptidase from rheumatoid synovial tissue culture. *Biochim. Biophys. Acta* 258, 566–576.

17. Sopata, I. and Dancewicz, A. M. (1974) Presence of a gelatin-specific proteinase and its latent form in human leucocytes. *Biochim. Biophys. Acta* 370, 510–523.

18. Galloway, W. A., Murphy, G., Sandy, J. D., Gavrilovic, J., Cawston, T. E., and Reynolds, J. J. (1983) Purification and characterization of a rabbit bone metalloproteinase that degrades proteoglycan and other connective-tissue components. *Biochem. J.* 209, 741–752.

19. Chin, J. R., Murphy, G., and Werb, Z. (1985) Stromelysin, a connective tissue-degrading metalloendopeptidase secreted by stimulated rabbit synovial fibroblasts in parallel with collagenase. Biosynthesis, isolation, characterization, and substrates. *J. Biol. Chem.* 260, 12367–12376.

20. Okada, Y., Nagase, H., and Harris, E. D., Jr. (1986) A metalloproteinase from human rheumatoid synovial fibroblasts that digests connective tissue matrix components. Purification and characterization. *J. Biol. Chem.* 261, 14245–14255.

21. Clark, I. M., and Cawston, T. E. (1989) Fragments of human fibroblast collagenase. Purification and characterization. *Biochem. J.* 263, 201–206.

22. Murphy, G., Allan, J. A., Willenbrock, F., Cockett, M. I., O'Connell, J. P., and Docherty, A. J. P. (1992) The role of the C-terminal domain in collagenase and stromelysin specificity. *J. Biol. Chem.* 267, 9612–9618.

23. Knäuper, V., Osthues, A., DeClerck, Y. A., Langley, K. E., Blaser, J., and Tschesche, H. (1993) Fragmentation of human polymorphonuclear-leucocyte collagenase. *Biochem. J.* 291, 847–854.

24. Knäuper, V., Cowell, S., Smith, B., López-Otín, C., O'Shea, M., Morris, H., et al. (1997) The role of the C-terminal domain of human collagenase-3 (MMP-13) in the activation of procollagenase-3, substrate specificity, and tissue inhibitor of metalloproteinase interaction. *J. Biol. Chem.* 272, 7608–7616.

25. Hirose, T., Patterson, C., Pourmotabbed, T., Mainardi, C. L., and Hasty, K. A. (1993) Structure-function relationship of human neutrophil collagenase: identification of regions responsible for substrate specificity and general proteinase activity. *Proc. Natl. Acad. Sci. USA* 90, 2569–2573.

26. Lovejoy, B., Hassell, A. M., Luther, M. A., Weigl, D., and Jordan, S. R. (1994) Crystal structures of recombinant 19-kDa human fibroblast collagenase complexed to itself. *Biochemistry* 33, 8207–8217.

27. Li, J., Brick, P., O'Hare, M. C., Skarzynski, T., Lloyd, L. F., Curry, V. A., et al. (1995) Structure of full-length porcine synovial collagenase reveals a C-terminal domain containing a calcium-linked, four-bladed beta-propeller. *Structure* 3, 541–549.

28. Bode, W. (1995) A helping hand for collagenases: the haemopexin-like domain. *Structure* 3, 527–530.

29. Welgus, H. G., Jeffrey, J. J., and Eisen, A. Z. (1981) Human skin fibroblast collagenase. Assessment of activation energy and deuterium isotope effect with collagenous substrates. *J. Biol. Chem.* 256, 9516–9521.

30. Gomis-Rüth, F. X., Gohlke, U., Betz, M., Knauper, V., Murphy, G., López-Otín, C., et al. (1996) The helping hand of collagenase-3 (MMP-13): 2.7 Å crystal structure of its C-terminal haemopexin-like domain. *J. Mol. Biol.* 264, 556–566.

31. de Souza, S. J., Pereira, H. M., Jacchieri, S., and Brentani, R. R. (1996) Collagen/collagenase interaction: Does the enzyme mimic the conformation of its own substrate? *FASEB J.* 10, 927–930.

32. Billinghurst, R. C., Dahlberg, L., Ionescu, M., Reiner, A., Bourne, R., Rorabeck, C., et al. (1997) Enhanced cleavage of type II collagen by collagenases in osteoarthritic articular cartilage. *J. Clin. Invest.* 99, 1534–1545.

33. Krane, S. M., Byrne, M. H., Lemaitre, V., Henriet, P., Jeffrey, J. J., Witter, J. P., et al. (1996) Different collagenase gene products have different roles in degradation of type I collagen. *J. Biol. Chem.* 271, 28509–28515.

34. Lemaître, V., Jungbluth, A., and Eeckhout, Y. (1997) The recombinant catalytic domain of mouse collagenase-3 depolymerizes type I collagen by cleaving its aminotelopeptides. *Biochem. Biophys. Res. Commun.* 230, 202–205.

35. Enghild, J. J., Salvesen, G., Brew, K., and Nagase, H. (1989) Interaction of human rheumatoid synovial collagenase (matrix metalloproteinase 1) and stromelysin (matrix metalloproteinase 3) with human α 2-macroglobulin and chicken ovostatin. Binding kinetics and identification of matrix metalloproteinase cleavage sites. *J. Biol. Chem.* 264, 8779–8785.

36. Okada, Y., Morodomi, T., Enghild, J. J., Suzuki, K., Yasui, A., Nakanishi, I., et al. (1990) Matrix metalloproteinase 2 from human rheumatoid synovial fibroblasts. Purification and activation of the precursor and enzymic properties. *Eur. J. Biochem.* 194, 721–730.

37. Morodomi, T., Ogata, Y., Sasaguri, Y., Morimatsu, M., and Nagase, H. (1992) Purification and characterization of matrix metalloproteinase 9 from U937 monocytic leukaemia and HT1080 fibrosarcoma cells. *Biochem. J.* 285, 603–611.

38. Senior, R. M., Griffin, G. L., Fliszar, C. J., Shapiro, S. D., Goldberg, G. I., and Welgus, H. G. (1991) Human 92- and 72-kilodalton type IV collagenases are elastases. *J. Biol. Chem.* 266, 7870–7875.

39. Gronski, T. J., Jr., Martin, R. L., Kobayashi, D. K., Walsh, B. C., Holman, M. C., Huber, M., et al. (1997) Hydrolysis of a broad spectrum of extracellular matrix proteins by human macrophage elastase. *J. Biol. Chem.* 272, 12189–12194.

40. Collier, I. E., Krasnov, P. A., Strongin, A. Y., Birkedal-Hansen, H., and Goldberg, G. I. (1992) Alanine scanning mutagenesis and functional analysis of the fibronectin-like collagen-binding domain from human 92-kDa type IV collagenase. *J. Biol. Chem.* **267,** 6776–6781.

41. Banyai, L., Tordai, H., and Patthy, L. (1994) The gelatin-binding site of human 72 kDa type IV collagenase (gelatinase A). *Biochem. J.* 298, 403–407.

42. Allan, J. A., Docherty, A. J. P., and Murphy, G. (1994) The binding of gelatinases A and B to type I collagen yields both high and low affinity sites. *Ann. N.Y. Acad. Sci.* 732, 365–366.

43. Steffensen, B., Wallon, U. M., and Overall, C. M. (1995) Extracellular matrix binding properties of recombinant fibronectin type II-like modules of human 72-kDa gelatinase/type IV collagenase. High affinity binding to native type I collagen but not native type IV collagen. *J. Biol. Chem.* 270, 11555–11566.

44. Allan, J. A., Docherty, A. J. P., Barker, P. J., Huskisson, N. S., Reynolds, J. J., and Murphy, G. (1995) Binding of gelatinases A and B to type-I collagen and other matrix components. *Biochem. J.* 309, 299–306.

45. Murphy, G., Nguyen, Q., Cockett, M. I., Atkinson, S. J., Allan, J. A., Knight, C. G., et al. (1994) Assessment of the role of the fibronectin-like domain of gelatinase A by analysis of a deletion mutant. *J. Biol. Chem.* 269, 6632–6636.

46. Shipley, J. M., Doyle, G. A., Fliszar, C. J., Ye, Q. Z., Johnson, L.L., Shapiro, S.D., et al. (1996) The structural basis for the elastolytic activity of the 92-kDa and 72-kDa gelatinases. Role of the fibronectin type II-like repeats. *J. Biol. Chem.* 271, 4335–4341.

47. Aimes, R. T., and Quigley, J .P. (1995) Matrix metalloproteinase-2 is an interstitial collagenase. Inhibitor-free enzyme catalyzes the cleavage of collagen fibrils and soluble native

type I collagen generating the specific 3/4- and 1/4-length fragments. *J. Biol. Chem.* 270, 5872–5876.

48. Giannelli, G., Falkmarzillier, J., Schiraldi, O., Stetler-Stevenson, W. G., and Quaranta, V. (1997) Induction of cell migration by matrix metalloprotease-2 cleavage of laminin-5. *Science* 277, 225–228.

49. Gunja-Smith, Z., Nagase, H., and Woessner, J. F., Jr. (1989) Purification of the neutral proteoglycan-degrading metalloproteinase from human articular cartilage tissue and its identification as stromelysin matrix metalloproteinase-3. *Biochem. J.* 258, 115–119.

50. Nicholson, R., Murphy, G., and Breathnach, R. (1989) Human and rat malignant-tumor-associated mRNAs encode stromelysin-like metalloproteinases. *Biochemistry* 28, 5195–5203.

51. Murphy, G., Cockett, M. I., Ward, R. V., and Docherty, A. J. P. (1991) Matrix metalloproteinase degradation of elastin, type IV collagen and proteoglycan. A quantitative comparison of the activities of 95 kDa and 72 kDa gelatinases, stromelysins-1 and -2 and punctuated metalloproteinase (PUMP). *Biochem. J.* 277, 277–279.

52. Nagase, H. (1995) Human stromelysins 1 and 2. *Methods Enzymol.* 248, 449–470.

53. Harrison, R. K., Chang, B., Niedzwiecki, L., and Stein, R. L. (1992) Mechanistic studies on the human matrix metalloproteinase stromelysin. *Biochemistry* 31, 10757–10762.

54. Suzuki, K., Enghild, J. J., Morodomi, T., Salvesen, G., and Nagase, H. (1990) Mechanisms of activation of tissue procollagenase by matrix metalloproteinase 3 (stromelysin). *Biochemistry* 29, 10261–10270.

55. Knäuper, V., Wilhelm, S. M., Seperack, P. K., DeClerck, Y. A., Langley, K. E., Osthues, A., et al. (1993) Direct activation of human neutrophil procollagenase by recombinant stromelysin. *Biochem. J.* 295, 581–586.

56. Knäuper, V., Murphy, G., and Tschesche, H. (1996) Activation of human neutrophil procollagenase by stromelysin 2. *Eur. J. Biochem.* 235, 187–191.

57. Nakamura, H., Fujii, Y., Ohuchi, E., Yamamoto, E., and Okada, Y. (1998) Activation of the precursor of human stromelysin 2 and its interactions with other matrix metalloproteinases. *Eur. J. Biochem.* 253, 67–75.

58. Ogata, Y., Enghild, J. J., and Nagase, H. (1992) Matrix metalloproteinase 3 (stromelysin) activates the precursor for the human matrix metalloproteinase 9. *J. Biol. Chem.* 267, 3581–3584.

59. Knäuper, V., López-Otín, C., Smith, B., Knight, G., and Murphy, G. (1996) Biochemical characterization of human collagenase-3. *J. Biol. Chem.* 271, 1544–1550.

60. Sato, H., Takino, T., Okada, Y., Cao, J., Shinagawa, A., Yamamoto, E., et al. (1994) A matrix metalloproteinase expressed on the surface of invasive tumour cells [see comments]. *Nature* 370, 61–65.

61. Butler, G. S., Will, H., Atkinson, S. J., and Murphy, G. (1997) Membrane-type-2 matrix metalloproteinase can initiate the processing of progelatinase A and is regulated by the tissue inhibitors of metalloproteinases. *Eur. J. Biochem.* 244, 653–657.

62. Takino, T., Sato, H., Shinagawa, A., and Seiki, M. (1995) Identification of the second membrane-type matrix metalloproteinase (MT-MMP-2) gene from a human placenta cDNA library. MT-MMPs form a unique membrane-type subclass in the MMP family. *J. Biol. Chem.* 270, 23013–23020.

63. Pei, D. (1999) Identification and characterization of the fifth membrane-type matrix metalloproteinase MT5-MMP. *J. Biol. Chem.* 274, 8925–8932.

64. Strongin, A. Y., Collier, I., Bannikov, G., Marmer, B. L., Grant, G. A., and Goldberg, G. I. (1995) Mechanism of cell surface activation of 72-kDa type IV collagenase. Isolation of the activated form of the membrane metalloprotease. *J. Biol. Chem.* 270, 5331–5338.

65. Butler, G. S., Butler, M. J., Atkinson, S. J., Will, H., Tamura, T., Vanwestrum, S. S., et al. (1998) The TIMP2 membrane type 1 metalloproteinase receptor regulates the concentration and efficient activation of progelatinase A—a kinetic study. *J. Biol. Chem.* 273, 871–880.

66. Kinoshita, T., Sato, H., Akiko, Okada, Ohuchi, E., Imai, K., Okada, Y., et al. (1998) TIMP-2 promotes activation of progelatinase A by membrane-type 1 matrix metalloproteinase immobilized on agarose beads. *J. Biol. Chem.* 273, 16098–16103.

67. Ohuchi, E., Imai, K., Fujii, Y., Sato, H., Seiki, M., and Okada, Y. (1997) Membrane type 1 matrix metalloproteinase digests interstitial collagens and other extracellular matrix macromolecules. *J. Biol. Chem.* 272, 2446–2451.

68. D'Ortho, M. P., Will, H., Atkinson, S., Butler, G., Messent, A., Gavrilovic, J., et al. (1997) Membrane-type matrix metalloproteinases 1 and 2 exhibit broad-spectrum proteolytic capacities comparable to many matrix metalloproteinases. *Eur. J. Biochem.* 250, 751–757.

69. Woessner, J. F., Jr., and Taplin, C. J. (1988) Purification and properties of a small latent matrix metalloproteinase of the rat uterus. *J. Biol. Chem.* 263, 16918–16925.

70. Murphy, G., Segain, J. P., O'Shea, M., Cockett, M., Ioannou, C., Lefebvre, O., et al. (1993) The 28-kDa N-terminal domain of mouse stromelysin-3 has the general properties of a weak metalloproteinase. *J. Biol. Chem.* 268, 15435–15441.

71. Nöel, A., Santavicca, M., Stoll, I., L'Hoir, C., Staub, A., Murphy, G., et al. (1995) Identification of structural determinants controlling human and mouse stromelysin-3 proteolytic activities. *J. Biol. Chem.* 270, 22866–22872.

72. Pei, D., Majmudar, G., and Weiss, S. J. (1994) Hydrolytic inactivation of a breast carcinoma cell-derived serpin by human stromelysin-3. *J. Biol. Chem.* 269, 25849–25855.

73. Banda, M. J., and Werb, Z. (1981) Mouse macrophage elastase. Purification and characterization as a metalloproteinase. *Biochem. J.* 193, 589–605.

74. Cossins, J., Dudgeon, T. J., Catlin, G., Gearing, A. J., and Clements, J. M. (1996) Identification of MMP-18, a putative novel human matrix metalloproteinase. *Biochem. Biophys. Res. Commun.* 228, 494–498.

75. Sedlacek, R., Mauch, S., Kolb, B., Schatzlein, C., Eibel, H., Peter, H. H., et al. (1998) Matrix metalloproteinase MMP-19 (RASI 1) is expressed on the surface of activated peripheral blood mononuclear cells and is detected as an autoantigen in rheumatoid arthritis. *Immunobiology* 198, 408–423.

76. Pendás, A. M., Knäuper, V., Puente, X. S., Llano, E., Mattei, M. G., Apte, S., et al. (1997) Identification and characterization of a novel human matrix metalloproteinase with unique structural characteristics, chromosomal location, and tissue distribution. *J. Biol. Chem.* 272, 4281–4286.

77. Fukae, M., Tanabe, T., Uchida, T., Lee, S. K., Ryu, O. H., Murakami, C., et al. (1998) Enamelysin (matrix metalloproteinase-20)—localization in the developing tooth and effects of pH and calcium on amelogenin hydrolysis. *J. Dent. Res.* 77, 1580–1588.

78. Llano, E., Pendás, A. M., Knäuper, V., Sorsa, T., Salo, T., Salido, E., et al. (1997) Identification and structural and functional characterization of human enamelysin (MMP-20). *Biochemistry* 36, 15101–15108.

79. Yang, M. Z., Murray, M. T., and Kurkinen, M. (1997) A novel matrix metalloproteinase gene (XMMP) encoding vitronectin-like motifs is transiently expressed in Xenopus laevis early embryo development. *J. Biol. Chem.* 272, 13527–13533.

80. Yang, M. Z. and Kurkinen, M. (1998) Cloning and characterization of a novel matrix metalloproteinase (MMP), CMMP, from chicken embryo fibroblasts—CMMP, Xenopus XMMP, and human MMP-19 have a conserved unique cysteine in the catalytic domain. *J. Biol. Chem.* 273, 17893–17900.

81. Gururajan, R., Lahti, J. M., Grenet, J., Easton, J., Gruber, I., Ambros, P. F., et al. (1998) Duplication of a genomic region containing the Cdc2l1-2 and MMP21-22 genes on human chromosome 1p36.3 and their linkage to d1z2. *Genome Res.* 8, 929–939.

82. Velasco, G., Pendás, A. M., Fueyo, A., Knäuper, V., Murphy, G., and López-Otín, C. (1999) Cloning and characterization of human MMP-23, a new matrix metalloproteinase predominantly expressed in reproductive tissues and lacking conserved domains in other family members. *J. Biol. Chem.* 274, 4570–4576.

83. Nagase, H., Enghild, J. J., Suzuki, K., and Salvesen, G. (1990) Stepwise activation mechanisms of the precursor of matrix metalloproteinase 3 (stromelysin) by proteinases and (4-aminophenyl)mercuric acetate. *Biochemistry* 29, 5783–5789.

84. Imper, V. and Van Wart, H. E. (1998) Substrate specificity and mechanisms of substrate recognition of the matrix metalloproteinases. *Matrix Metalloproteinases* (Parks, W. C., and Mecham, R. P., eds) pp. 219–242, Academic Press, San Diego.

85. Grams, F., Reinemer, P., Powers, J. C., Kleine, T., Pieper, M., Tschesche, H., et al. (1995) X-ray structures of human neutrophil collagenase complexed with peptide hydroxamate and peptide thiol inhibitors. Implications for substrate binding and rational drug design. *Eur. J. Biochem.* 228, 830–841.

86. Netzel-Arnett, S., Sang, Q. X., Moore, W. G., Navre, M., Birkedal-Hansen, H., and Van Wart, H. E. (1993) Comparative sequence specificities of human 72- and 92-kDa gelatinases (type IV collagenases) and PUMP (matrilysin). *Biochemistry* 32, 6427–6432.

87. Welch, A. R., Holman, C. M., Huber, M., Brenner, M. C., Browner, M. F., and Van Wart, H. E. (1996) Understanding the P1' specificity of the matrix metalloproteinases: effect of S1' pocket mutations in matrilysin and stromelysin-1. *Biochemistry* 35, 10103–10109.

88. Massova, I., Fridman, R., and Mobashery, S. (1997) Structural insights into the catalytic domains of human matrix metalloprotease-2 and human matrix metalloprotease-9: implications for substrate specificities. *J. Mol. Model.* 3, 17–30.

89. Nagai, Y., Masui, Y., and Sakakibara, S. (1976) Substrate specificity of vetebrate collagenase. *Biochim. Biophys. Acta* 445, 521–524.

90. Masui, Y., Takemoto, T., Sakakibara, S., Hori, H., and Nagai, Y. (1977) Synthetic substrates for vertebrate collagenase. *Biochem. Med.* 17, 215–221.

91. Weingarten, H., Martin, R., and Feder, J. (1985) Synthetic substrates of vertebrate collagenase. *Biochemistry* 24, 6730–6734.

92. Weingarten, H., and Feder, J. (1986) Cleavage site specificity of vertebrate collagenases. *Biochem. Biophys. Res. Commun.* 139, 1184–1187.

93. Seltzer, J. L., Weingarten, H., Akers, K. T., Eschbach, M. L., Grant, G. A., and Eisen, A. Z. (1989) Cleavage specificity of type IV collagenase (gelatinase) from human skin. Use of synthetic peptides as model substrates. *J. Biol. Chem.* 264, 19583–19586.

94. Seltzer, J. L., Akers, K. T., Weingarten, H., Grant, G. A., McCourt, D. W., and Eisen, A. Z. (1990) Cleavage specificity of human skin type IV collagenase (gelatinase). Identification of cleavage sites in type I gelatin, with confirmation using synthetic peptides. *J. Biol. Chem.* 265, 20409–20413.

95. Fields, G. B., Van Wart, H. E., and Birkedal-Hansen, H. (1987) Sequence specificity of human skin fibroblast collagenase. Evidence for the role of collagen structure in determining the collagenase cleavage site. *J. Biol. Chem.* 262, 6221–6226.

96. Netzel-Arnett, S., Fields, G. B., Birkedal-Hansen, H., and Van Wart, H. E. (1991) Sequence specificities of human fibroblast and neutrophil collagenases [published erratum appears in J Biol Chem 1991 Nov 5; 266(31):21326]. *J. Biol. Chem.* 266, 6747–6755.

97. Niedzwiecki, L., Teahan, J., Harrison, R. K., and Stein, R. L. (1992) Substrate specificity of the human matrix metalloproteinase stromelysin and the development of continuous fluorometric assays. *Biochemistry* 31, 12618–12623.

98. Gomis-Rüth, F. X., Maskos, K., Betz, M., Bergner, A., Huber, R., Suzuki, K., et al. (1997) Mechanism of inhibition of the human matrix metalloproteinase stromelysin-1 by TIMP-1. *Nature* 389, 77–81.

99. Meng, Q., Malinovskii, V., Huang, W., Hu, Y., Chung, L., Nagase, H., et al. (1999) Residue 2 of TIMP-1 is a major determinant of affinity and specificity for matrix metalloproteinases but effects of substitutions do not correlate with those of the corresponding P1' residue of substrate. *J. Biol. Chem.* 274, 10184–10189.

100. Benbow, U., Butticè, G., Nagase, H., and Kurkinen, M. (1996) Characterization of the 46-kDa intermediates of matrix metalloproteinase 3 (stromelysin 1) obtained by site-directed mutation of phenylalanine 83. *J. Biol. Chem.* 271, 10715–10722.

101. Reinemer, P., Grams, F., Huber, R., Kleine, T., Schnierer, S., Piper, M., et al. (1994) Structural implications for the role of the N terminus in the 'superactivation' of collagenases. A crystallographic study. *FEBS Lett.* 338, 227–233.

102. Lark, M. W., Bayne, E. K., Flanagan, J., Harper, C. F., Hoerrner, L. A., Hutchinson, N. I., et al. (1997) Aggrecan degradation in human cartilage—evidence for both matrix metalloproteinase and aggrecanase activity in normal, osteoarthritic, and rheumatoid joints. *J. Clin. Invest.* 100, 93–106.

103. Hollander, A. P., Heathfield, T. F., Webber, C., Iwata, Y., Bourne, R., Rorabeck, C., et al. (1994) Increased damage to type II collagen in osteoarthritic articular cartilage detected by a new immunoassay. *J. Clin. Invest.* 93, 1722–1732.

104. Nicholls, A., Sharp, K. A., and Honig, B. (1991) Protein folding and association: insights from the interfacial and thermodynamic properties of hydrocarbons. *Proteins* 11, 281–296.

105. Sang, Q. A. and Douglas, D. A. (1996) Computational sequence analysis of matrix metalloproteinases. *J. Protein Chem.* 15, 137–160.

106. Sage, H., Balian, G., Vogel, A. M., and Bornstein, P. (1984) Type VIII collagen. Synthesis by normal and malignant cells in culture. *Lab. Invest.* 50, 219–231.

107. Gadher, S. J., Eyre, D. R., Duance, V. C., Wotton, S. F., Heck, L. W., Schmid, T. M. et al. (1988) Susceptibility of cartilage collagens type II, IX, X, and XI to human synovial collagenase and neutrophil elastase. *Eur. J. Biochem.* 175, 1–7.

108. Menzel, E. J. and Smolen, J. S. (1978) [Degradation of C1q, the first subcomponent of the complement sequence, by synovial collagenase from patients with rheumatoid arthritis (author's transl)]. [German]. *Wien. Klin. Wochenschr.* 90, 727–730.

109. Nguyen, Q., Murphy, G., Hughes, C. E., Mort, J. S., and Roughley, P. J. (1993) Matrix metalloproteinases cleave at two distinct sites on human cartilage link protein. *Biochem. J.* 295, 595–598.

110. Fukai, F., Ohtaki, M., Fujii, N., Yajima, H., Ishii, T., Nishizawa, Y., et al. (1995) Release of biological activities from quiescent fibronectin by a conformational change and limited proteolysis by matrix metalloproteinases. *Biochemistry* 34, 11453–11459.

111. Imai, K., Shikata, H., and Okada, Y. (1995) Degradation of vitronectin by matrix metalloproteinases-1, -2, -3, -7 and -9. *FEBS Lett.* 369, 249–251.

112. Chandler, S., Coates, R., Gearing, A., Lury, J., Wells, G., and Bone, E. (1995) Matrix metalloproteinases degrade myelin basic protein. *Neurosci. Lett.* 201, 223–226.

113. Desrochers, P. E., Jeffrey, J. J., and Weiss, S. J. (1991) Interstitial collagenase (matrix metalloproteinase-1) expresses serpinase activity. *J. Clin. Invest.* 87, 2258–2265.

114. Ito, A., Mukaiyama, A., Itoh, Y., Nagase, H., Thogersen, I. B., Enghild, J. J., et al. (1996) Degradation of interleukin 1beta by matrix metalloproteinases. *J. Biol. Chem.* 271, 14657–14660.

115. Gearing, A. J., Beckett, P., Christodoulou, M., Churchill, M., Clements, J. M., Crimmin, M., et al. (1995) Matrix metalloproteinases and processing of pro-TNF-alpha. *J. Leukoc. Biol.* 57, 774–777.

116. Fowlkes, J. L., Enghild, J. J., Suzuki, K., and Nagase, H. (1994) Matrix metalloproteinases degrade insulin-like growth factor-binding protein-3 in dermal fibroblast cultures. *J. Biol. Chem.* 269, 25742–25746.

117. Cawston, T. E. and Tyler, J. A. (1979) Purification of pig synovial collagenase to high specific activity. *Biochem. J.* 183, 647–656.

118. Siri, A., Knäuper, V., Veirana, N., Caocci, F., Murphy, G., and Zardi, L. (1995) Different susceptibility of small and large human tenascin-C isoforms to degradation by matrix metalloproteinases. *J. Biol. Chem.* 270, 8650–8654.

119. Sasaki, T., Gohring, W., Mann, K., Maurer, P., Hohenester, E., Knäuper, V., et al. (1997) Limited cleavage of extracellular matrix protein BM-40 by matrix metalloproteinases increases its affinity for collagens. *J. Biol. Chem.* 272, 9237–9243.

120. Imai, K., Hiramatsu, A., Fukushima, D., Pierschbacher, M. D., and Okada, Y. (1997) Degradation of decorin by matrix metalloproteinases: identification of the cleavage sites, kinetic analyses and transforming growth factor-beta1 release. *Biochem. J.* 322, 809–814.

121. Mast, A. E., Enghild, J. J., Nagase, H., Suzuki, K., Pizzo, S. V., and Salvesen, G. (1991) Kinetics and physiologic relevance of the inactivation of α 1-proteinase inhibitor, α 1-antichymotrypsin, and antithrombin III by matrix metalloproteinases-1 (tissue collagenase), -2 (72-kDa gelatinase/type IV collagenase), and -3 (stromelysin). *J. Biol. Chem.* 266, 15810–15816.

122. Nakagawa, H. and Debuchi, H. (1992) Inactivation of substance P by granulation tissue-derived gelatinase. *Biochem.Pharmacol.* 44, 1773–1777.

123. Mayer, U., Mann, K., Timpl, R., and Murphy, G. (1993) Sites of nidogen cleavage by proteases involved in tissue homeostasis and remodelling. *Eur. J. Biochem.* 217, 877–884.

124. Harrison, R., Teahan, J., and Stein, R. (1989) A semicontinuous, high-performance liquid chromatography-based assay for stromelysin. *Anal. Biochem.* 180, 110–113.

125. Sakamoto, W., Fujie, K., Kaga, M., Handa, H., Gotoh, K., Nishihira, J., et al. (1996) Degradation of T-kininogen by cathepsin D and matrix metalloproteinases. *Immunopharmacology* 32, 73–75.

126. Miyazaki, K., Hattori, Y., Umenishi, F., Yasumitsu, H., and Umeda, M. (1990) Purification and characterization of extracellular matrix-degrading metalloproteinase, matrin (pump-1), secreted from human rectal carcinoma cell line. *Cancer Res.* 50, 7758–7764.

127. Quantin, B., Murphy, G., and Breathnach, R. (1989) Pump-1 cDNA codes for a protein with characteristics similar to those of classical collagenase family members. *Biochemistry* 28, 5327–5334.

128. Sires, U. I., Murphy, G., Baragi, V. M., Fliszar, C. J., Welgus, H. G., and Senior, R. M. (1994) Matrilysin is much more efficient than other matrix metalloproteinases in the proteolytic inactivation of α 1-antitrypsin. *Biochem. Biophys. Res. Commun.* 204, 613–620.

129. Fletcher, D. S., Williams, H. R., and Lin, T.-Y. (1978) Effects of human polymorphonuclear leukocyte collagenase on sub-component C1q of the first component of human complement. *Biochim. Biophys. Acta* 540, 270–277.

130. Murphy, G., Reynolds, J. J., Bretz, U., and Baggiolini, M. (1982) Partial purification of collagenase and gelatinase from human polymorphonuclear leucocytes. Analysis of their actions on soluble and insoluble collagens. *Biochem. J.* 203, 209–221.

131. Kudo, K., Saito, A., Sudo, K., Adachi, M., Ikai, A., Ofuji, Y., et al. (1988) [The inhibitory effects of chicken ovomacroglobulin on collagenolytic activity in Bacteroides gingivalis culture supernatant, human PMN and human gingival crevicular fluid]. [Japanese]. *Nippon Shishubyo Gakkai Kaishi* 30, 1061–1069.

132. Desrochers, P. E., Mookhtiar, K., Van Wart, H. E., Hasty, K. A., and Weiss, S. J. (1992) Proteolytic inactivation of α 1-proteinase inhibitor and alpha 1-antichymotrypsin by oxidatively activated human neutrophil metalloproteinases. *J. Biol. Chem.* 267, 5005–5012.

133. Diekmann, O., and Tschesche, H. (1994) Degradation of kinins, angiotensins and substance P by polymorphonuclear matrix metalloproteinases MMP 8 and MMP 9. *Braz. J. Med. Biol. Res.* 27, 1865–1876.

134. Hirose, T., Reife, R. A., Smith, G. N., Jr., Stevens, R. M., Mainardi, C. L., and Hasty, K. A. (1992) Characterization of type V collagenase (gelatinase) in synovial fluid of patients with inflammatory arthritis. *J. Rheumatol.* 19, 593–599.

135. Sires, U. I., Dublet, B., Aubert-Foucher, E., van der Rest, M., and Welgus, H. G. (1995) Degradation of the COL1 domain of type XIV collagen by 92-kDa gelatinase. *J. Biol. Chem.* 270, 1062–1067.

136. Gijbels, K., Proost, P., Masure, S., Carton, H., Billiau, A., and Opdenakker, G. (1993) Gelatinase B is present in the cerebrospinal fluid during experimental autoimmune encephalomyelitis and cleaves myelin basic protein. *J. Neurosci. Res.* 36, 432–440.

137. Lyons, J. G., Birkedal-Hansen, B., Moore, W. G., O'Grady, R. L., and Birkedal-Hansen, H. (1991) Characteristics of a 95-kDa matrix metalloproteinase produced by mammary carcinoma cells. *Biochemistry* 30, 1449–1456.

138. Sanchez-Lopez, R., Alexander, C. M., Behrendtsen, O., Breathnach, R., and Werb, Z. (1993) Role of zinc-binding- and hemopexin domain-encoded sequences in the substrate specificity of collagenase and stromelysin-2 as revealed by chimeric proteins. *J. Biol. Chem.* 268, 7238–7247.

139. Chandler, S., Cossins, J., Lury, J., and Wells, G. (1996) Macrophage metalloelastase degrades matrix and myelin proteins and processes a tumour necrosis factor-α fusion protein. *Biochem. Biophys. Res. Commun.* 228, 421–429.

140. Banda, M. J., Rice, A. G., Griffin, G. L., and Senior, R. M. (1988) α 1-proteinase inhibitor is a neutrophil chemoattractant after proteolytic inactivation by macrophage elastase. *J. Biol. Chem.* 263, 4481–4484.

141. Welgus, H. G., Kobayashi, D. K., and Jeffrey, J. J. (1983) The collagen substrate specificity of rat uterus collagenase. *J. Biol. Chem.* 258, 14162–14165.

142. Welgus, H. G., Grant, G. A., Sacchettini, J. C., Roswit, W. T., and Jeffrey, J. J. (1985) The gelatinolytic activity of rat uterus collagenase. *J. Biol. Chem.* 260, 13601–13606.

143. Eeckhout, Y., Riccomi, H., Cambiaso, C., Vaes, G., and Masson, P. (1976) Studies on properties common to collagen and C1q. *Arch. Int. Physiol. Biochim.* 84, 611–612.

144. Fosang, A. J., Last, K., Knauper, V., Murphy, G., and Neame, P. J. (1996) Degradation of cartilage aggrecan by collagenase-3 (MMP-13). *FEBS Lett.* 380, 17–20.

145. Nethery, A., and O'Grady, R. L. (1991) Interstitial collagenase from rat mammary carcinoma cells: interaction with substrates and inhibitors. *Invasion Metastasis* 11, 241–248.

146. Imai, K., Ohuchi, E., Aoki, T., Nomura, H., Fujii, Y., Sato, H., et al. (1996) Membrane-type matrix metalloproteinase 1 is a gelatinolytic enzyme and is secreted in a complex with tissue inhibitor of metalloproteinases 2. *Cancer Res.* 56, 2707–2710.

147. Stolow, M. A., Bauzon, D. D., Li, J., Sedgwick, T., Liang, V. C., Sang, Q. A., et al. Identification and characterization of a novel collagenase in Xenopus laevis: possible roles during frog development. *Mol. Biol. Cell.* 7, 1996 1471–1483.

148. Sasaki, T., Mann, K., Murphy, G., Chu, M. L., and Timpl, R. (1996) Different susceptibilities of fibulin-1 and fibulin-2 to cleavage by matrix metalloproteinases and other tissue proteases. *Eur. J. Biochem.* 240, 427–434.

149. Murphy, G., Knäuper, V., Cowell, S., Hembry, R., Stanton, H., Butler, G., et al. (1999) Evaluation of some newer matrix metalloproteinases. In *Ann. N.Y. Acad. Sci.* 878, 25–39.

150. Welgus, H. G., Jeffrey, J. J., and Eisen, A. Z. (1981) The collagen substrate specificity of human skin fibroblast collagenase. *J. Biol. Chem.* 256, 9511–9515.

151. Hasty, K. A., Jeffrey, J. J., Hibbs, M. S., and Welgus, H. G. (1987) The collagen substrate specificity of human neutrophil collagenase. *J. Biol. Chem.* 262, 10048–10052.

152. Mitchell, P. G., Magna, H. A., Reeves, L. M., Lopresti-Morrow, L. L., Yocum, S. A., Rosner, P. J., et al. (1996) Cloning, expression, and type II collagenolytic activity of matrix metalloproteinase-13 from human osteoarthritic cartilage. *J. Clin. Invest.* 97, 761–768.

3 The Tissue Inhibitors of Metalloproteinases (TIMPs)

Biology and Regulation

Dylan R. Edwards, *PhD*

CONTENTS

1. INTRODUCTION

The Tissue Inhibitors of Metalloproteinases (TIMPs) are a family of secreted proteins whose primary function is to limit the degradative actions of the matrix metalloproteinases (MMPs) during tissue remodeling *(1)*. This ability to neutralize the collagenases, stromelysins, gelatinases, and membrane-type-MMPs that destroy basement membranes and tissue matrices is central to their potency as suppressors of tumor invasion, metastasis, and angiogenesis. It is also consistent with their involvement in the orchestrated remodeling that occurs during wound repair and embryogenesis. However, TIMPs may be multifunctional, since additional effects on cell growth and apoptosis have been reported, and in some cases these activities appear to be distinct from their MMP inhibitory capabilities. To date, four TIMPs, numbered TIMP-1 through TIMP-4 based on their order of discovery *(2)* have been identified in mammals,

From: *Cancer Drug Discovery and Development:*
Matrix Metalloproteinase Inhibitors in Cancer Therapy
Edited by: Neil J. Clendeninn and Krzysztof Appelt © Humana Press Inc., Totowa, NJ

Table 1
Properties of the Tissue Inhibitors of Metalloproteinases

	TIMP-1	TIMP-2	TIMP-3	TIMP-4
Gene (human)	Xp11.3-11.23	17q2.3-2.5	22q12.1-13.2	3p25
Protein (kDa)	28	21	24	22
N-Glycosylation	yes, two	no	yes, one	no
Protein localization	diffusible	diffusible	ECM bound	diffusible
RNA (kb)	0.9–1.0	3.5, 1.0	4.5 (2.8, 2.4)	1.2
Expression in vivo	ovary, bone, uterus	placenta, lung, brain	kidney, lung, uterus, brain	brain, heart, skel. Muscle
Expression in vitro	inducible	constitutive (largely)	inducible and constitutive	? constitutive (restricted)
MT-MMP inhibition	no	yes	yes	yes
Pro-MMP-2/9 association	MMP-9	MMP-2	MMP2/9	MMP-2
Erythroid potentiation	yes	yes	?	?
Mitogenicity	yes	yes	yes	?
Apoptosis	inhibition (lymphoid)	inhibition (melanoma)	promotion (diverse)	?

and at least one TIMP gene has been found in invertebrates *(3)*. Although all four mammalian TIMPs have many similarities, individual family members have distinctive structural features, biochemical properties, and expression patterns, suggesting that each TIMP has a preferred set of tasks in vivo, and some roles may be unique to a particular TIMP. This is highlighted by the identification of one family member, TIMP-3, as the gene responsible for an autosomal dominant macular degeneration syndrome (Sorsby's fundus dystrophy) that leads to early blindness *(4)*. Thus, the functions of TIMPs may be complex and multifaceted. This chapter will focus on recent progress in understanding TIMP actions and regulation, building on knowledge discussed in several excellent earlier reviews *(5–7)*.

Table I summarizes basic information on the TIMP family and exposes several important similarities and differences. TIMPs are 20–30kDa secreted proteins that form tight, 1:1 complexes with the active forms of MMPs, in general with relatively low selectivity. An exception to this rule is the inability of TIMP-1 to associate with MT-MMPs 1–3 (MMP14–16) *(8,9)*. At the gene level, protein-coding information is held in 5 exons and intron-exon boundaries are conserved, suggesting that all of the genes likely emerged from a single ancestor via gene duplication *(10)*. This is supported by conservation of the rather curious organization of *timp* genes, which are embedded intragenically in intron 5 of the synapsin genes, an organization that is also found in *Drosophila Timp (3)*. The *timp*1 genes have an additional sixth exon at the 5′-end that does not encode protein; this has significance for regulation of *timp*1 expression, as will be discussed in a subsequent section, *"Timp* Gene Expression."

2. TIMPs AND ADAMs

A new area of interest has emerged with the recognition that certain TIMPs are functionally relevant inhibitors of the adamalysin metalloproteinases, that possess both a disintegrin and metalloproteinase (ADAM) domains *(11,12)*. The ADAMs also have Cys-rich, epidermal growth factor (EGF)-like regions, followed in most by transmembrane and cytoplasmic domains. They are related to snake venom proteins that cause hemorrhage via disruption of platelet integrin function and dissolution of basement membranes. Biological roles of the mammalian ADAMs are starting to emerge in the areas of fertlization, cell adhesion and fusion, ectodomain shedding of cell surface receptors or adhesion molecules, and proteolytic activation of cytokines and growth factors. To date 28 ADAMs have been identified, but we know of the substrates and binding partners for only a very few. One family member is tumor necrosis factor-α (TNFα) converting enzyme (TACE, ADAM-17), that is important in inflammation, since it processes cell-associated pro-TNFα to the mature 17kDa soluble form *(13)*. Another enzyme, ADAM-10 or kuzbanian, is involved in signaling through the Notch pathway, likely via activation of ligands such as Delta *(14)*.

Alone among the TIMPs, TIMP-3 can inhibit ADAM-17 and prevent TNF-α shedding from monocytes *(15,16)*. As shown in Table 2, TIMP-3 can also block interleukin-6 receptor shedding from myeloma cells *(17)* and release of L-selectin from leukocytes *(16)*. These observations are consistent with ADAM-17 inhibition, since ADAM-17-null cells are deficient in shedding all of these molecules, as well as TGFα and TNF receptors *(18)*, thus implying that this enzyme is either a sort of "pan-sheddase" or an upstream regulator of the functions of other ADAMs. It is likely that a number of metalloproteinases function in ectodomain shedding, since Lombard et al. *(19)* have reported that TIMP-2 and synthetic hydroxamate MP inhibitors (but not TIMP-1) block release of p55 TNFα-RI and p75 TNFαRII from colon adenocarcinoma cells. Also, ectodomain cleavage of HER2/neu from breast adenocarcinoma cells is sensitive to TIMP-1, but not TIMP-2 *(20)* which suggests the involvement of a novel MP activity. These observations have important implications. They significantly expand the repertoire of TIMP actions and they emphasize the unique capabilities of particular family members. Moreover, they may shed light on the

Table 2
Inhibition of Protein Ectodomain Shedding by TIMP[a]

Substrate	TIMP-1	TIMP-2	TIMP-3	TIMP-4	Reference
pro TNFα	−	−	+	−	Amour et al., *(15)*
					Borland et al., *(16)*
TNFRI	−	+	ND	ND	Lombard et al., *(19)*
TNFRI	ND	ND	+	ND	Smith et al., *(64)*
TNFRII	−	+	ND	ND	Lombard et al., *(19)*
L-selectin	−	−	+	ND	Borland et al., *(16)*
HER2/neu	+	−	ND	ND	Codony-Servat et al., *(20)*
IL6R	−	−	+	ND	Hargreaves et al., *(17)*

[a]ND, not determined; +, inhibition; −, no inhibition.

mechanisms by which TIMPs can selectively affect cell growth and apoptosis in addition to their more readily interchangeable actions as suppressors of MMP-mediated ECM degradation.

3. TIMP STRUCTURE

The conserved signature of mammalian TIMPs is the 12 cysteine residues responsible for folding the proteins into a 6-looped, two-domain structure (Fig. 1). The N-terminal domain (residues 1–126 in TIMP-1), comprising the first three disulfide-bonded loops, can fold independently of the C-terminal domain and is necessary and sufficient for MMP inhibition *(21)*. The structures of TIMP-1 and TIMP-2 have been solved by a combination of NMR and X-ray crystallography studies *(22–24)*. The N-terminal domain is a 5-stranded β-sheet that is folded over to form a barrel, a structure that is homologous to the oligonucleotide/ oligosaccharide-binding (OB) fold of several bacterial enterotoxins and nucleases and yeast apartyl-tRNA synthetase *(22)*. Solution of the X-ray crystal structures of full-length TIMPs in MMP-3/TIMP-1 and MT1-MMP/TIMP-2 complexes *(23,24)* shows the TIMP molecule as an elongated, continuous wedge that occupies the entire length of the active site cleft of the MMP. Six separate polypeptide segments of TIMP-1 make contact with MMP-3, four coming from the N-terminal domain and two from the C-terminal domain *(23)*. Cys 1 coordinates the Zn atom in the MMP active site bidentally through its N-terminal α-amino group and its carbonyl group. The critical nature of the α-amino group is shown by the observation that extension of TIMP-2 by one Ala residue renders the molecule inactive as an MMP inhibitor *(25)*.

The Cys 1/Cys 70 disulfide bond in TIMP-1 creates a surface ridge involving residues from Cys 1 to Val 4 and Met 66 to Val 70 that contacts the active site. This explains the large influence of mutations in this area *(26,27)*. In par-

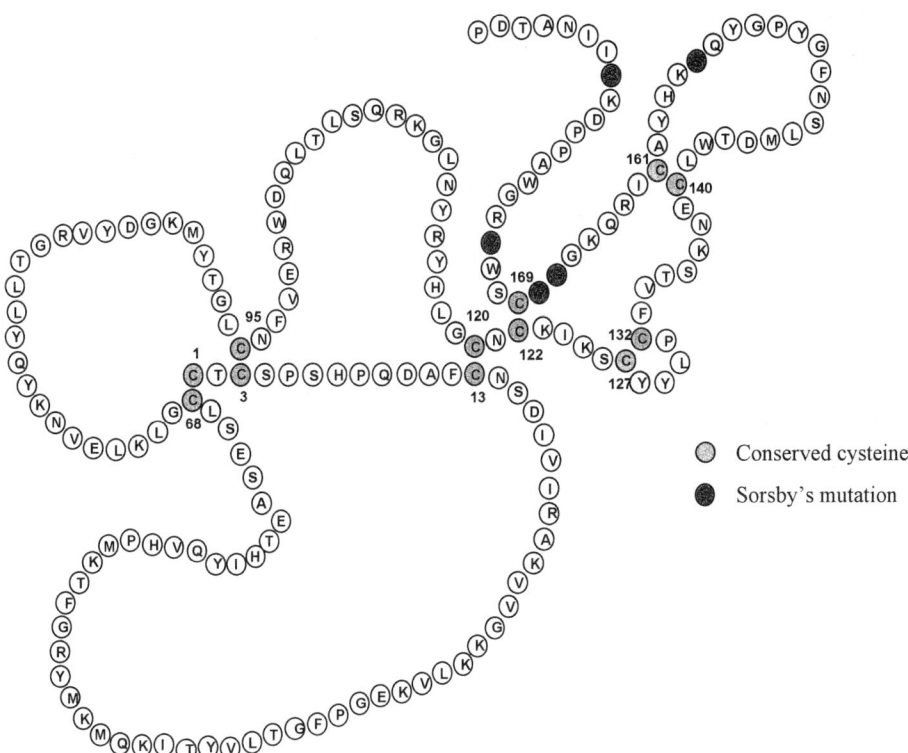

Fig. 1. TIMP Structure. The structure of human TIMP-3 is shown, with the positions of the conserved Cys residues indicated, as well as the mutations in the C-terminal domain that give rise to Sorsby's fundus dystrophy.

ticular, Thr 2 interacts with the S1′ pocket of the MMP, which is a critical determinant of substrate specificities of the enzymes. Mutation of Thr 2 in TIMP-1 to Ala generates a molecule that is 17-fold more effective against MMP-3 than MMP-1 *(26)*. In TIMP-2, mutation of the analgous Ser 2 residue to Lys profoundly reduced effectiveness against MMP-3, but did not influence action on MMP-2 or MMP-14 *(28)*.

Another major region of the molecule contributing to the specificity of TIMPs is the loop between the A and B strands in the β-barrel. In TIMP-1 this loop is very short, whereas TIMP-2 (and TIMP-4) have much longer AB loops. In TIMP-2, this long loop folds over the edge of the active site cleft in MT1-MMP and extends into a surface pocket caused by a structural feature known as the "MT-loop" that is unique to MT1-3 MMPs. This loop is formed by an 8-residue insertion in the MT-MMPs relative to other MMPs *(24)*. Mutation of Tyr 36 in the TIMP-2 AB loop severely compromises its ability to inhibit MT1-MMP, without significantly affecting actions on other MMPs *(28)*. The short AB loop may go a long way toward explaining the inability of TIMP-1 to inhibit MT-MMPs. However, TIMP-3 also has a relatively short AB loop and it binds MT-MMPs as well as TIMP-2, so other parts of the molecule probably make important contributions. These likely involve the other zones of contact between the TIMP extended wedge and MMPs, including the C-terminal domain interactions *(23)*.

These data indicate that it will be possible to engineer TIMPs with altered specificities for MMPs. Such "Designer TIMPs" may be valuable for gene therapy for diseases such as cancer or arthritis since selective MMP inhibition might not elicit the side-effects such as tendinitis that are seen with broad-range synthetic hydroxamate MP inhibitors in clinical use *(29)*.

One aspect of TIMP function for which the C-terminal domain is critical is the formation of specific complexes with gelatinases, which involve interactions with the hemopexin-like C-terminal domains of the MMPs *(30,31)*. These C-terminal domain interactions are very tight for TIMP-1 and TIMP-3 with MMP-9 (gelatinase-B) and TIMP-2, -3 and -4 with MMP-2 *(32–35)*. These interactions appear to serve several purposes. First, they provide a means by which the initial docking of TIMP with an active MMP speeds up the interaction of the N-terminal part of the TIMP with the catalytic site of the MMP. Secondly, association of TIMPs with the latent forms of the gelatinases regulates activation of the enzymes. Pro-MMP-9 that is complexed with TIMP-1 is less susceptible to activation by other MMPs such as MMP-3 and MMP-2, because stoichiometric amounts of the activator are needed to overcome the exposed TIMP-1 N-terminal MMP inhibitory domain *(36)*. In a very different fashion, the TIMP-2/pro-MMP-2 interaction regulates activation of pro-MMP-2 by MT1-, 2- and 3-MMPs. Here, inhibition of active MT-MMP on the cell surface by N-terminal domain interactions with TIMP-2 creates a "receptor" for pro-MMP-2 *(32)*. The relative levels of TIMP-2 and MT-MMPs are critical, since excess TIMP-2 blocks MT-MMP function, preventing pro-MMP-2 activation, whereas a surplus of MT-MMP allows activation to occur. Since MT1-MMP and TIMP-2 show similar spatio-temporal patterns of expression in vivo *(37)*, this mechanism is physiologically relevant.

The highly acidic exposed C-terminal "tail" of TIMP-2 is a significant factor in the association of TIMP-2 with pro-MMP-2 *(30)*. However, the corresponding tails of both TIMP-3 and TIMP-4 do not have the same acidic flavor, so it is possible that these TIMPs cannot substitute for TIMP-2 to form a pro-MMP-2 receptor, and they may not support pro-MMP-2 activation *(35)*. Thus subtle control over pro-MMP-2 activation may be provided via the levels of specific TIMPs in the pericellular environment.

4. TIMPs AND CELL GROWTH

The links between TIMPs and effects on cell growth go back over a decade to the initial cloning of human TIMP-1 as erythroid potentiating activity (EPA,

38). There have since been numerous reports of both stimulation and inhibition of growth of various cell types by TIMP-1, TIMP-2, and TIMP-3 (reviewed in *5–7*). In particular, Hayakawa and colleagues have shown that depletion of TIMP-1 from fetal calf serum reduces the ability of the serum to stimulate growth of a large number of cell lines, which could be restored upon adding back the stripped TIMP-1 *(39)*. Subsequently, TIMP-2 at subnanomolar concentrations has been shown to stimulate growth of Raji Burkitt's lymphoma cells *(40)* and Hs68 fibroblasts and HT1080 fibrosarcoma cells *(41)*, with some studies suggesting a comitogenic action with insulin *(42)*. The implication from these studies is that TIMPs can act via specific, saturable, high-affinity receptors (Kd = 0.15n*M, 40*), perhaps linking to G-protein signaling pathways and cAMP elevation *(41)*. Moreover it is proposed that these actions are distinct from MMP inhibitory action, since reduced and alkylated TIMP-2 retains its mitogenic actions *(40)* and the inactive Ala+TIMP-2 extended at the N-terminus is still able to promote fibroblast growth *(25)*. The N-terminal domain of TIMP-1 was effective as an EPA, but erythroid precursor growth stimulation and MMP inhibition could be uncoupled using point mutants in this domain *(43)*. Increases in MAP (Mitogen Activated Protein) kinase activities and tyrosine phosphorylation have been observed in TIMP-1 and TIMP-2-treated osteosarcoma cells *(44)*.

To this catalog we must add observations that elevated expression of TIMP-1 has been linked with increased malignancy in human lymphomas *(45,46)* and in colorectal cancer *(47)* and the same is true for TIMP-2 in bladder cancer *(48)*. High TIMP-1 levels are to be found in plasma from patients with advanced breast or colorectal cancer *(49)*. This suggests that in at least some tumors, TIMPs may be linked with the promotion of malignancy rather than its suppression, and these paradoxical effects may involve growth promotion. But if so, how do TIMPs promote growth? It is possible that TIMP-specific receptors exist, which recognize different aspects of the molecule than those involved in MMP inhibition. However, none has yet been cloned. Recently, fluorescence tagged-TIMP-1 has been visualized binding to the membrane of MCF-7 cells, with subsequent translocation to the nucleus *(50)*. Nuclear accumulation of TIMP-1-immunoreactivity has also been seen in human gingival fibroblasts, with peak levels in S-phase *(51)*. TIMP-1 activated responses may thus involve direct transfer of the inhibitor to the nucleus.

The selective effects of TIMPs on ADAM-mediated ectodomain shedding of signaling receptors may indirectly enhance cell growth by potentiating mitogenic signal transduction. MMPs have also been proposed roles in the control of growth factor bioavailability. For instance, cleavage of insulin-like growth factor binding protein-3 (IGFBP-3) by MMP-2, -3 and -9 can liberate IGF for binding to the IGF-1 receptor, leading to growth stimulation *(52,53)*. MMP-2 may itself "shed" fibroblast growth factor receptors *(54)*, and a decoy receptor for interleukin-1 (IL-1), thereby potentiating IL-1 actions *(55)*. However, all of these actions would seem to depend upon retention of antiproteolytic activity, and as we have seen, in at least some instances growth effects have been segregated from this property *(40,43)*.

A complex characterized as TIMP-1/procathepsin-L has been reported to stimulate steroidogenesis in Leydig and granulosa cells *(56)*. Recombinant TIMP-1 increased estradiol-17beta levels in granulosa cell media in vitro, but no impact on steroidogenesis in TIMP-1-null mice has been observed *(57)*. Thus, at present there is no clear unifying explanation for the effects of TIMPs on cell growth, and it is likely that multiple cell-specific mechanisms underlie these intriguing observations.

5. TIMPs AND APOPTOSIS

Closely linked with proposed mitogenic actions are reports that TIMPs can selectively promote or inhibit apoptosis. Guedez et al. *(58)* have shown that in Burkitt's lymphoma cell lines high TIMP-1 expression correlates with increased expression of activation and survival markers such as CD40, and that retrovirus-driven expression of TIMP-1 in otherwise low-TIMP-1-expressing cells induced this antiapoptotic phenotype. The same authors went on to show that TIMP-1, but not the hydroxamate BB-94 or TIMP-2, conferred resistance to CD95/Fas-dependent and -independent apoptosis in the lymphoma cells *(59)*. This resistance was paralleled by induction of Bcl-X$_L$ expression. However, other data indicate that TIMP-2 and BB-94 (but not TIMP-1) can promote apoptosis in activated T-cells, probably via inhibition of Fas-ligand shedding (M. Lim, personal communication). TIMP-2 overexpression in B16F10 melanoma cells has been reported to inhibit apoptosis *(60)*.

Some of the most powerful effects on cell growth and apoptosis have been seen with adenoviral delivery of TIMPs. As expected, adenovirus-mediated over-expression of TIMP-1, -2 or -3 in rat aortic smooth muscle cells (SMC) inhibited invasion through Matrigel, but TIMP-2 reduced cell proliferation, whereas TIMP-3 promoted apoptosis *(61)*. The TIMP-3 effect was replicated by exogenous recombinant TIMP-3. Subsequent studies have shown that TIMP-3-induced apoptosis in melanoma cells *(62)* and HT1080 and HeLa cells *(63)*. These effects on cell death were not seen with BB-94 or other TIMPs *(61)*. The mechanism involved is as yet unknown, though stabilization of cell surface TNF receptors has been reported *(64)*. This may involve a TIMP-3 selective effect on an ADAM, as discussed earlier in "TIMPs and ADAMs", though if that were the case, BB-94 ought to give an analogous response. Alternatively, it is possible that high levels of TIMP-3 may indirectly induce cell death via effects on cell attachment. TIMP-3 is unique among the TIMPs in being ECM-associated, and it is possible that high-level expression of TIMP-3 might interfere with cell-ECM interactions, essentially by "squelching" matrix binding sites. Indeed, chicken TIMP-3 was originally identified on the basis of its association with transformation of chick fibroblasts, including promotion of cell rounding and detachment (65,66).

It is not clear whether TIMP-3-induced apoptosis has any physiological parallel, though Chapter 4 discusses one possibility. In fact, the opposite may be true in normal development, because high level TIMP-3 expression in uterine decidual cells between 4.5–7.5 days post coitum of embryo implantation in the mouse has been linked with survival of these differentiated cells (67). However, whatever the mechanism involved, the ability of TIMP-3 to induce cell death makes it very attractive for gene therapy of cancer, particularly when combined with its other properties of ECM-association (and hence optimal local tissue retention) and antiinvasive and antiangiogenic actions (68).

6. TIMP-3 AND SORSBY'S FUNDUS DYSTROPHY

The C-terminal domain of TIMP-3 has been suggested to be responsible for the ability of the protein to associate with ECM, since its deletion generated a soluble activity, and a TIMP-2/TIMP-3 N-C domain chimera displayed matrix binding (69). The C-terminal domain also has great biological significance since, as shown in Figure 1, it is here that the mutations that give rise to Sorsby's Fundus Dystrophy (SFD) are found (4). SFD is an autosomal dominant macular disorder, characterized by subretinal neovascularization and atrophy of the choriocapillaris, retinal pigmented epithelium, and retina (70). An important component is Bruch's membrane, a multilayered ECM located between the choroid and the retinal pigmented epithelium (71), which expands and becomes lipid-rich in SFD. TIMP-3 is expressed by the retinal pigmented epithelium and ciliary epithelium of the eye and is a normal component of Bruch's membrane (72). The SFD TIMP-3 mutations seem only to affect the function of the eye, as no other pathologies in other organs have been reported.

All five published SFD mutations result in the introduction of an additional Cys residue (at positions Ser156, Gly167, Tyr168, Tyr172, and Ser181). As might be anticipated, these mutations do not have a profound effect on MMP inhibition and ECM localization. However, these SFD TIMP-3s form additional protein-protein complexes, including multimers that retain TIMP activity. At this time it is not clear how these mutations relate to the pathogenesis of SFD. One possibility is that the metabolism of SFD TIMP-3 differs from wild-type protein, leading to a chronic disturbance of the MP/TIMP balance. However, given the proapoptotic actions of TIMP-3 discussed above, it is possible that an accumulation of TIMP-3 in Bruch's membrane may induce the death of retinal pigmented epithelial (RPE) cells. It is also possible that SFD mutant TIMP-3 has reduced potency in the control of angiogenesis, allowing blood vessels to move into Bruch's membrane from the choroid, ultimately leading to hemorrhage (68).

7. TUMOR GROWTH, METASTASIS, AND ANGIOGENESIS

There is a wealth of literature documenting a tumor suppressive role for TIMPs in in vitro and in vivo model systems, which has been well-covered elsewhere *(5,7,73)*. The classical interpretation of these findings, based on TIMP suppression of MMP-mediated invasion and metastatic spread of malignant cells, is currently under review, based on a number of findings (73). For instance, intravital video microscopy of cells in the process of extravasation has shown that cells with very different tumor-forming abilities extravasate equally well *(74)*. This was also true for control and TIMP-1-overexpressing B16F10 melanoma cells, though the latter showed greatly reduced tumor formation using classical "end-point" metastasis assays *(75)*. This suggests that the effects of TIMPs on tumor growth may be more important than invasion suppression *(73)*.

So if not through inhibition of tumor cell invasion/extravasation, how do TIMPs prevent tumor growth? A major contribution may come from the preservation of epithelial tissue organization by blocking the actions of enzymes such as MMP-3 that can destroy E-cadherin at cell-cell attachment sites *(76)*. As discussed earlier in "TIMPs and Cell Growth", control of growth factor bioavailability must also be important. There is good evidence that the suppression of SV40T-antigen-induced hepatocarcinomas seen in transgenic TIMP-1-overexpressing mice compared to control or antisense TIMP-1-expressing mice *(77)* involves stabilization of IGFBP-3 and thus inhibition of IGF signaling *(78)*. TIMP-1 inhibition of HER2/neu shedding may also be significant in limiting tumor growth, since truncation of HER2/neu leaves a membrane-associated remnant that may promiscuously associate with and stimulate other EGFR family members *(20)*. Furthermore, metalloproteinases are involved in release of cell-surface EGFR ligands, which leads to autocrine growth stimulation of some tumor cell lines *(79)*.

It is clear that synthetic MP inhibitors and TIMP-1, -2 and -3 can suppress angiogenesis, and this will likely be the case for TIMP-4 also *(80)*. An important part of neovascularization involves endothelial cell (EC) invasion through stroma, in which MT1-MMP has been suggested to be a key player *(81)*. This is consistent with the reported abilities of TIMP-2 and TIMP-3 to block EC tube formation in three-dimensional collagen gels, whereas TIMP-1 could not *(68)*. However, angiogenesis during development and tumorigenesis likely involves many MMPs, particularly MMP-2 and MMP-9 *(82,83)*, so TIMP-1 would be expected to have a significant suppressive effect in vivo.

Once again, though, I return to the enigma of TIMP effects on growth, because these may be very relevant in the context of tumorigenesis. Soloway et al. *(84)* derived coisogenic ras-transformed cell lines from fibroblasts isolated from TIMP-1-null mice and control littermates. When these cells were reintroduced into mice, the picture that emerged was that the TIMP-1 expression of the cell lines was an important determinant of phenotype, regardless of the genotype of the host. Some pairs of cell lines showed the expected increase in metastatic ability for the TIMP-1-deficient partner, but at least one cell pair showed increased tumor formation for the control, TIMP-1 expressing line. This suggests that in the context of some cellular phenotypes, the presence of TIMP-1 can enhance tumor growth. In other studies, TIMP-1 overexpressing rat mammary carcinoma cell lines have been shown to generate larger tumors in nude mice than corresponding control lines, without any impact on in vitro growth *(85)*. Tumors from the TIMP-1-overexpressing cells showed higher vascularity than controls, which was paralleled by increased expression of vascular endothelial growth factor by the TIMP-1-expressing cells in vitro. TIMP-1 over-expression led to increased production of type IV collagen and laminin and a more extensive connective tissue stroma in the resulting tumors, perhaps creating a more favorable environment for attachment-dependent tumor cells to grow *(86)*. In *Min* mice, which carry a defective copy of the adenomatous polyposis coli (APC) gene and spontaneously develop gastrointestinal tract lesions, treatment with BB-94 reduced tumor formation by 48% *(87)*. However, forced overexpression of TIMP-1 in Min mice either had no effect on tumor formation, or in one case augmented Min-induced tumors by 32%. These observations underscore the need to understand the multifunctionality of TIMPs, particularly in the context of tumor biology.

8. TIMP GENE EXPRESSION

Each *timp* has a characteristic expression pattern in vivo and in vitro, with *timp*-1 and *timp*-3 being frequently responsive to stimuli such as growth factors, cytokines, tumor promoters, and inflammatory mediators, whereas *timp*-2 and -4 are expressed in a more constitutive fashion (Table 1; *2,88,89*). The organization of the promoter regions of the genes (*see* Fig. 2) reflects these substantial differences, with *timp*-2 and -4 showing more features characteristic of housekeeping genes than *timp*-1 and *timp*-3, where binding sites for transcription factors such as AP1 (activator protein -1), Ets/PEA3, and STAT have been shown to be involved in transcriptional activation *(90–94)*. The *timp*-1 promoter region also has at least two binding sites for a single-stranded DNA binding protein (termed ssT1) that contribute to basal promoter activity *(95)*. Both the untranslated exon 1 and intron1 in *timp*-1 genes contain important regulatory elements *(92)*. In fact, intron 1 is a mosaic of positive and negative regulatory elements, at least one of the latter involving a combination of Ets/PEA3 and Sp1 binding motifs. Intron 1 overall has a negative impact on transcription in vitro, which may be important for correct spatio-temporal expression of *timp*-1 in vivo.

Given the expanded knowledge of the particular attributes of individual TIMPs summarized in Tables 1 and 2, understanding the expression patterns of TIMPs becomes of increasing importance. We need to know whether rela-

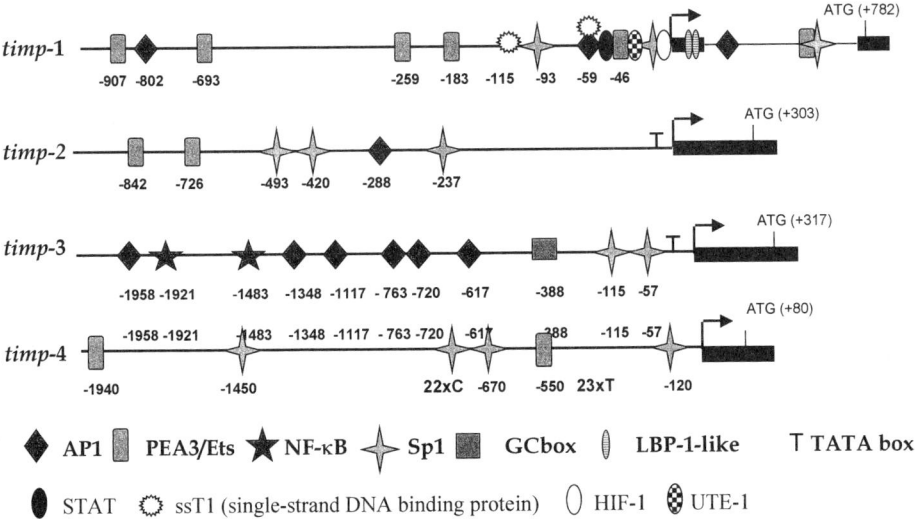

Fig. 2. Organization of the promoter regions of *timp* genes. The figure shows the relative organization (not to scale) from studies of the human and mouse *timp*-1, human *timp*-2, and mouse *timp*-3 and *timp*-4. HIF-1, hypoxia-inducible factor-1; UTE-1, upstream TIMP element-1.

tionships recognized in in vitro systems, such as TIMP-2 and its role in pro-MMP-2 activation, or TIMP-3 and its inhibition of ADAM-17, are reflected in integrated expression of the partners in physiological and pathological settings. It will therefore be valuable in the future for attention to be given to analysis of expression of all of the TIMP family members when studying a particular biological problem, instead of looking at a single gene.

9. FUTURE DIRECTIONS

The TIMPs are fascinating molecules that are involved in many aspects of biology. Although we now understand a lot about their structure and the mechanisms by which they inhibit MMPs, the basis of their multifunctional effects on cell growth and death remain enigmatic. This needs to be resolved urgently, particularly if the results of structure-function studies are to be exploited to develop "Designer TIMPs" for gene therapeutics. We need also to understand the relationships between TIMPs and ADAMs and the basis for the apparently greater selectivity of inhibition of these metalloproteinases compared to their more interchangeable character with the MMPs. In parallel, there is a dearth of information on the functions of ADAMs, which needs to be addressed by defining their substrates and sites of expression. Finally, functional genomics approaches using transgenic and gene knockout technology are as yet in their infancy with regard to the TIMPs. We need to assemble a full complement of mouse models deficient in TIMPs-1 through -4, and pursue the impact of single and compound gene ablation in disease models.

ACKNOWLEDGMENTS

This work was supported by the Norfolk and Norwich Big C Appeal and the Leukaemia Research Fund.

REFERENCES

1. Nagase, H. and Woessner, J. F. Jr. (1999) Matrix metalloproteinases. *J. Biol. Chem.* 274, 21491–21494.
2. Greene, J., Wang, M., Liu, Y. E., Raymond, L. A., Rosen, C., and Shi, Y. E. (1996) Molecular cloning and characterization of human Tissue Inhibitor of Metalloproteinases 4. *J. Biol. Chem.* 271, 30375–30380.
3. Pohar, N., Godenschwege, T. A., and Buchner, E. (1999) Invertebrate tissue inhibitor of metalloproteinase: structure and nested gene organization within the synapsin locus is conserved from Drosophila to human. *Genomics* 57, 293–296.
4. Weber, B. H., Vogt, G., Pruett, R. C., Stohr, H., and Felbor, U. (1994) Mutations in the tissue inhibitor of metalloproteinases-3 (TIMP3) in patients with Sorsby's fundus dystrophy. *Nature Genetics* 8, 352–356.
5. Denhardt, D. T., Feng, B., Edwards, D. R., Cocuzzi, E. T., and Malyankar, U. M. (1993) Tissue inhibitor of metalloproteinases (TIMP, aka EPA): structure, control of expression and biological functions. *Pharmac. Ther.* 59, 329–341.
6. Edwards, D. R., Beaudry, P. P., Laing, T. D., Kowal, V., Leco, K. J., Leco, P. A., and Lim, M. S. (1996) The roles of tissue inhibitors of metalloproteinases in tissue remodeling and cell growth. *Int. J. Obes.* 20, S9–S15.
7. Gomez, D. E., Alonso, D. F., Yoshiji, H., and Thorgeirsson, U. P. (1997) Tissue inhibitors of metalloproteinases: structure, regulation and biological functions. *Eur. J. Cell Biol.* 74, 111–122.
8. Strongin, A. Y., Marmer, B. L., Grant, G. A., and Goldberg, G. I. (1993) Plasma membrane-dependent activation of the 72-kDa type IV collagenase is prevented by complex formation with TIMP-2. *J. Biol. Chem.* 268, 14033–14039.
9. Will, H., Atkinson, S. J., Butler, G., Smith, B., and Murphy, G. (1996) The soluble catalytic domain of membrane type 1 matrix metalloproteinase cleaves the propeptide of progelatinase A and initiates autoproteolytic activation- Regulation by TIMP-2 and TIMP-3. *J. Biol. Chem.* 271, 17119–17123.
10. Apte, S. S., Murphy, G., and Olsen, B. R. (1995) The gene structure of Tissue Inhibitor of Metalloproteinases-3 (TIMP-3) and its inhibitory activities define the distinct TIMP family. *J. Biol. Chem.* 270, 14313–14318.
11. Black, R. A. and White, J. M. (1998) ADAMs: focus on the protease domain. *Curr. P. Cell Biol.* 10, 654–659.
12. Blobel C. P. (1997) Metalloprotease-Disintegrins: Links to cell adhesion and cleavage of TNFα and Notch. *Cell* 90, 589–592.
13. Black, R. A., Rauch, C. T., Kozlosky, C. J., et al. (1997) A metalloproteinase disintegrin that releases tumor-necrosis factor-alpha from cells. *Nature* 385, 729–733.
14. Qi, H., Rand, M. D., Wu, X., Sestan, N., Wang, W., Rakic, P., et al. (1999) Processing of the Notch ligand Delta by the metalloprotease kuzbanian. *Science* 283, 91–94.

15. Amour, A., Slocombe, P. M., Webster, A., Butler, M., Knight, C. G., Smith, B. J., et al. (1998) TNF-α converting enzyme (TACE) is inhibited by TIMP-3. *FEBS Letts.* 435, 39–44.
16. Borland, G., Murphy, G., and Ager, A. (1999) Tissue inhibitor of metalloproteinase-3 inhibits shedding of L-selectin from leukocytes. *J. Biol. Chem.* 274, 2810–2815.
17. Hargreaves, P. G., Wang, F., Antcliff, J., Murphy, G., Lawry, J., Russell, G. G., et al. (1998) Human myeloma cells shed the interleukin-6 receptor: inhibition by tissue inhibitor of metalloproteinase-3 and a hydroxamate-based metalloproteinase inhibitor. *Br. J. Haematol.* 101, 694–702.
18. Peschon, J. J., Slack, J. L., Reddy, P., et al. (1998) An essential role for ectodomain shedding in mammalian development. *Science* 282, 1281–1284.
19. Lombard, M. A., Wallace, T. L., Kubicek, M. F., Petzold, G. L., Mitchell, M. A., Hendges, S. K., et al. (1998) Synthetic matrix metalloproteinase inhibitors and tissue inhibitor of metalloproteinase -2 (TIMP-2), but not TIMP-1, inhibit shedding of tumor necrosis factor-α receptors in a human colon adenocarcinoma (Colo205) cell line. *Cancer Res.* 58, 4001–4007.
20. Codony-Servat, J., Albanell, J., Lopez-Talavera, J. C., Arribas, J., and Baselga, J. (1999) Cleavage of the HER2 ectodomain is a pervanadate-activable process that is inhibited by the Tissue Inhibitor of Metalloproteinases-1 in breast cancer cells. *Cancer Res.* 59, 1196–1201.
21. Murphy, G., Houbrechts, A., Cockett, M. I., Williamson, R. A., O'Shea M., and Docherty, A. J. P. (1991) The N-terminal domain of tissue inhibitor of metalloproteinase retains metalloproteinase inhibitory activity. *Biochemistry* 30, 8097–8102.
22. Williamson, R. A., Martorell, G., Carr, M. D., Murphy, G., Docherty, A. J. P., Freedman, R. B., et al. (1994) Solution structure of the active domain of tissue inhibitor of metalloproteinases-2: A new member of the OB fold protein family. *Biochemistry* 33, 11745–11759.
23. Gomis-Ruth, F-X., Maskos, K., Betz, M., Bergner, A., Huber, R., Suzuki, K., et al. (1997) Mechanism of inhibition of the human matrix metalloproteinase stromelysin-1 by TIMP-1. *Nature* 389, 77–81.
24. Fernandez-Catalan, C., Bode, W., Huber, R., Turk, D., Calvete, J. J., Lichte, A., et al. (1998) Crystal structure of the complex formed by the membrane type-1-matrix metalloproteinase with the tissue inhibitor of metalloproteinases-2, the soluble progelatinase A receptor. *EMBO J.* 17, 5238–5248.
25. Wingfield, P. T., Sax, J. K., Stahl, S. J., Kaufman, J., Palmer, I., Chung, V., et al. (1999) Biophysical and functional characterization of full length recombinant human tissue inhibitor of metalloproteinases-2 (TIMP-2) produced in *Escherischia coli*. *J. Biol. Chem.* 274, 21362–21368.
26. Huang, W., Meng, Q., Suzuki, K., Nagase, H., and Brew, K. (1997) Mutational study of the amino-terminal domain of human tissue inhibitor of metalloproteinase 1 (TIMP-1) locates an inhibitory region for matrix metalloproteinases. *J. Biol. Chem.* 272, 22086–22091.
27. Meng, Q., Malinovskii, V., Huang, W., Chung, L., Nagase, H., Bode, W., et al. (1999) Residue 2 of TIMP-1 is a major determinant of affinity and specificity for matrix metalloproteinases but effects of substitutions do not correlate with those of the corresponding P1′ residue of substrate. *J. Biol. Chem.* 274, 10184–10189.
28. Butler, G. S., Hutton, M., Wattam, B. A., Williamson, R. A., Knäuper, V., Willenbrock, F., et al. (1999) The specificity of TIMP-2 for matrix metalloproteinases can be modified by single amino acid mutations. *J. Biol. Chem.* 274, 20391–20396.
29. Nemunaitis, J., Poole, C., Primrose, J., Rosemurgy, A., Malfetano, J., Brown, P., et al. (1998) Combined analysis of studies of the effects of the matrix metalloproteinase inhibitor marimastat on serum tumor markers in advanced cancer: selection of a biologically active and tolerable dose for longer-term studies. *Clin. Cancer Res.* 4, 1101–1109.
30. Murphy, G. and Knäuper, V. (1997) Relating matrix metalloproteinase structure to function: Why the "hemopexin" domain? *Matrix Biol.* 15, 511–518.
31. Overall, C. M., King, A. E., Sam, D. K., Ong, A. D., Lau, T. T., Wallon, U. M., et al. (1999) Identification of the tissue inhibitor of metalloproteinases-2 (TIMP-2) binding site on the he-

mopexin carboxyl domain of human gelatinase A by site-directed mutagenesis. The hierarchical role in binding TIMP-2 of the unique cationic clusters of hemopexin modules II and IV. *J. Biol. Chem.* 274, 4421–4429.

32. Butler, G. S., Butler, M. J., Atkinson, S. A., Will, H., Tamura, T., Schade van Westrum, S., et al. (1998). The TIMP2 membrane type 1 metalloproteinase "receptor" regulates the concentration and efficient activation of progelatinase A. *J. Biol. Chem.* 273, 873–880.

33. O'Connell, J. P., Willenbrock, F., Docherty, A. J. P., Eaton, D., and Murphy, G. (1994) Analysis of the role of the COOH-terminal domain in the activation, proteolytic activity and tissue inhibitor of metalloproteinase interactions of gelatinase B. *J. Biol. Chem.* 269, 14967–14973.

34. Bigg, H. F., Shi, Y. E., Liu, Y. E., Steffenson, B., and Overall, C. M. (1997) Specific, high affinity binding of tissue inhibitor of metalloproteinases-4 (TIMP-4) to the COOH-terminal hemopexin-like domain of human gelatinase A. *J. Biol. Chem.* 272, 15496–15500.

35. Butler, G. S., Apte, S. S., Willenbrock, F., and Murphy, G. (1999) Human tissue inhibitor of metalloproteinases 3 interacts with both N- and C-terminal domains of gelatinases A and B. *J. Biol. Chem.* 274, 10846–10851.

36. Itoh, Y. and Nagase, H. (1995) Preferential inactivation of tissue inhibitor of metalloproteinases-1 that is bound to the precursor of matrix metalloproteinase 9 (progelatinase B) by human neutrophil elastase. *J. Biol. Chem.* 270, 16518–16521.

37. Apte, S. S., Fukai, N., Beier, D. R., and Olsen, B. R. (1997) The matrix metalloproteinase-14 (MMP-14) gene is structurally distinct from other MMP genes and is co-expressed with the TIMP-2 gene during mouse embryogenesis. *J. Biol. Chem.* 272, 25511–25517.

38. Gasson, J. C., Golde, D. W., Kaufman, S. E., Westbrook, C. A., Hewick, R. M., Kaufman, R. J., et al. (1985) Molecular characterization and expression of the gene encoding human erythroid-potentiating activity. *Nature* 315, 768–771.

39. Hayakawa, T., Yamashita, K., Tanzawa, K., Uchijima, E., and Iwata, K. (1992) Growth promoting activity of tissue inhibitor of metalloproteinases-1 (TIMP-1) for a wide range of cells. *FEBS Letts.* 298, 29–32.

40. Hayakawa, T., Yamashita, K., Ohuchi, E., and Shinagawa, A. (1994) Cell growth-promoting activity of tissue inhibitor of metalloproteinases-2 (TIMP-2). *J. Cell Sci.* 107, 2373–2379.

41. Corcoran, M. L. and Stetler-Stevenson, W. G. (1995) Tissue inhibitor of metalloproteinases-2 (TIMP-2) stimulates fibroblast proliferation via a cyclic adenosine 3′,5′-monophosphate (cAMP)-dependent mechanism. *J. Biol. Chem.* 270, 13453–13459.

42. Nemeth, J. A., Rafe, A., Steiner, M., and Goolsby, C. L. (1996) TIMP-2 growth-stimulatory activity: a concentration- and cell type-specific response in the presence of insulin. *Exp. Cell Res.* 224, 110–115.

43. Chesler, L., Golde, D. W., Bersch, N., and Johnson, M. D. (1995) Metalloproteinase inhibition and erythroid potentiation are independent activities of tissue inhibitor of metalloproteinases-1. *Blood* 86, 4506–4515.

44. Yamashita, K., Suzuki, M., Iwata, H., Koike, T., Hamaguchi, M., Shinagawa, A., et al. (1996) Tyrosine phosphorylation is crucial for growth signaling by tissue inhibitors of metalloproteinases (TIMP-1 and TIMP-2). *FEBS Letts.* 396, 103–107.

45. Kossakowska, A. E., Urbanski, S., and Edwards, D. R. (1991) Tissue inhibitor of metalloproteinases (TIMP) RNA is expressed at elevated levels in malignant non-Hodgkin's lymphomas. *Blood* 77, 2475–2481.

46. Stetler-Stevenson, M., Mansoor, A., Lim, M. S., Fukushima, P., Kerhl, J., Marti, G., et al. (1997) Expression of matrix metalloproteinases and tissue inhibitors of metalloproteinases (TIMPs) in reactive and neoplastic lymph nodes. *Blood* 89, 1708–1715.

47. Zeng, Z. S., Cohen, A. M., Zhang, Z. F., Stetler-Stevenson, W., and Guillem, J. G. (1995) Elevated tissue inhibitor of metalloproteinase 1 RNA in colorectal cancer stroma correlates with lymph node and distant metastases. *Clin. Cancer Res.* 1, 899–906.

48. Grignon, D. J., Sakr, W., Toth, M., Ravery, V., Angulo, J., Shamsa, F., et al. (1996) High levels of tissue inhibitor of metalloproteinase-2 (TIMP-2) expression are associated with poor outcome in invasive bladder cancer. *Cancer Res.* 56, 1654–1659.

49. Holten-Andersen, M. N., Murphy, G., Nielsen, H. J., Pedersen, A. N., Christensen, I. J., Høyer-Hansen, G., et al. (1999) Quantitation of TIMP-1 in plasma of healthy blood donors and patients with advanced cancer. *Br. J. Cancer* 80, 495–503.

50. Ritter, L. M., Garfield, S. H., and Thorgeirsson, U. P. (1999) Tissue inhibitor of metalloproteinases-1 (TIMP-1) binds to the cell surface and translocates to the nucleus of human MCF-7 breast carcinoma cells. *Biochim. Biophys. Res. Comm.* 257, 494–499.

51. Zhao, W. Q., Li, H., Yamashita, K., Guo, X. K., Hoshino, T., Yoshida, S., et al. (1998) Cell cycle-associated accumulation of tissue inhibitor of metalloproteinases-1 (TIMP-1) in the nuclei of human gingival fibroblasts. *J. Cell Sci.* 111, 1147–1153.

52. Fowlkes, J. L., Enghild, J. J., Suzuki, K., and Nagase, H. (1994) Matrix metalloproteinases degrade insulin-like growth factor-binding protein-3 in dermal fibroblast cultures. *J. Biol. Chem.* 269, 25742–25746.

53. Mañes, S., Llorente, M., Lacalle, R. A., Gómez-Moutón, C., Kremer, L., Mira, E., et al. (1999) The matrix metalloproteinase-9 regulates the insulin-like growth factor-triggered autocrine response in DU-145 carcinoma cells. *J. Biol. Chem.* 274, 6935–6945.

54. Levi, E., Fridman, R., Miao, H-Q., Ma, Y-S., Yayon, A., and Voldoavsky, I. (1996) Matrix metalloproteinase 2 releases active soluble ectodomain of fibroblast growth factor receptor 1. *Proc. Natl. Acad. Sci. USA* 93, 7069–7074.

55. Orlando, S., Sironi, M., Bianchi, G., Drummond, A. H., Boraschi, D., Yabes, D., et al. (1997) Role of Metalloproteases in the Release of the IL-1 type II Decoy Receptor. *J. Biol. Chem.* 272, 31764–31769.

56. Boujrad, N., Ogwuegbu, S. O., Garnier, M., Lee, C-H., Martin, B. M., and Papadopoulos, V. (1995) Identification of a stimulator of steroid hormone synthesis isolated from testis. *Science* 268, 1609–1612.

57. Nothnick, W. B., Soloway, P., and Curry, T. E. Jr. (1997) Assessment of the role of tissue inhibitor of metalloproteinases-1 (TIMP-1) during the periovulatory period in female mice lacking a functional TIMP-1 gene. *Biol. Reprod.* 56, 1181–1188.

58. Guedez, L., Courtemanch, L., and Stetler-Stevenson, M. (1998) Tissue Inhibitor of Metalloproteinase (TIMP-1) induces differentiation and an antiapoptotic phenotype in germinal center B cells. *Blood* 92, 1342–1349.

59. Guedez, L., Stetler-Stevenson, W. G., Wolff, L., Wang, J., Fukushima, P., Mansoor, A., et al. (1998) In vitro suppression of programmed cell death of B cells by tissue inhibitor of metalloproteinases-1. *J. Clin. Invest.* 102, 2002–2010.

60. Valente, P., Fassina, G., Melchiori, A., Masiello, L., Cilli, M., Vacca, A., et al. (1998) TIMP-2 over-expression reduces invasion and angiogenesis and protects B16F10 melanoma cells from apoptosis. *Int. J. Cancer* 75, 246–253.

61. Baker, A. H., Zaltsman A. B., George, S. J., and Newby, A. C. (1998) Divergent effects of tissue inhibitors of metalloproteinase-1, -2 and -3 overexpression on rat vascular smooth muscle cell invasion, proliferation and death in vitro. *J. Clin. Invest.* 101, 1478–1487.

62. Ahonen, M., Baker, A. H., and Kahari, V. M. (1998) Adenovirus-mediated gene delivery of tissue inhibitor of metalloproteinases-3 inhibits invasion and induces apoptosis in melanoma cells. *Cancer Res.* 58, 2310–2315.

63. Baker, A. H., George, S. J., Zaltsman, A. B., Murphy, G., and Newby, A. C. (1999) Inhibition f invasion and induction of apoptotic cell death of cancer cell lines by overexpression of TIMP-3. *Br. J. Cancer* 79, 1347–1355.

64. Smith, M. R., Kung, H-F., Durum, S. K., Colburn, N. H., and Sun, Y. (1997) TIMP-3 induces cell death by stabilizing TNF-α receptors on the surface of human colon carcinoma cells. *Cytokine* 9, 770–780.

65. Blenis, J. and Hawkes, S. P. (1983) Transformation-sensitive protein associated with the cell substratum of chicken embryo fibroblasts. *Proc. Natl. Acad. Sci. USA* 80, 770–774.
66. Yang, T-T. and Hawkes, S. P. (1992) Role of the 21-kDa protein TIMP-3 in oncogenic transformation of cultured chicken embryo fibroblasts. *Proc. Natl. Acad. Sci. USA* 89, 10,676–10,680.
67. Alexander, C. M., Hansell, E. J., Behrendtsen, O., Flannery, M. L., Kishnani, N. S., Hawkes, S. P., et al. (1996) Expression and function of matrix metalloproteinases and their inhibitors at the maternal-embryonic boundary during mouse embryo implantation. *Development* 122, 1723–1736.
68. Anand-Apte, B., Pepper, M. S., Voest, E., Montesano, R., Olsen, B., Murphy, G., et al. (1997) Inhibition of angiogenesis by tissue inhibitor of metalloproteinas-3. *Invest. Opthalmol.* 38, 817–823.
69. Langton, K. P., Barker, M. D., and McKie, N. (1998). Localization of the functional domains of human tissue inhibitor of metalloproteinase-3 and the effects of a Sorsby's fundus dystrophy mutation. *J. Biol. Chem.* 273, 16778–16781.
70. Polkinghorne, P. J., Capon, M. R. C., Berninger, T., Lyness, A. L., Sehmi, K., and Bird, A. C. (1989) Sorsby's fundus dystrophy: a clinical study. *Opthalmology* 96, 1763–1768.
71. Capon, M. R. C., Marshall, J., Krafft, J. I., Alexander, R. A., Hiscott, P. S., and Bird, A. C. (1989) Sorsby's fundus dystrophy: a light and electron microscopy study. *Opthalmology* 96, 1769–1777.
72. Fariss, R. N., Apte, S. S., Olsen, B. R., Iwata, K., and Milam, A. H. (1997) Tissue inhibitor of metalloproteinases-3 is a component of Bruch's membrane of the eye. *Am. J. Pathol.* 150, 323–328.
73. Chambers, A. F. and Matrisian, L. M. (1997) Changing views of the role of matrix metalloproteinases in metastasis. *J. Natl. Cancer. Inst.* 89, 1260–1270.
74. Koop, S., Schmidt, E. E., MacDonald, I. C., Morris, V. L., Khokha, R., Grattan, M., et al. (1996) Independence of metastatic ability and extravasation: metastatic ras-transformed and control fibroblasts extravasate equally well. *Proc. Natl. Acad. Sci. USA* 93, 11080–11084.
75. Koop, S., Khokha, R., Schmidt, E. E., MacDonald, I. C., Morris, V. L., Chambers, A. F., et al. (1994) Overexpression of metalloproteinase inhibitor in B16F10 cells does not affect extravastion but reduces tumor growth. *Cancer Res.* 54, 4791–4797.
76. Lochter, A., Galosy, S., Muschler, J., Freedman, N., Werb, Z., and Bissell, M. J. (1997) Matrix metalloproteinase stromelysin-1 triggers a cascade of molecular alterations that leads to stable epithelial-to-mesenchymal conversion and a premalignant phenotype in mammary epithelial cells. *J. Cell Biol.* 139, 1861–1872.
77. Martin, D. C., Rüther, U., Sanchez-Sweatman, O. H., Orr, F. W., and Khokha, R. (1996) Inhibition of SV40 T antigen-induced hepatocellular carcinoma in TIMP-1 transgenic mice. *Oncogene* 13, 569–576.
78. Martin, D.C., Fowlkes, J.L., Babic, B., and Khokha, R. (1999) Insulin-like growth factor II signaling in neoplastic proliferation is blocked by transgenic expression of the metalloproteinase inhibitor TIMP-1. J. Cell Biol. 146, 881–892.
79. Ong, J., Opresko, L. K., Dempsey, P. J., Lauffenburger, D. A., Coffey, R. J., and Wiley, H. S. (1999) Metalloprotease-mediated ligand release regulates autocrine signaling through the epidermal growth factor receptor. *Proc. Natl. Acad. Sci. USA* 96, 6235–6240.
80. Zetter, B. R. (1998) Angiogenesis and tumor metastasis. *Ann. Rev. Med.* 49, 407–424.
81. Hiraoka, N., Allen, E., Apel, I. J., Gyetko, M. R., and Weiss, S. J. (1998) Matrix metalloproteinases regulate neovascularization by acting as pericellular fibrinolysins. *Cell* 95, 365–377.
82. Vu, T. H., Shipley, J. M., Bergers, G., Berger, J. E., Helms, J. A., Hanahan, D., et al. (1998) MMP-9/gelatinase B is a key regulator of growth plate angiogenesis and apoptosis of hypertrophic chondrocytes. *Cell* 93, 411–422.
83. Itoh, T., Tanioka, M., Yoshida, H., Yoshioka, T., Nishimoto, H., and Itohara, S. (1998) Reduced angiogenesis and tumor progression in gelatinase A-deficient mice. *Cancer Res.* 58, 1048–1051.

84. Soloway, P. D., Alexander, C. M., Werb. Z., and Jaenisch, R. (1996) Targeted mutagenesis of Timp-1 reveals that lung tumor invasion is influenced by Timp-1 genotype of the tumor but not by that of the host. *Oncogene* 13, 2307–2314.

85. Yoshiji, H., Harris, S. R., Raso, E., Gomez, D. E., Lindsay, C. K., Shibuya, M., et al. (1998) Mammary carcinoma cells over-expressing tissue inhibitor of metalloproteinases-1 show enhanced vascular endothelial growth factor expression. *Int. J. Cancer* 75, 81–87.

86. Yoshijy, H., Buck, T. B., Harris, S. R., Ritter, L. M., Lindsay, C. K., and Thorgeirsson, U. P. (1998) Stimulatory effect of endogenous tissue inhibitor of metalloproteinases-1 (TIMP-1) overexpression on type IV collagen and laminin gene expression in rat mammary carcinoma cells. *Biochem. Biophys. Res. Comm.* 247, 605–609.

87. Heppner Goss, K. J., Brown, P. D., and Matrisian, L. M. (1998) Differing effects of endogenous and synthetic inhibitors of metalloproteinases on intestinal tumorigenesis. *Int. J. Cancer* 78, 629–635.

88. Leco, K. J., Khokha, R., Pavloff, N., Hawkes, S. P., and Edwards, D. R. (1994) Tissue inhibitor of metalloproteinases-3 (TIMP-3) is an extracellular matrix-associated protein with a distinctive pattern of expression in mouse cells and tissues. *J. Biol. Chem.* 269, 9352–9360.

89. Leco, K. J., Apte, S. S., Taniguchi, G. T., Hawkes, S. P., Choke, R., Schultz, G. A., et al. (1997) Murine tissue inhibitor of metalloproteinases-4 (Timp-4): cDNA isolation and expression in adult mouse tissues. *FEBS Letts.* 401, 213–217.

90. Bugno, M., Graeve, L., Gatsios, P., Koj, A., Heinrich, P. C., Travis, J., et al. (1995) Identification of the interleukin-6/oncostatin M response element in the rat tissue inhibitor of metalloproteinases-1 (TIMP-1) promoter. *Nuc. Acids Res.* 23, 5041–5047.

91. Logan, S. K., Garabedian, M. J., Campbell, C. E., and Werb, Z. (1996) Synergistic transcriptional activation of the tissue inhibitor of metalloproteinases-1 promoter via functional interaction of AP-1 and Ets-1 transcription factors. *J. Biol. Chem.* 271, 774–782.

92. Clark, I. M., Rowan, A. D., Edwards, D. R., Bech-Hansen, T., Mann, D. A., Bahr, M. J., et al. (1997) Transcriptional activity of the human tissue inhibitor of metalloproteinases 1(TIMP-1) gene in fibroblasts involves elements in the promoter, exon 1 and intron 1. *Biochem. J.* 324, 611–617.

93. Botelho, F. M., Edwards, D. R., and Richards, C. D. (1998) Oncostatin M stimulates c-fos to bind a transcriptionally responsive AP-1 element within the tissue inhibitor of metalloproteinase-1 promoter. *J. Biol. Chem.* 273, 5211–5218.

94. Kim, H., Pennie, W. D., Sun, Y., and Colburn, N. H. (1997) Differential functional significance of AP-1 binding sites in the promoter of the gene encoding mouse tissue inhibitor of metalloproteinases-3. *Biochem. J.* 324, 547–553.

95. Phillips, B. W., Sharma, R., Leco, P. A., and Edwards, D. R. (1999) A Sequence-selective Single-strand DNA-binding Protein Regulates Basal Transcription of the Murine Tissue Inhibitor of Metalloproteinases-1 (Timp-1) Gene. *J. Biol. Chem.* 274, 22197–22207.

4 Matrix Metalloproteinases in Cancer

Barbara Fingleton, *PhD*
and Lynn M. Matrisian, *PhD*

CONTENTS

1. INTRODUCTION

The production of proteinase activity has long been thought to be an essential property of tumor cells that allow them to invade and metastasize to distant sites. The "three step theory of invasion" proposed by Liotta and colleagues *(1)* suggests that potentially invasive cells must first attach to basement membrane proteins via cell-surface receptors, i.e., the integrins. Localized, extracellular proteolytic activity then clears a path for the cell. Finally, the cell has to move into the cleared region, a locomotive process which probably depends on specific chemotactic factors. This invasion process first occurs as a tumor cell breaches the basement membrane at the primary tumor site—an event which signifies a malignant lesion. In order to result in a growth at a secondary site, the process has to be repeated as tumor cells penetrate blood vessels through a process referred to as intravasation. They can be carried to a new location, where a third invasive event must occur to extravasate into the parenchyma of the distant organ. Thus, proteolysis of basement membrane (BM) and extracellular matrix (ECM) components has been viewed as an essential step in tumor invasion and metastasis. Since metastasis is the principal cause of cancer-

From: *Cancer Drug Discovery and Development:*
Matrix Metalloproteinase Inhibitors in Cancer Therapy
Edited by: Neil J. Clendeninn and Krzysztof Appelt © Humana Press Inc., Totowa, NJ

associated mortality, the tumor proteases responsible for BM and ECM degradation have been viewed as accessible targets for therapeutic intervention.

There has been considerable progress over the last decade in identifying the specific proteases contributing to tumor invasion and metastasis. The contribution of members of the matrix metalloproteinase (MMP) family is the topic of this volume, although it must be noted that endoproteases of the serine, cysteine, and aspartyl classes have been associated with invasion and metastasis as well and are likely to have overlapping functions in tumor-mediated matrix degradation. Nevertheless, there have been compelling reports of "proof-of-principle" experiments in which the invasive and metastatic ability of tumor cells has been altered by manipulating the levels of a MMP or the endogenous tissue MMP inhibitors, the TIMPs. It was these observations that provided the driving force behind the development of synthetic MMP inhibitors for cancer therapy.

As the field has matured however, it has become clear that the biology of MMPs in cancer is more complex than originally envisioned. Most of these proteinases are produced by stromal fibroblasts or by infiltrating inflammatory cells as a response to tumor-produced factors. In addition, it has become evident that MMP activity can contribute to early-stage tumorigenesis and to angiogenesis, as well as to the late stage events of invasion and metastasis. In this chapter, we explore the roles played by MMPs in multiple stages of tumor progression, and the preclinical data suggesting a therapeutic benefit to inhibiting these enzymes.

2. MMP EXPRESSION IN HUMAN TUMORS

A striking feature of the MMPs is the abundant expression of multiple family members in malignant disease. In contrast to the absence or relatively low levels of MMP transcripts or protein noted in normal tissues, including those resected with a malignant lesion, a wide variety of human tumors have been reported to express high levels of specific MMP family members. A survey of the current literature on the expression of MMPs by human tumors is shown in Table 1. Many of the studies in which MMP levels have been measured in human tumors demonstrate a positive correlation between MMP levels and tumor grade (2–4). Concomitantly, a number of researchers also examined endogenous levels of inhibitors produced by tumors and found that tumor aggressiveness tends to be related not only to an overall increase in MMP levels but also a decrease in TIMP levels (5,6). This leads to the theory that the aggressive, invasive, and ultimately metastatic nature of a tumor is due, at least in part, to an imbalance between proteases and their inhibitors resulting in excessive proteolytic degradation (7–10).

Although studies in which multiple MMP family members have been examined in a single cohort of specimens are relatively rare, the coexpression of several members of the family appears to be a common occurrence in many cancer types (*11,12* for example). The functional significance of this is currently unclear. A mechanism for coordinate expression of redundant enzymes may have been evolutionarily selected, for example in reproductive tissues, and conserved in pathological situations such as cancer. The expression of multiple enzymes may also reflect a program of events leading to the expression of MMPs with slightly different substrate specificities so that all possible basement membrane components can be cleaved. Alternatively, it may indicate that different members of the family play very distinct roles in tumor progression. In this case, the apparent coexpression may be the result of examining primarily advanced tumors which represent the accumulation of multiple events in tumor progression. In support of this possibility, an examination of colonic adenomas revealed a more restricted pattern of MMP expression relative to that observed in colorectal carcinomas *(13)*.

Since many of the original studies associating MMP activity with tumor aggressiveness were carried out in established tumor cell lines, examination of actual tumor specimens yielded some initially surprising results. Localization of either mRNA or protein revealed that most MMPs are produced largely by the stroma surrounding tumors as opposed to being expressed by the malignant cells themselves (*14–16,* for examples). This production appears to be in response to signals from tumor cells, either through soluble factors *(17),* or by direct cell contact *(18).* There are some exceptions to this stromal association; matrilysin for example is produced almost exclusively by cells of epithelial origin and is thus expressed by the malignant epithelium of adenocarcinomas (*19,* for review). Additionally, there is evidence that MT1-MMP, produced by tumor cells, can act as a receptor for, and activator of, gelatinase A produced by surrounding stromal cells *(20,21).* It is interesting to note that advanced tumors that undergo an epithelial to mesenchymal transition also often express an expanded range of MMPs *(22–25),* perhaps suggesting a tight association between cell-type specific gene regulatory mechanisms and MMP expression.

Although studies characterizing MMP and TIMP levels have yielded and continue to yield much valuable information, the limitations in the methodology used to measure MMPs levels as an indication of the presence of proteolytically-active enzyme should be realized. Methods that detect specific mRNA transcripts have been widely used because of their ability to distinguish different MMP and TIMP family members. Reverse transcription polymerase chain reaction (RT-PCR) provides a sensitive, but rarely quantitative approach, whereas Northern analysis is relatively insensitive but quantitative. *In situ* hybridization has been valuable as it is relatively sensitive and provides localization data. Measurement of mRNA levels falls short of determining the relative protein levels, or the levels of activated enzyme. MMP protein levels have been assayed by zymography, immunoblotting, ELISAs, and immunohistochemistry. The first three of these methods requires that protein be extracted from the tumor tissue

Table 1
Tumor-Associated Expression of MMPs

MMP	Tumor/Tissue	Reference(s)
Interstitial collagenase (MMP-1)	Breast	(8,117)
	Cholangiocarcinoma	(118)
	Colorectal	(119)
	Gastrointestinal	(120,121)
	Head and Neck	(122,123)
	Hepatocellular	(124)
	Oesophagus	(125)
	Prostate	(4)
Gelatinase A (MMP-2)	Bladder	(126)
	Breast	(2,8,117,127–129)
	Bronchopulmonary	(130)
	Cervical	(131)
	Colon	(15,132,133)
	Glioma/Glioblastoma	(134,135)
	Laryngeal/Hypnopharyngeal	(136,137)
	Lung	(138,139)
	Melanoma	(140)
	Myeloma	(141)
	Oesophagus	(142)
	Ovary	(143–145)
	Pancreas	(146,147)
	Prostate	(148–151)
	Skin	(152)
	Stomach/Gastric	(120,153,154)
Stromelysin-1 (MMP-3)	Brain/Glioma	(155,156)
	Breast	(117)
	Cholangiocarcinoma	(118)
	Cholesteatoma	(157)
	Colorectal	(133)
	Gastric	(120)
	Lung	(25)
	Oesophagus	(142)
	Oral SCC	(158)
	Pancreas	(147)
	Prostate	(4)
	Skin	(159)
Matrilysin (MMP-7)	Breast	(11)
	Colorectal	(13,160–164)
	Glioma	(156)
	Lung	(25,138)
	Prostate	(165)
	Stomach	(161,166–168)

Table 1 *(continued)*

MMP	Tumor/Tissue	Reference(s)
Gelatinase B (MMP-9)	Bone (Giant Cell Tumor)	*(169)*
	Breast	*(2,12,117,127,129,170)*
	Cholesteatoma	*(157)*
	Colorectal	*(12,133,171,174)*
	Gastrointestinal	*(175,176)*
	Glioma	*(134)*
	Hepatocellular	*(177)*
	Lung	*(12,178)*
	Lymphoma	*(12)*
	Myeloma	*(141)*
	Ovary	*(144)*
	Pancreas	*(179)*
	Prostate	*(150)*
	Skin	*(152,180,181)*
	Stomach	*(154)*
Stromelysin-2 (MMP-10)	Head and Neck	*(122,182)*
Stromelysin-3 (MMP-11)	Breast	*(12,23,183,184)*
	Bronchopulmonary	*(130)*
	Colorectal	*(12,185–188)*
	Head and Neck	*(182)*
	Lung	*(12,25)*
	Oesophagus	*(189)*
	Skin (BCC)	*(190–193)*
Collagenase-3 (MMP-13)	Breast	*(194)*
	Head and Neck	*(195)*
	Skin	*(196)*
MT1-MMP (MMP-14)	Breast	*(123,197,198)*
	Bronchopulmonary	*(130)*
	Cervical	*(199)*
	Colorectal	*(123)*
	Head and Neck	*(123)*
	Liver	*(200)*
	Lung	*(198)*
	Ovary	*(145)*
	Pancreas	*(201)*
	Stomach	*(202)*

prior to analysis, which thus prevents the identification of the cell types responsible for the production of protease or inhibitor. Additionally, the measurement of active forms of the enzymes, which is considered to be of ultimate importance, may not be accurately achieved as extraction methods may result in activation of inactive zymogens. Enzyme-inhibitor complexes may also not be detected as the complexes can be disrupted by the analysis procedure. Immunohistochemistry has the advantage of providing information as to the localization of these proteins, but depends on the availability of useful antibodies, is not suitable for quantification, and provides little information on activity as very few of the currently available immunological reagents can accurately distinguish between latent and active MMPs. More recently, a combination of zymography and *in situ* techniques has been developed. A suitable enzyme substrate such as gelatin can be mixed with a photographic emulsion or labeled with fluorescent markers and then laid over a tissue section and incubated. Protease activity results in lysis of the substrate and formation of clear zones *(26,27)*. This technique is being further refined to make use of substrates specific to one particular, or one subgroup, of MMPs whereas labels are also being further improved to increase sensitivity. Ultimately, these refinements in approach should be useful in determining the identity of the enzyme which is functionally contributing to increased proteolytic degradation in a specific tumor type.

It has become evident that excessive proteolysis associated with tumor progression is not always associated with a decrease in TIMP levels *(10,28)*. TIMP levels may increase as a physiological, but inadequate, mechanism to control rising MMP levels. However, it has also become clear that TIMPs are multifunctional molecules. TIMP-2 is required by MT-MMP to activate gelatinase A *(20,21)* and its expression can therefore be a proinvasive event. TIMPs-1 and -2 also appear to be homologous to a growth factor activity termed "erythroid potentiating activity" (EPA) and have been shown to possess growth promoting qualities in some models *(29,30)*. TIMP-2 may aid tumor growth in a different manner, by protecting against apoptotic cell death *(31)*. Thus, some of the functions of TIMPs may complement the actions of MMPs in promoting tumor progression.

3. MMPS IN TUMOR INVASION AND METASTASIS

3.1 A Role for MMPs in Invasion

The invasive ability of tumor cells, which has been correlated with metastatic potential *(32–35),* can be measured in vitro using a number of different models. These include the embryonic chick heart invasion assay *(36)* in which tumor cells are placed in three-dimensional culture with fragments of embryonic chick heart tissue; the amnion invasion assay in which tumor cells are placed on one side of a human amniotic membrane that has been stripped of its epithelium in such a way as to leave the basement membrane intact *(37);* and the "matrigel" invasion assay which is similar to the amnion-based assay except that basement membrane components are provided in a commercially available gel form *(38,39)*. In all cases, the number of cells which invade through basement membrane can be stained and quantified. Studies using such assays have found a strong correlation between invasive ability and MMP expression in a variety of cell lines *(32,34,35,40,41)*. For example, one of the earliest of these studies examined increasingly metastatic varients of the murine melanoma cell line B16 for expression of type IV collagenase *(32)*. The collagenase activity was measured using a collagen degradation assay and was shown to increase with the metastatic potential of the cells. This study did not, however, establish whether the increase in MMP activity was a direct cause of the enhanced invasive ability of the melanoma cells.

More direct evidence was obtained using the naturally occurring inhibitors of MMPs, the TIMPs. For example, using an amnion invasion assay, Thorgeirsson and colleagues demonstrated that addition of either a bovine cartilage extract containing inhibitors of both serine and metalloproteinases or of a purified collagenase inhibitor dramatically reduced invasion by a highly invasive sarcoma cell line *(37)*. The protease inhibitors specifically blocked invasion as tumor cell proliferation, attachment to amnion, and migration through noncoated filters were not affected by their presence. Using recombinant TIMP-1, Schultz and colleagues demonstrated that the invasive murine melanoma cell line B16-F10 depended on metalloproteinase activity for its invasive ability in an amnion invasion assay *(42)*. This was similar to results obtained by Mignatti et al. with purified natural TIMP *(43)*. In a manner similar to TIMP, SC-44463, one of the first described synthetic MMP inhibitors, was shown to reduce invasion of malignant cell lines through a reconstituted basement membrane *(44)*. Purified recombinant TIMP-2, when added to invasive tumor cell lines HT 1080 and Ha-*ras*-transformed-4R, inhibited degradation of smooth muscle cell matrices by approx 70% *(45)*. The inhibitor had no effect on cell growth or attachment. As these researchers had previously determined that the TIMPs are secreted by endothelial cells, they concluded that the TIMPs may play a role in protecting large blood vessels from invasion. The availability of cDNAs encoding the proteases or their inhibitors has been useful in directly determining effects of these molecules on tumor invasion. For example, antisense technology allowed Khokha et al. to demonstrate that down-modulation of TIMP-1 in a noninvasive, nontumorigenic fibroblast cell line resulted in the acquisition of an invasive, tumorigenic, and metastatic phenotype *(46)*. The complementary experiment in which malignant B16-F10 melanoma cells were transfected so as to overexpress TIMP-1 protein demonstrated a reduction in in vitro invasive ability which correlated with the level of TIMP-1 overexpression observed in different clones of the transfected cells *(47)*. Using embryonic stem cells in culture, Alexander and Werb generated a cell line by homologous recombination, which was null for the TIMP-1 gene *(45)*. Although this was not specifically a cancer model, the enhanced invasive ability of the TIMP-1-null cells when compared to wild-type cells also demonstrated the antiinvasive function of TIMP. Addition of exogenous TIMP-1 protein to the TIMP-1-null cultures resulted in a reversion to a noninvasive phenotype. Some studies have demonstrated that the expression of a specific MMP is sufficient to increase invasion. The expression of matrilysin in the prostate cell line DU-145 resulted in an invasive phenotype when the cells were implanted into nude mice *(48)*. In addition, the expression of MT1-MMP, the activator of gelatinase A, in three different human tumor cell lines resulted in increased invasive capacity *(49)*.

3.2 Determining a Role for MMPs in Metastasis

Many studies in which MMP activity was modified by the introduction of recombinant or transfected TIMPs demonstrate a role for MMPs in in vivo models of metastasis (reviewed in *50*). Both experimental metastasis models, which require that the injected cells are capable of lodging and growing in a foreign environment, and spontaneous metastasis models, which require invasion and extravasation of the injected cells in addition, have been used. For example, recombinant TIMP (rTIMP) was administered to mice in which B16-F10 melanoma cells were injected into the tail vein and the number of lung deposits counted. A significant decrease in number but not size of metastases was seen in this model indicating that inhibition of proteinase activity had no effect on growth rate of the tumor cells *(42)*. A similar study with a Ha-*ras* transformed cell line also showed that rTIMP is a potent inhibitor of lung metastases when tumor cells are introduced into nude mice *(51)*. Subcutaneous injection of a TIMP-2-transfected cell line demonstrated that the TIMP-2 markedly reduced tumor growth rate in vivo and partially suppressed hematogenous metastasis *(52)*. The effect on growth rate was suggested to be the result of suppressed local invasion thus inhibiting expansion of the tumor mass. The most recently described TIMP, TIMP-4, has also been shown to act as an inhibitor of metastasis in a mouse model of breast cancer *(50)*. The use of transgenic animal models, in which TIMP-1 was overexpressed, further demonstrated that an antimetastatic function can be attributed to this protein *(53,54)*.

Other studies have demonstrated a role for specific MMPs in tumor metastasis. For example, Gelatinase B was stably transfected into a tumorigenic but nonmetastatic cell line. Unlike control-transfected cells, these gelatinase B-positive cells were capable of generating metastatic lesions in nude mice in which the cells were introduced via tail vein injection *(55)*. Interestingly, a bladder carcinoma cell line, MYU3L, which already secretes progelatinase B was found to be tumorigenic but not metastatic in an orthotopic model in nude mice unless progelatinase A was overexpressed *(56)*.

The broad-spectrum British Biotechnology MMPI, batimastat [BB-94], has been used extensively in in vitro and in vivo systems to demonstrate the effect of MMP inhibition. Intraperitoneal administration of BB-94 significantly reduced the number of lung metastases when murine malignant melanoma B16-bl6 cells were injected intravenously into syngeneic mice *(57)*. By radiolabeling the melanoma cells prior to injection, the organ distribution and site of arrest of the cells could be followed. The batimastat did not appear to affect arrest in the lung but did prevent retention, possibly by blocking extravasation. In a model of spontaneous metastasis whereby tumor cells were injected into the foot pad, allowed to grow into a tumor mass and then surgically excised, batimastat treatment did not reduce the number of lung metastases but significantly reduced their weight, i.e., secondary tumor growth *(57)*. No difference in proliferation rate or in vascularization between the untreated and batimastat-treated animals was apparent in these studies.

In an ovarian carcinoma model, treatment with batimastat significantly reduced the size of xenografts in nude mice which translated into a five- to six-fold increase in survival time compared to untreated animals *(58)*. As the principal pathology associated with untreated xenografted mice was extensive ascitic disease, it was suggested that the batimastat treatment caused the transition of ascites to solid tumors which grew more slowly and which became encapsulated by stroma. Batimastat has also been used in a Phase I trial in the treatment of human ascitic disease and appeared to cause a similar transition to solid tumor *(59,60)*.

Another MMPI, CT1746, which is orally-active and which has a greater specificity for gelatinase A, gelatinase B, and stromelysin-1 than for interstitial collagenase and matrilysin, has been tested in a nude mouse model that mimics the clinical development of colon cancer *(61)*. Treatment with this compound significantly prolonged survival time from 51 to 78 days, decreased primary tumor growth by 32%, and resulted in a significant reduction in total spread and metastasis of the tumor. As the authors assert, the result of treatment with this compound was "conversion of an aggressive cancer to a more controlled indolent disease." Such control of aggressiveness is a realistic expectation for MMPI therapy and is probably the most reasonable marker of successful treatment. A more extensive range of examples of MMPI activity is presented in Chapters 5–10 of this volume.

In summary, there are multiple examples of tumor invasion and resultant metastasis being mediated through MMPs which can, in various in vitro and in vivo animal models, be controlled by inhibitors of metalloproteinases, both natural and synthetic.

4. EXTENDED ROLES FOR MMPS IN TUMOR DEVELOPMENT AND PROGRESSION

In recent years, it has become clear that the effects of MMPs extend to the earliest stages of tumor development in addition to being focused on tumor invasion and metastasis (reviewed in *62*). One exciting development has been the realization that angiogenesis, like tumor invasion, requires ECM degradation, thus expanding the potential of MMPIs as therapeutic agents into this arena. In addition, it has become apparent that MMPs can influence the development and

Table 2
MMP-and TIMP-Null Mice and Tumor Development

Deleted MMP	Effect on tumors
Gelatinase A (MMP-2)	Reduction in tumor-induced angiogenesis and in experimental metastasis (68)
Stromelysin-1 (MMP-3)	Enhanced tumor growth following carcinogen treatment[a]
Matrilysin (MMP-7)	Reduction in tumor formation in Min mice (84)
Gelatinase B (MMP-9)[b]	Aberrant angiogenesis and apoptosis in developing bone (71)
Stromelysin-3 (MMP-11)	Decreased tumorigenesis following application of a carcinogen; Decreased implantation of a malignant epithelial cell line (78)
Metalloelastase (MMP-12)[b]	Macrophages have diminished invasive capacity (203)
TIMP-1	No effect on metastasis when host is null for TIMP-1 but TIMP-1 −/− tumor cells demonstrated either increased or reduced metastatic capacity (87)

[a]Unpublished results H.C. Crawford, J. Mudgett and L.M. Matrisian.
[b]No specific tumor-related phenotype has yet been reported. Phenotypes described relate to healthy animals.

growth of benign tumors, as well as the establishment of malignant tumors, and regulate apoptosis. Many of these insights have come with the ability to distinguish the effects of individual MMPs on specific stages of tumor progression. This has been accomplished primarily by the development of transgenic and "knock-out" mice in which the levels of a specific MMP are modulated genetically. The phenotypes of these animals that are related to tumor progression are summarized in Tables 2 and 3.

4.1 A Role for MMPs in Angiogenesis

Angiogenesis, the process by which new blood vessels are formed, is considered essential if tumors larger than a few millimeters are to survive (63, and references therein). Indeed, it has been asserted that both tumor growth and metastasis are angiogenesis-dependent, as the blood flow is required to carry oxygen and nutrients into the growing tumor mass and also acts as a conduit by which metastatic cells can be carried to a secondary site (64). In order for a blood vessel to form, localized degradation of capillary basement membranes is required as an early event (65). Transformed endothelial cells can begin a process of forming vessels which is associated with morphological changes and attendant protease activity (66). Inhibition of endothelial cell migration can be

Table 3
MMP- & TIMP-Transgenic Animals and Tumor Development

MMP	Targeted tissue	Promoter	Effect on tumors
Collagenase (MMP-1)	Skin	Haptoglobin	Acanthosis,[a] Hyperkeratosis[a] and basal cell hyperproliferation. Increased tumor formation after DMBA/TPA treatment (82)
Collagenase (MMP-1)	Lung	Haptoglobin	Emphysema[a] (204)
Stromelysin-1 (MMP-3)	Mammary Gland	Whey Acidic Protein (WAP)	Precocious maturation of gland; Increased proliferation and apoptosis; Development of adenocarcinoma (81,90,201)
Stromelysin-1 (MMP-3)	Mammary Gland	Mouse Mammary Tumor Virus (MMTV)	Precocious maturation of gland; Significant increase in apoptosis; Decreased tumor formation following DMBA treatment. (88,205)
Matrilysin (MMP-7)	Mammary Gland	MMTV	Milk protein (β-casein) production in virgin gland; Formation of HANs in multiparous females; Acceleration of *neu*-induced tumorigenesis in bigenic animals (88,206)
TIMP-1	Global	β-actin	No phenotype but when crossed with WAP-stromelysin-1 transgenics, rescued apoptotic and BM degradative phenotype (91)
TIMP-1	Liver	Major histocompatibility complex-1 (MHC-1)	When crossed with TAg mice, a significant decrease in incidence of hepatocellular carcinoma resulted (83)
	Skin-Liver		20–40% reduction in primary tumor incidence following intradermal injection of T cell lymphoma line (53)
TIMP-1	Brain	Metallothionein	75% reduction in number of brain metastases in an experimental metastasis model (53)

[a]Not specifically tumor-related phenotypes.

achieved by TIMP-1 *(67)*. Additionally, cells which acquire an angiogenic phenotype demonstrate a significant down-regulation of TIMP mRNA *(67)* indicating that both up-regulation of positive factors and down-regulation of inhibitors are features of the angiogenic process.

Tube formation by human umbilical vein endothelial cells grown on matrigel has been shown to require gelatinase A activity, as the addition of a specific antigelatinase A function-perturbing antibody or TIMP prevented this morphological change *(68)*. Interestingly, the gelatinase A inhibition was only effective in blocking the initial stages of tube formation and had no effect on subsequent morphological changes. The use of gelatinase-A-deficient mice support the requirement of this enzyme for tumor-related angiogenesis, as tumors of significantly reduced volumes compared to those in wild-type mice resulted following implantation of tumorigenic cell lines *(69)*. Gelatinase A-deficient mice are born and develop normally, however, indicating that ablation of the enzyme does not effect the angiogenic process during fetal development. It has been proposed that interactions of the hemopexin-like domain of gelatinase A with the integrin $\alpha_v\beta_3$ are important for angiogenesis *(70)*. A soluble fragment of this domain of gelatinase A, denoted PEX, blocks gelatinase A binding to the integrin and inhibits the amount of angiogenesis occurring at a particular site.

Gelatinase B has also been implicated in the remodeling of capillary basement membranes that occurs during the angiogenic process. Its accumulation in an active form within vesicles of microvascular endothelial cells has led to the suggestion that it facilitates migration of this particular cell type *(71)*. Analysis of the gelatinase B-null mouse has revealed a role for gelatinase B in the release of an angiogenic factor from cartilage matrix as vascularization of cartilage is delayed in these animals *(72)*. Capillary invasion, however, does not appear to be significantly affected by the lack of gelatinase B. Similarily, interstitial collagenase has been found to be expressed in microvascular but not macrovascular endothelial cells and is thought to aid the invasive process *(73)*.

Paradoxically, the MMPs gelatinase B and matrilysin have been proposed to act as negative regulators of angiogenesis by virtue of their effects on angiostatin, a potent physiological angiogenesis inhibitor. These MMPs could cleave plasminogen to yield angiostatin *(74)*, although as this was an in vitro reaction, it is not clear if the same process occurs physiologically. Macrophage metalloelastase has, however, been demonstrated to be important in angiostatin production in vivo *(75)*. In this case, Lewis lung carcinoma cells were implanted into syngeneic mice. Macrophage infiltration of the graft resulted in the generation of angiostatin from plasminogen and growth inhibiton of the tumor.

Due to the recognized involvement of MMPs in angiogenesis, synthetic MMPIs have also been promoted as angiogenesis inhibitors *(76)*. In a rat corneal model of angiogenesis, treatment with GM6001, an hydroxymate inhibitor produced by Glycomed, significantly reduced both blood vessel number and area following six days of continuous treatment *(77)*. Batimastat (BB-94) was shown to significantly reduce in vivo growth of an hemangioma, a particularly well-vascularized tumor which was used to test the antiangiogenic effect of this drug *(78)*.

4.2 Effects of MMPs on Tumor Growth

Although there are several examples in the early literature which indicate an effect of MMPs on tumor growth, the recognition that the rate limiting step in metastasis was establishment or growth of metastatic nodules rather than tumor cell extravasation, as detected by intravital microscopic technology, strongly reinforced this idea (reviewed in *62*). When B16F10 melanoma cells were engineered to overexpress TIMP and introduced into the chick embryo chorioallantoic membrane (CAM) model, no differences in the rate of extravasation was observed between TIMP-expressing and parental cells *(79)*. By seven days, however, a significant reduction in size and number of tumors was observed with the TIMP-expressing clones compared to parental cells. In a different study with a tumorigenic, metastatic rat bladder cell line transfected with TIMP-1 or TIMP-2 cDNA, researchers could show that these inhibitors only slightly affected primary tumor growth and local invasion *(80)*. Their major effect was inhibition of extravascular growth at a distant metastatic site. Both of these studies would suggest that metalloproteinase activity is more relevant to the establishment and growth of tumor deposits than in the invasive steps associated with blood-borne metastasis.

The role of MMPs in tumor growth has been reinforced by studies using genetically-modified mice (*see* Tables 2 and 3). For example, stromelysin-3 deficient mice demonstrated decreased implantation of a malignant epithelial cell line, as well as decreased mammary and ovarian tumorigenesis following application of the chemical carcinogen 7,12 dimethylbenz[2]anthracene (DMBA) *(81)*. Earlier work had established that stromelysin-3 could facilitate "tumor take" when human tumor cells were introduced into nude mice *(82)*. This occurred without any effect on the invasive ability of the tumors. The overexpression of stromelysin-1 and matrilysin in mammary glands also appears to aid the tumorigenic process. The direct result of matrilysin overexpression is the development of lesions that resemble preneoplastic hyperplastic alveolar nodules (HANs) *(83)*. More strikingly, when matrilysin over-expressing mice are crossed with mice transgenic for the *neu* oncogene, accelerated tumor formation and growth occurs. Overexpression of another MMP, stromelysin-1, in the mammary gland has also been reported to result in tumor formation *(78,84)*. However, this effect may be dependent on the strain of mouse used as not all stromelysin-1 transgenics develop tumors *(78)*. The overexpression of collagenase in mouse skin resulted in an epidermal hyperplasia *(85)*, which is not, in itself, a neoplasia. However, increased susceptibility of the skin to tumor formation in a two-stage carcinogenesis protocol was then observed in these mice, again reinforcing the idea that metalloproteinase activity in an early lesion can potentiate tumor progression. As further evidence, implantation of tumor cells into TIMP-1 transgenic mice has demonstrated that overexpression of this endogenous MMP inhibitor results in slower-growing tumors (53,86).

Studies in which matrilysin-deficient animals were crossed with Min mice, a model system in which multiple benign intestinal tumors are produced, demonstrated that matrilysin contributes to the growth and development of these benign neoplasias since its deletion resulted in a 58% reduction in tumor number (87). In addition, a significant reduction in the number of lesions was observed following treatment of Min mice with the synthetic MMPI batimastat (88). Since the Min mouse is a model of human Familial Adenomatous Polyposis (89), these studies suggest the possibility that MMPIs may have some value as chemopreventative agents in high-risk patients.

There are several examples of experiments in which evidence is presented that refutes the prevailing assumption that all MMPs play a causal role in tumor progression. TIMP-1 transgenic and "knock-out" animals have, for example, generated some conflicting data. In TIMP-1-null mice, results of experimental metastasis assays were unchanged from wild-type controls indicating that TIMP-1 status had no bearing on the metastatic process (90). Additionally, when pairs of cell lines with either a wild-type or a TIMP-1-null genotype were injected into tail veins of wildtype mice, mixed results were observed when the lungs were analyzed two weeks later. In two cases, the TIMP-1-null lines resulted in an increased number of metastases as expected, however, in another pair, ablation of TIMP-1 decreased the metastatic ability of the tumor cells (90). These results suggest that TIMP-1, either by itself or through its action on MMPs, has both tumor-promoting and growth- or invasion-suppressive functions. Transgenic mice expressing stromelysin-1 in the mammary gland, under control of the MMTV promoter, produced fewer tumors than wild-type controls following DMBA treatment (91). In this case, it was determined that expression of stromelysin-1 had altered both the proliferation and apoptosis rates of the normal mammary epithelium which negatively influenced the effects of carcinogen treatment. This is in contrast to the apparent tumor-promoting effects of stromelysin-1 overexpression in differentiated mammary cells as occurred when the whey acidic protein (WAP) promoter was used to drive expression (92). More puzzling is the observation that ablation of stromelysin-1 enhanced the formation and growth of benign tumors following chemical carcinogen treatment*. In this case, a protective effect of stromal stromelysin which influenced only the earliest stage tumors was surmised. Lack of stromelysin-1 appeared not to hin-

*Unpublished results H. C. Crawford, J. Mudgett and L. M. Matrisian

der advanced, malignant tumors. These results suggest that dermal stromelysin-1 activity is part of a wound healing effect which functions in the host response to tumors, but has limited ability to alter the progression of advanced tumors. It might be expected that the lack of metalloelastase in a tumor setting may also promote tumor growth, as it would prevent macrophage infiltration and thus limit host immunological responses. These type of studies support the need to understand the roles of MMPs in normal defense mechanisms so that selective synthetic MMPIs can be applied in appropriate therapeutic settings.

4.3 Possible Mechanisms

Possible mechanisms for effects of MMPs at early stages of tumorigenesis are only beginning to be explored, but potentially include roles in both cellular proliferation and apoptosis. Alterations in basement membrane and ECM substrates can contribute to both of these processes *(93–95)*. However, along with the awareness that MMPs play extended roles in tumor progression comes the realization that basement membrane and ECM components are not the only potential substrates for MMPs. An expansion of MMP substrates to biological modifiers such as growth and apoptosis factors provides potential mechanisms for the observed effects of MMPs on cellular processes contributing to the establishment and growth of tumors. The potential role of MMPs in processing or releasing such factors needs to be seriously evaluated.

The processing of growth factors or their receptors into active forms by various MMP activities, often determined by MMPI inhibition of processing, has been reported *(96)*. Shedding of the fibroblast growth factor (FGF) type 1 receptor, for example, can be accomplished by the activity of gelatinase A *(97)*. Such release of a soluble receptor, which maintains its ligand-binding ability, may then modulate growth- and angiogenesis-related activities of FGF. Epidermal growth factor (EGF)-receptor ligands such as amphiregulin, TGF-α and HB-EGF have all been reported as MMP substrates *(96,98,99)*. Tumor necrosis factor (TNF)-α can also be processed to its soluble form by a number of MMPs in vitro *(100)*, although a specific enzyme known as tumor necrosis factor-α converting enzyme (TACE) has been identified as the principal processor of TNF-α in vivo *(101,102)*. A mouse model engineered so as not to express enzymatically competent TACE demonstrated that TGF-α, TNF-α receptor, and L-selectin are other important substrates for this enzyme *(103)*. TACE is a member of the adamalysin family of proteins, a family of transmembrane proteins characterized by the presence of both disintegrin and metalloproteinase domains *(104)*. The members of this family that are enzymatically active can be inhibited by many of the synthetic MMPIs, thus increasing the number of potential targets of such compounds.

Growth factor activity can also be regulated by processing of sequestering or binding proteins. The insulin-like growth factor binding proteins (IGF-BPs) regulate bioavailability of IGF by preventing its interaction with receptors. There is accumulating evidence to demonstrate that cleavage of IGF-BPs can be achieved by various MMPs *(105–107)*, thus releasing free IGF which can then result in increased tumor cell proliferation *(108,109)*. Some extracellular matrix proteins are also known to be sequestors of growth factors *(110)*. For example decorin, an ECM protein involved in collagen fibril alignment, is known to bind the growth factor TGF-β1. Decorin has been shown to be a substrate of matrilysin, stromelysin-1, and gelatinase A and its cleavage by these enzymes results in the release of TGF-β1 *(111)*. The growth inhibitor, growth promoting, and angiogenic activities of TGF-β make this an attractive candidate to explain some of the effects of MMP manipulation.

The action of MMPs on ECM proteins can also result in death signals being transmitted to cells, a process mediated through a family of cell:matrix adhesion molecules known as integrins *(112,113)*. Alternatively, the integrins themselves can be substrates of these enzymes *(114)*, which could also result in the activation of a signaling pathway within a tumor cell. The cell:cell adhesion molecule E-cadherin has been implicated in the control of tumor growth, and loss of this molecule may overcome the normal contact inhibition of cellular proliferation *(115)*. It has been reported that expression of stromelysin-1 in mammary epithelial cells results in cleavage of E-cadherin and the gain of a more mesenchymal phenotype, although it is not clear if stromelysin-1 is the enzyme directly responsible for the E-cadherin cleavage *(116)*.

Although there is much evidence to support roles for MMPs in early tumor growth and potential mechanisms have been suggested, there are still many pathways which have yet to be fully investigated.

5. SUMMARY AND CONCLUSION

The envisioned role of proteolysis in tumor invasion and metastasis, the identification of members of the MMP family as secreted enzymes with ECM components as their substrates, and the elevated expression of a number of MMP family members in advanced cancer provided the incentive for a number of laboratories to design proof of principle experiments to test the role of MMPs in tumor progression. The initial experiments in which MMP activity was modulated by manipulation in the levels of TIMPs, the endogenous MMP inhibitors, were highly promising and provided further justification for increased knowledge and more sophisticated approaches. With these advances, we have obtained abundant encouragement for pursuing MMPs as therapeutic targets, but we have also been forced to appreciate the complexity of the system: the number of MMPs has expanded to greater than 20 and is unlikely yet to be complete; the expression pattern demonstrates cell- and tissue-specificity which may influence function; the role of MMPs has expanded to effects on angiogenesis and growth of benign as well as malignant tumors; and the range of potential relevant substrates has been substantially broadened. Irrespective of the daunting realization that there is much we do *not* know about MMPs, we have come a long way. With the development of pharmaceutical reagents and the initiation of clinical trials, the ultimate goal of determining if there is a therapeutic benefit to cancer patients by inhibition of MMPs is being realized. This too is fraught with challenges, as the mechanisms for evaluating the efficacy of modulators of tumor progression as opposed to a cytotoxic agents are in their infancy. Nevertheless, there is much cause for optimism, not only for MMPIs but also for the discovery process. The combined efforts of biochemists and structural biologists, cell and molecular biologists, organic chemists, pharmacologists, and clinicians has resulted in an exciting example of basic science observations that have been translated into clinical practice. Further advances on the basic science front and additional preclinical experimentation will continue to contribute by "fine tuning" the system, resulting in improved inhibitors and the most appropriate application. Work in this field is likely to continue to serve as a model for the development of a whole new generation of modulators of cancer behavior for many years to come.

REFERENCES

1. Liotta, L., Thorgeirsson, U., and Garbisa, S. (1982) Role of collagenases in tumor cell invasion. *Cancer Metast. Rev.* 1, 277–297.
2. Davies, B., Miles, D. W., Happerfield, L. C., Naylor, M. S., Bobrow, L. G., Rubens, R. D., and Balkwill, F. R. (1993) Activity of type IV collagenases in benign and malignant breast disease. *Brit. J. Cancer* 67, 1126–1131.
3. Davies, B., Waxman, J., Wasan, H., et al. (1993) Levels of matrix metalloproteases in bladder cancer correlate with tumor grade and invasion. *Cancer Res.* 53, 5365–5369.
4. Jung, K., Nowak, L., Lein, M., Priem, F., Schnorr, D., and Loening, S. A. (1997) Matrix metalloproteinases 1 and 3, tissue inhibitor of metalloproteinase-1 and the complex of metalloproteinase-1 tissue inhibitor in plasma of patients with prostate cancer. *Int. J. Cancer* 74, 220–223.
5. Halaka, A., Bunning, R., Bird, C., Gibson, M., and Reynolds, J. (1983) Production of collagenase and inhibitor (TIMP) by intracranial tumors and dura in vitro. *J. Neurosurg.* 59, 444–461.
6. Hicks, N., Ward, R., and Reynolds, J. (1984) A fibrosarcoma model derived from mouse embryo cells: growth properties and secretion of collagenase and metalloproteinase inhibitor (TIMP) by tumor cell lines. *Int. J. Cancer* 33, 834–844.
7. Gohji, K., Fujimoto, N., Okawa, J., Fujii, A., and Nakajima, M. (1998) Imbalance between serum matrix metalloproteinase 2 and its inhibitor as a predictor of recurrence of urothelial cancer. *Brit. J. Cancer* 77, 650–655.
8. Polette, M., Clavel, C., Cockett, M., Girod de Bentzmann, S., Murphy, G., and Birembaut, P. (1993) Detection and localization of mRNAs encoding matrix metalloproteinases and their tissue inhibitor in human breast pathology. *Invas. Metast.* 13, 31–37.
9. Ponton, A., Coulombe, B., and Skup, D. (1991) Decreased expression of tissue inhibitor of metalloproteinases in metastatic tumor cells leading to increased levels of collagenase activity. *Cancer Res.* 51, 2138–2143.
10. Grignon, D. J., Sakr, W., Toth, M., Ravery, V., Angulo, J., Shamsa, F., Pontes, J. E., Crissman, J. C., and Fridman, R. (1996) High levels of tissue inhibitor of metalloproteinase-

2 (timp-2) expression are associated with poor outcome in invasive bladder cancer. *Cancer Res.* 56, 1654–1659.

11. Heppner, K. J., Matrisian, L. M., Jensen, R. A., and Rodgers, W. H. (1996) Expression of most matrix metalloproteinase family members in breast cancer represents a tumor-induced host response. *Am. J. Pathol.* 149, 273–282.

12. Kossakowska, A. E., Huchcroft, S. A., Urbanski, S. J., and Edwards, D. R. (1996) Comparative analysis of the expression patterns of metalloproteinases and their inhibitors in breast neoplasia, sporadic colorectal neoplasia, pulmonary carcinomas and malignant non-Hodgkin's lymphomas in humans. *Brit. J. Cancer* 73, 1401–1408.

13. Newell, K. J., Witty, J. P., Rodgers, W. H., and Matrisian, L. M. (1994) Expression and localization of matrix-degrading metalloproteinases during colorectal tumorigenesis. *Mol. Carcinogen.* 10, 199–206.

14. Basset, P., Bellocq, J. P., Wolf, C., Stoll, I., Hutin, P., Limacher, J. M., et al. (1990) A novel metalloproteinase gene specifically expressed in stromal cells of breast carcinomas. *Nature* 348, 699–704.

15. Grigioni, W., D'Errico, A., Fiorentino, M., Baccarini, P., Onisto, M., Caenazzo, C., et al. (1994) Gelatinase A (MMP-2) and its mRNA detected in both neoplastic and stromal cells of tumors with different invasive and metastatic properties. *Diagn. Mol. Pathol.* **3**, 163–169.

16. Poulsom, R., Pignatelli, M., Stetler-Stevenson, W. G., Liotta, L. A., Wright, P. A., Jeffery, R. E., et al. (1992) Stromal expression of 72 kda Type IV collagenase (MMP-2) and TIMP-2 mRNAs in colorectal neoplasia. *Am. J. Pathol.* 141, 389–396.

17. Biswas, C., Zhang, Y., DeCastro, R., Guo, H., Nakamura, T., Kataoka, H., et al. (1995) The human tumor cell-derived collagenase stimulatory factor (renamed EMMPRIN) is a member of the immunoglobulin superfamily. *Cancer Res.* 55, 434–439.

18. Himelstein, B. P., Canete-Soler, R., Bernhard, E. J., and Muschel, R. J. (1994) Induction of fibroblast 92 kDa gelatinase/type IV collagenase expression by direct contact with metastatic tumor cells. *J. Cell Sci.* 107, 477–486.

19. Wilson, C. L. and Matrisian, L. M. (1996) Matrilysin: An epithelial matrix metalloproteinase with potentially novel functions. *Int. J. Biochem. Cell Biol.* 28, 123–136.

20. Strongin, A. Y., Collier, I. E., Bannikov, G., Marmer, B. L., Grant, G. A., and Goldberg, G. I. (1995) Mechanism of cell surface activation of 72-kDa type IV collagenase. Isolation of the activated form of the membrane metalloprotease. *J. Biol. Chem.* 270, 5331–5338.

21. Kinoshita, T., Sato, H., Okada, A., Ohuchi, E., Imai, K., Okada, Y., et al. (1998) TIMP-2 promotes activation of progelatinase A by membrane type 1 matrix metalloproteinase immobilized on agarose beads. *J. Biol. Chem.* 273, 16098–16103.

22. Wright, J. H., McDonnell, S., Portella, G., Bowden, G. T., Balmain, A., and Matrisian, L. M. (1994) A switch from stromal to tumor cell expression of stromelysin-1 mRNA associated with the conversion of squamous to spindle carcinomas during mouse skin tumor progression. *Mol. Carcinogen,* 10, 207–215.

23. Ahmed, A., Hanby, A., Dublin, E., Poulsom, R., Smith, P., Barnes, D., et al. (1998) Stromelysin-3: an independent prognostic factor for relapse-free survival in node-positive breast cancer and demonstration of novel breast carcinoma cell expression. *Am. J. Pathol.* 152, 721–728.

24. Pulyaeva, H., Bueno, J., Polette, M., Birembaut, P., Sato, H., Seiki, M., et al. (1997) MT1-MMP correlates with MMP-2 activiation potential seen after epithelial to mesenchymal transition in human breast cancer cells. *Clin. Exp. Metastas.* 15, 111–120.

25. Bolon, I., Devouassoux, M., Robert, C., Moro, D., Brambilla, C., and Brambilla, E. (1997) Expression of urokinase-type plasminogen activator, stromelysin 1, stromelysin 3, and matrilysin genes in lung carcinomas. *Am. J. Path.* 150, 1619–1629.

26. Galis, Z. S., Sukhova, G. K., and Libby, P. (1995) Microscopic localization of active proteases by in situ zymography: Detection of matrix metalloproteinase activity in vascular tissue. *FASEB J.* 9, 974–980.

27. Knox, J., Sukhova, G., Whittemore, A., and Libby, P. (1997) Evidence for altered balance between matrix metalloproteinases and their inhibitors in human aortic diseases. *Circulation* 95, 205–212.

28. Zucker, S., Lysik, R., Malik, M., Bauer, B., Caamano, J., and Klein-Szanto, A. (1992) Secretion of gelatinases and tissue inhibitors of metalloproteinases by human lung cancer cell lines and revertant cell lines: not an invariant correlation with metastasis. *Int. J. Cancer* 52, 366–371.

29. Docherty, A., Lyons, A., Smith, B., Wright, E., Stephens, P., Harris, T., et al. (1985) Sequence of human tissue inhibitor of metalloproteinases and its identity to erythroid-potentiating activity. *Nature* 315, 761–768.

30. Stetler-Stevenson, W. G., Bersch, N., and Golde, D. W. (1992) Tissue inhibitor of metalloproteinase-2 (TIMP-2) has erythroid-potentiating activity. *FEBS Lett.* 296, 231–234.

31. Valente, P., Fassina, G., Melchiori, A., Masiello, L., Cilli, M., Vacca, A., et al. (1998) TIMP-2 over-expression reduces invasion and angiogenesis and protects B16 F10 melanoma cells from apoptosis. *Int. J. Cancer* 75, 246–253.

32. Liotta, L. A., Tryggvason, K., Garbisa, S., Hart, I., Foltz, C. M., and Shafie, S. (1980) Metastatic potential correlates with enzymatic degradation of basement membrane collagen. *Nature* 284, 67–68.

33. Yagel, S., Khokha, R., Denhardt, D., Kerbel, R., Parhar, R., and Lala, P. (1989) Mechanisms of cellular invasiveness: a comparison of amnion invasion in vitro and metastatic behavior in vivo. *J. Natl. Cancer Inst.* 81, 768–775.

34. Nakajima, M., Welch, D. R., Belloni, P. N., and Nicolson, G. L. (1987) Degradation of basement membrane type IV collagen and lung subendothelial matrix by rat mammary adenocarcinoma cell clones of differing metastatic potentials. *Cancer Res.* 47, 4869–4876.

35. Bernhard, E., Muschel, R., and Hughes, E. (1990) Mr 92,000 gelatinase release correlates with the metastatic phenotype in transformed rat embryo cells. *Cancer Res.* 50, 3872–3877.

36. Mareel, M., Kint, J., and Meyvisch, C. (1979) Methods of study of the invasion of malignant C3H mouse fibroblasts into embryonic chick heart in vitro. *Virchows Arch. B* 30, 95–111.

37. Thorgeirsson, U., Liotta, L., Kalebic, T., Margulies, I., Thomas, K., Rios-Candelore, M., et al. (1982) Effect of natural protease inhibitors and a chemoattractant on tumor cell invasion in vitro. *J. Natl. Cancer Inst.* 69, 1049–1054.

38. Repesh, L. (1989) A new in vitro assay for quantitiating tumor cell invasion. *Invas. Metast.* 9, 192–208.

39. Hendrix, M., Seftor, E., Seftor, R., and Fidler, I. (1987) A simple quantitative assay for studying the invasive potential of high and low metastatic variants. *Cancer Lett.* 38, 137–147.

40. Kossakowska, A., Hinek, A., Edwards, D., Lim, M., Zhang, C., Breitman, D., et al. (1998) Proteolytic activities of human non-Hodgkins lymphoma. *Am. J. Pathol.* 152, 565–576.

41. Sreenath, T., Matrisian, L. M., Stetler-Stevenson, W., Gattoni-Celli, S., and Pozzatti, R. O. (1992) Expression of matrix metalloproteinase genes in transformed rat cell lines of high and low metastatic potential. *Cancer Res.* 52, 4942–4947.

42. Schultz, R., Silberman, S., Persky, B., Bajkowski, A., and Carmichael, D. (1988) Inhibition by human recombinant tissue inhibitor of metalloproteinases of human amnion invasion and lung colonization by murine B16-F10 melanoma cells. *Cancer Res.* 48, 5539–5545.

43. Mignatti, P., Robbins, E., and Rifkin, D. B. (1986) Tumor invasion through the human amniotic membrane: requirement for a proteinase cascade. *Cell* 47, 487–498.

44. Reich, R., Thompson, E. W., Iwamoto, Y., Martin, G. R., Deason, J. R., Fuller, G. C., et al. (1988) Effects of inhibitors of plasminogen activator, serine proteases, and collagenase IV on the invasion of basement membranes by metastatic cells. *Cancer Res.* 48, 3307–3312.

45. DeClerck, Y., Yean, T., Chan, D., Shimada, H., and Langley, K. (1991) Inhibition of tumor invasion of smooth muscle cell layers by recombinant human metalloproteinases inhibitor. *Cancer Res.* 51, 2151–2157.

46. Khokha, R., Waterhouse, P., Yagel, S., Lala, P., Overall, C., Norton, G., et al. (1989) Antisense RNA-induced reduction in murine TIMP levels confers oncogenicity on Swiss 3T3 cells. *Science* 244, 947–950.

47. Khokha, R., Zimmer, M. J., Graham, C. H., Lala, P. K., and Waterhouse, P. (1992) Suppression of invasion by inducible expression of tissue inhibitor of metalloproteinase-1 (TIMP-1) in B16-F10 melanoma cells. *J. Natl. Cancer Inst.* 84, 1017–1022.

48. Powell, W. C., Knox, J. D., Navre, M., Grogan, T. M., Kittelson, J., Nagle, R. B., et al. (1993) Expression of the metalloproteinase matrilysin in DU-145 cells increases their invasive potential in severe combined immunodeficient mice. *Cancer Res.* 53, 417–422.

49. Deryugina, E., Luo, G., Reisfeld, R., Bourdon, M., and Strongin, A. (1997) Tumor cell invasion through matrigel is regulated by activated matrix metalloproteinase-2. *Anticancer Res.* 17, 3201–3210.

50. Gomez, D., Alonso, D., Yoshiji, H., and Thorgeirsson, U. (1997) Tissue inhibitors of metalloproteinases: structure, regulation and biological function. *Eur. J. Cell Biol.* 74, 111–122.

51. Alvarez, O. A., Carmichael, D. F., and DeClerck, Y. A. (1990) Inhibition of collagenolytic activity and metastasis of tumor cells by a recombinant human tissue inhibitor of metalloproteinases. *J. Natl. Cancer Inst.* 82, 589–595.

52. De Clerck, Y. A., Perez, N., Shimada, H., Boone, T. C., Langley, K. E., and Taylor, S. M. (1992) Inhibition of invasion and metastasis in cells transfected with an inhibitor of metalloproteinases. *Cancer Res.* 52, 701–708.

53. Kruger, A., Sanchez-Sweatman, O., Martin, D., Fata, J., Ho, A., Orr, F., et al. (1998) Host TIMP-1 overexpression confers resistance to experimental brain metastasis of a fibrosarcoma cell line. *Oncogene* 16, 2419–2423.

54. Kruger, A., Fata, J., and Khokha, R. (1997) Altered tumor growth and metastasis of a T-cell lymphoma in TIMP-1 transgenic mice. *Blood* 90, 1993–2000.

55. Bernhard, E., Gruber, S., and Muschel, R. (1994) Direct evidence linking expression of matrix metalloproteinase-9 (92 kDa gelatinase/collagenase) to the metastatic phenotype in transformed rat embryo cells. *Proc. Natl. Acad. Sci. USA.* 91, 4293–4297.

56. Kawamata, H., Kameyama, S., Kawai, K., Tanaka, Y., Nan, L., Barch, D. H., et al. (1995) Marked acceleration of the metastatic phenotype of a rat bladder carcinoma cell line by the expression of human gelatinase A. *Int. J. Cancer* 63, 568–575.

57. Chirivi, R. G. S., Garofalo, A., Crimmin, M. J., Bawden, L. J., Stoppacciaro, A., Brown, P. D., et al. (1994) Inhibition of the metastatic spread and growth of B16-BL6 murine melanoma by a synthetic matrix metalloproteinase inhibitor. *Int. J. Cancer* 58, 460–464.

58. Davies, B., Brown, P. D., East, N., Crimmin, M. J., and Balkwill, F. R. (1993) A synthetic matrix metalloproteinase inhibitor decreases tumor burden and prolongs survival of mice bearing human ovarian carcinoma xenografts. *Cancer Res.* 53, 2087–2091.

59. Parsons, S., Watson, S., and Steele, R. (1997) Phase I/II trial of batimastat, a matrix metalloproteinase inhibitor, in patients with malignant ascites. *Eur. J. Surg. Oncol.* 23, 526–531.

60. Beattie, G. and Smyth, J. (1998) Phase I study of intraperitoneal metalloproteinase inhibitor BB-94 in patients with malignant ascites. *Clin. Cancer Res.* 4, 1899–1902.

61. An, Z. L., Wang, X. E., Willmott, N., Chander, S. K., Tickle, S., Docherty, A. J. P., et al. (1997) Conversion of highly malignant colon cancer from an aggressive to a controlled disease by oral administration of a metalloproteinase inhibitor. *Clin. Exp. Metastas.* 15, 184–195.

62. Chambers, A. F. and Matrisian, L. M. (1997) Changing views of the role of matrix metalloproteinases in metastasis. *J. Natl. Cancer Inst.* 89, 1260–1270.

63. Holmgren, L. (1996) Antiangiogenesis restricted tumor dormancy. *Cancer Metast. Rev.* 15, 241–245.

64. Folkman, J. and Shing, Y. (1992) Angiogenesis. *J. Biol. Chem.* 267, 10,931–10,934.

65. Ingber, D. (1992) Extracellular matrix as a solid-state regulator in angiogenesis: identification of new targets for anti-cancer therapy. *Semin. Cancer Biol.* 3, 57–63.

66. Schnaper, H. W., Grant, D. S., Stetler-Stevenson, W. G., Fridman, R., D'Orazi, G., Murphy, A. N., et al. (1993) Type IV collagenase(s) and TIMPs modulate endothelial cell morphogenesis in vitro. *J. Cell. Physiol.* 156, 235–246.

67. Johnson, M. D., Kim, H.-R.C., Chesler, L., Tsao-Wu, G., Bouck, N., and Polverini, P. J. (1994) Inhibition of angiogenesis by tissue inhibitor of metalloproteinase. *J. Cell. Physiol.* 160, 194–202.

68. Montesano, R. and Orci, L. (1985) Tumor-promoting phorbol esters induce angiogenesis in vitro. *Cell* 42, 469–477.

69. Itoh, T., Tanioka, M., Yoshida, H., Yoshioka, T., Nishimoto, H., and Itohara, S. (1998) Reduced angiogenesis and tumor progression in gelatinase A-deficient mice. *Cancer Res.* 58, 1048–1051.

70. Brooks, P., Silletti, S., von Schalscha, T., Friedlander, M., and Cheresh, D. (1998) Disruption of angiogenesis by PEX, a noncatalytic metalloproteinase fragment with integrin binding activity. *Cell* 92, 391–400.

71. Nguyen, M., Arkell, J., and Jackson, C. (1998) Active and tissue inhibitor of matrix metalloproteinase-free gelatinase B accumulates within human microvascular endothelial vesicles. *J. Biol. Chem.* 273, 5400–5404.

72. Vu, T., Shipley, J., Bergers, G., Berger, J., Helms, J., Hanahan, D., et al. (1998) MMP-9/Gelatinase B is a key regulator of growth plate angiogenesis and apoptosis of hypertrophic chondrocytes. *Cell* 93, 411–422.

73. Jackson, C. and Nguyen, M. (1997) Human microvascular endothelial cells differ from macrovascular endothelial cells in their expression of matrix metalloproteinases. *Int. J. Biochem. Cell Biol.* 29, 1167–1177.

74. Patterson, B. and Sang, Q. (1997) Angiostatin-converting enzyme activities of human matrilysin (MMP-7) and gelatinase B/ type IV collagenase (MMP-9). *J. Biol. Chem.* 272, 28823–28825.

75. Dong, Z., Kumar, R., Yang, X., and Fidler, I. J. (1997) Macrophage-derived metalloelastase is responsible for the generation of angiostatin in Lewis lung carcinoma. *Cell* 88, 801–810.

76. Brown, P. (1997) Matrix metalloproteinase inhibitors. *Angiogenesis* 1, 142–154.

77. Galardy, R. E., Grobelny, D., Foellmer, H. G., and Fernandez, L. A. (1994) Inhibition of angiogenesis by the matrix metalloprotease inhibitor *N*-[2R-2-(hydroxamidocarbonymethyl)-4-methylpentanoyl)]-L-tryptophan methylamide. *Cancer Res.* 54, 4715–4718.

78. Taraboletti, G., Garofalo, A., Belotti, D., Drudis, T., Borsotti, P., Scanziani, E., et al. (1995) Inhibition of angiogenesis and murine hemangioma growth by batimastat, a synthetic inhibitor of matrix metalloproteinases. *J. Natl. Cancer Inst.* 87, 293–298.

79. Koop, S., Khokha, R., Schmidt, E. E., MacDonald, I. C., Morris, V. L., Chambers, A. F., et al. (1994) Overexpression of metalloproteinase inhibitor in B16F10 cells does not affect extravasation but reduces tumor growth. *Cancer Res.* 54, 4791–4797.

80. Kawamata, H., Kawai, K., Kameyama, S., Johnson, M. D., Stetler-Stevenson, W. G., and Oyasu, R. (1995) Over-expression of tissue inhibitor of matrix metalloproteinases (timp1 and timp2) suppresses extravasation of pulmonary metastasis of a rat bladder carcinoma. *Int. J. Cancer* 63, 680–687.

81. Masson, R., Lefebvre, O., Noel, A., El Fahime, M., Chenard, M., Wendling, C., et al. (1998) In vivo evidence that the stromelysin-3 metalloproteinase contributes in a paracrine manner to epithelial cell malignancy. *J. Cell Biol.* 140, 1535–1541.

82. Noel, A. C., Lefebvre, O., Maquoi, E., Van Hoorde, L., Chenard, M. P., Mareel, M., et al. (1996) Stromelysin-3 expression promotes tumor take in nude mice. *J. Clin. Invest.* 97, 1924–1930.

83. Rudolph-Owen, L., Chan, R., Muller, W., and Matrisian, L. (1998) The matrix metalloproteinase matrilysin influences early-stage mammary tumorigenesis. *Cancer Res.* 58, 5500–5506.

84. Sternlicht, M. D., Xie, J., Sympson, C., Bissell, M., and Werb, Z. (1997) Mice that express an autoactivating stromelysin-1 transgene develop progressive mammary gland lesions. *Proc. Am. Assoc. Cancer Res.* 38, 257.

85. D'Armiento, J., DiColandrea, T., Dalal, S. S., Okada, Y., Huang, M. T., Conney, A. H., et al. (1995) Collagenase expression in transgenic mouse skin causes hyperkeratosis and acanthosis and increases susceptibility to tumorigenesis. *Mol. Cell. Biol.* 15, 5732–5739.

86. Martin, D. C., Ruther, U., Sanchez-Sweatman, O. H., Orr, F. W., and Khokha, R. (1996) Inhibition of SV40 T antigen-induced hepatocellular carcinoma in TIMP-1 transgenic mice. *Oncogene* 13, 569–576.

87. Wilson, C. L., Heppner, K. J., Labosky, P. A., Hogan, B. L. M., and Matrisian, L. M. (1997) Intestinal tumorigenesis is suppressed in mice lacking the metalloproteinase matrilysin. *Proc. Natl. Acad. Sci. USA.* 94, 1402–1407.

88. Heppner Goss, K. J., Brown, P. D., and Matrisian, L. M. (1998) Differing effects of endogenous and synthetic inhibitors of metalloproteinases on intestinal tumorigenesis. *Int. J. Cancer* 78:(5)629–635.

89. Moser, A. R., Pitot, H. C., and Dove, W. F. (1990) A dominant mutation that predisposes to multiple intestinal neoplasia in the mouse. *Science* 247, 322–324.

90. Soloway, P. D., Alexander, C. M., Werb, Z., and Jaenisch, R. (1996) Targeted mutagenesis of Timp-1 reveals that lung tumor invasion is influenced by *Timp-1* genotype of the tumor but not by that of the host. *Oncogene* 13, 2307–2314.

91. Witty, J. P., Lempka, T., Coffey, R. J., Jr., and Matrisian, L. M. (1995) Decreased tumor formation in 7,12-dimethylbenzanthracene-treated stromelysin-1 transgenic mice is associated with alterations in mammary epithelial cell apoptosis. *Cancer Res.* 55, 1401–1406.

92. Lochter, A., Srebrow, A., Sympson, C. J., Terracio, N., Werb, Z., and Bissell, M. J. (1997) Misregulation of stromelysin-1 expression in mouse mammary tumor cells accompanies acquisition of stromelysin-1-dependent invasive properties. *J. Biol. Chem.* 272, 5007–5015.

93. Boudreau, N., Sympson, C. J., Werb, Z., and Bissell, M. J. (1995) Suppression of ICE and apoptosis in mammary epithelial cells by extracellular matrix. *Science* 267, 891–893.

94. Alexander, C. M., Howard, E. W., Bissell, M. J., and Werb, Z. (1996) Rescue of mammary epithelial cell apoptosis and entactin degradation by a tissue inhibitor of metalloproteinase-1 transgene. *J. Cell. Biol.* 135, 1667–1677.

95. Damsky, C. H. and Werb, Z. (1992) Signal transduction by integrin receptors for extracellular matrix: cooperative processing of extracellular information. *Curr. Op. Cell Biol.* 4, 772–781.

96. Arribas, J., Coodly, L., Vollmer, P., Kishimoto, T. K., Rosejohn, S., and Massague, J. (1996) Diverse cell surface protein ectodomains are shed by a system sensitive to metalloprotease inhibitors. *J. Biol. Chem.* 271, 11376–11382.

97. Levi, E., Fridman, R., Miao, H., Ma, Y., Yayon, A., Vlodavsky, I., et al. (1996) Matrix metalloproteinase 2 releases active soluble ectodomain of fibroblast growth factor receptor 1. *Proc. Natl. Acad. Sci. USA* 93, 7069–7074.

98. Dempsey, P., Meise, K., Yoshitake, Y., Nishikawa, K., and Coffey, R. (1997) Apical enrichment of human EGF precursor in Madin-Darby Canine Kidney cells involves preferential basolateral ectodomain cleavage sensitive to a metalloprotease inhibitor. *J. Cell Biol.* 138, 747–758.

99. Suzuki, M., Raab, G., Moses, M., Fernandez, C., and Klagsbrun, M. (1997) Matrix metalloproteinase-3 releases active heparin-binding EGF-like growth factor by cleavage at a specific juxtamembrane site. *J. Biol. Chem.* 272, 31730–31737.

100. Gearing, A. J. H., Beckett, P., Christodoulou, M., Churchill, M., Clements, J., Davidson, A. H., et al. (1994) Processing of tumour necrosis factor-α precursor by metalloproteinases. *Nature* 370, 555–557.

101. Black, R. A., Rauch, C. T., Kozlosky, C. J., Peschon, J. J., Slack, J. L., Wolfson, M. F., et al. (1997) A metalloproteinase disintegrin that releases tumour-necrosis factor-alpha from cells. *Nature* 385, 729–733.

102. Moss, M. L., Jin, S. L. C., Milla, M. E., Burkhart, W., Carter, H. L., Chen, W. J., et al. (1997) Cloning of a disintegrin metalloproteinase that processes precursor tumour-necrosis factor-alpha. *Nature* 385, 733–736.

103. Peschon, J., Slack, J., Reddy, P., Stocking, K., Sunnarborg, S., Lee, D., et al. (1998) An essential role for ectodomain shedding in mammalian development. *Science* 282, 1281–1284.
104. Wolfsberg, T. G., Primakoff, P., Myles, D. G., and White, J. M. (1995) ADAM, a novel family of membrane proteins containing a disintegrin and metalloprotease domain: Multipotential functions in cell-cell and cell-matrix interactions. *J. Cell. Biol.* 131, 275–278.
105. Fowlkes, J. L., Enghild, J. J., Suzuki, K., and Nagase, H. (1994) Matrix metalloproteinases degrade insulin-like growth factor-binding protein-3 in dermal fibroblast cultures. *J. Biol. Chem.* 269, 25742–25746.
106. Thrailkill, K. M., Quarles, L. D., Nagase, H., Suzuki, K., Serra, D. M., and Fowlkes, J. L. (1995) Characterization of insulin-like growth factor-binding protein 5-degrading proteases produced throughout murine osteoblast differentiation. *Endocrinology* 136, 3527–3533.
107. Rajah, R., Nunn, S. E., Herrick, D. J., Grunstein, M. M., and Cohen, P. (1996) Leukotriene d-4 induces MMP-1, which functions as an IGFBP protease in human airway smooth muscle cells. *Am. J. Physiol.* 15, L1014–L1022.
108. Macauley, V. (1992) Insulin-like growth factors and cancer. *Brit. J. Cancer* 65, 311–320.
109. Lahm, H., Suardet, L., Laurent, P., Fischer, J., Ceyhan, A., Givel, J., et al. (1992) Growth regulation and co-stimulation of human colorectal cancer cell lines by insulin-like growth factors I, II and transforming growth factor alpha. *Brit. J. Cancer* 65, 341–346.
110. Vlodavsky, I., Korner, G., Ishai-Michaeli, R., Bashkin, P., Bar-Shavit, R., and Fuks, Z. (1990) Extracellular matrix-resident growth factors and enzymes: possible involvement in tumor metastasis and angiogenesis. *Cancer Metast. Rev.* 9, 203–226.
111. Imai, K., Hiramatsu, A., Fukushima, D., Pierschbacher, M. D., and Okada, Y. (1997) Degradation of decorin by matrix metalloproteinases: identification of the cleavage sites, kinetic analyses and transforming growth factor-beta1 release. *Biochem. J.* 322, 809–814.
112. Strater, J., Wedding, U., Barth, T. F., Koretz, K., Elsing, C., and Moller, P. (1996) Rapid onset of apoptosis in vitro follows disruption of beta 1 integrin/matrix interactions in human colonic crypt cells. *Gastroenterology* 110, 1776–1784.
113. Frisch, S. M. and Francis, H. (1994) Disruption of epithelial cell-matrix interactions induces apoptosis. *J. Cell. Biol.* 124, 619–626.
114. von Bredow, D., Nagle, R., Bowden, G., and Cress, A. (1997) Cleavage of beta 4 integrin by matrilysin. *Exp. Cell Res.* 236, 341–345.
115. StCroix, B., Sheehan, C., Rak, J., Florenes, V., Slingerland, J., and Kerbel, R. (1998) E-Cadherin-dependent growth suppression is mediated by the cyclin-dependent kinase inhibitor p27[Kip1]. *J. Cell Biol.* 142, 557–571.
116. Lochter, A., Galosy, S., Muschler, J., Freedman, N., Werb, Z., and Bissell, M. (1997) Matrix metalloproteinase stromelysin-1 triggers a cascade of molecular alterations that leads to stable epithelial-to-mesenchymal conversion and a premalignant phenotype in mammary epithelial cells. *J. Cell Biol.* 139, 1861–1872.
117. Remacle, A., Noel, A., Duggan, C., McDermott, E., O'Higgins, N., Foidart, J., et al. (1998) Assay of matrix metalloproteinases types 1,2,3 and 9 in breast cancer. *Brit. J. Cancer* 77, 926–931.
118. Terada, T., Okada, Y., and Nakanuma, Y. (1996) Expression of immunoreactive matrix metalloproteinases and tissue inhibitors of matrix metalloproteinases in human normal livers and primary liver tumors. *Hepatology* 23, 1341–1344.
119. Murray, G. I., Duncan, M. E., Oneil, P., Melvin, W. T., and Fothergill, J. E. (1996) Matrix metalloproteinase-1 is associated with poor prognosis in colorectal cancer. *Nat. Med.* 2, 461–462.
120. Nomura, H., Fujimoto, N., Seiki, M., Mai, M., and Okada, Y. (1996) Enhanced production of matrix metalloproteinases and activation of matrix metalloproteinase 2 (gelatinase A) in human gastric carcinomas. *Int. J. Cancer* 69, 9–16.
121. Sakurai, Y., Otani, Y., Kameyama, K., Hosoda, Y., Okazaki, I., Kubota, T., et al. (1997) Expression of interstitial collagenase (matrix metalloproteinase-1) in gastric cancers. *Jap. J. Cancer Res.* 88, 401–406.

122. Muller, D., Breathnach, R., Engelmann, A., Millon, R., Bronner, G., Flesch, H., et al. (1991) Expression of collagenase-related metalloproteinase genes in human lung or head and neck tumours. *Int. J. Cancer* 48, 550–556.
123. Okada, A., Bellocq, J., Chenard, M., Rio, M., Chambon, P., and Basset, P. (1995) Membrane-type matrix metalloproteinase (MT-MMP) gene is expressed in stromal cells of human colon, breast and head and neck carcinomas. *Proc. Natl. Acad. Sci. USA* 92, 2730–2734.
124. Okazaki, I., Wada, N., Nakano, M., Saito, A., Takasaki, K., Doi, M., et al. (1997) Difference in gene expression for matrix metalloproteinase-1 between early and advanced hepatocellular carcinomas. *Hepatology* 25, 580–584.
125. Murray, G., Duncan, M., O'Neil, P., McKay, J., Melvin, W., and Fothergill, J. (1998) Matrix metalloproteinase-1 is associated with poor prognosis in oesophageal cancer. *J. Pathol.* 185, 256–261.
126. Kanayama, H., Yokota, K., Kurokawa, Y., Murakami, Y., Nishitani, M., and Kagawa, S. (1998) Prognostic values of matrix metalloproteinase-2 and tissue inhibitor of metalloproteinase-2 expression in bladder cancer. *Cancer* 82, 1359–1366.
127. Rha, S., Yang, W., Kim, J., Roh, J., Min, J., Lee, K., et al. (1998) Different expression patterns of MMP-2 and MMP-9 in breast cancer. *Oncol. Rep.* 5, 875–879.
128. Kurizaki, T., Toi, M., and Tominaga, T. (1998) Relationship between matrix metalloproteinase expression and tumor angiogenesis in human breast carcinoma. *Oncol. Rep.* 5, 673–677.
129. Soini, Y., Hurskainen, T., Höyhtyä, M., Oikarinen, A., and Autio-Harmainen, H. (1994) 72 KD and 92 KD type IV collagenase, type IV collagen, and laminin mRNAs in breast cancer: A study by in situ hybridization. *J. Histochem. Cytochem.* 42, 945–951.
130. Nawrocki, B., Polette, M., Marchand, V., Monteau, M., Gillery, P., Tournier, J. M., et al. (1997) Expression of matrix metalloproteinases and their inhibitors in human bronchopulmonary carcinomas—quantificative and morphological analyses. *Int. J. Cancer* 72, 556–564.
131. Garzetti, G. G., Ciavattini, A., Lucarini, G., Goteri, G., Romanini, C., and Biagini, G. (1996) The 72-kda metalloproteinase immunostaining in cervical carcinoma—relationship with lymph nodal involvement. *Gynecol. Oncol.* 60, 271–276.
132. Levy, A. T., Cioce, V., Sobel, M. E., Garbisa, S., Grigioni, W. F., Liotta, L. A., et al. (1991) Increased expression of the M_r 72,000 type IV collagenase in human colonic adenocarcinoma. *Cancer Res.* 51, 439–444.
133. Gallegos, N. C., Smales, C., Savage, F. J., Hembry, R. M., and Bolos, P. B. (1995) The distribution of matrix metalloproteinases and tissue inhibitor of metalloproteinases in colorectal cancer. *Surg. Oncol.* 4, 111–119.
134. Nakano, A., Tani, E., Miyazaki, K., Yamamoto, Y., and Furuyama, J. (1995) Matrix metalloproteinases and tissue inhibitors of metalloproteinases in human gliomas. *J. Neurosurg.* 83, 298–307.
135. Forsyth, P., Laing, T., Gibson, A., Rewcastle, N., Brasher, P., Sutherland, G., et al. (1998) High levels of gelatinase-B and active gelatinase-A in metastatic glioblastoma. *J. Neurooncol.* 36, 21–29.
136. Repassy, G., Forster-Horvath, C., Juhasz, A., Adany, R., Tamassy, A., and Timar, J. (1998) Expression of invasion markers CD44v6/v3, NM23 and MMP2 in laryngeal and hypopharyngeal carcinoma. *Pathol. Oncol. Res.* 4, 14–21.
137. Miyajima, Y., Nakano, R., and Morimatsu, M. (1995) Analysis of expression of matrix metalloproteinases-2 and -9 in hypopharyngeal squamous cell carcinoma by in situ hybridization. *Ann. Oto. Rhinol. Laryngol.* 104, 678–684.
138. Kawano, N., Osawa, H., Ito, T., Nagashima, Y., Hirahara, F., Inayama, Y., et al. (1997) Expression of gelatinase A, tissue inhibitor of metalloproteinases-2, matrilysin, and trypsin(ogen) in lung neoplasms—an immunohistochemical study. *Hum. Pathol.* 28, 613–622.

139. Brown, P. D., Bloxidge, R. E., Stuart, N. S. A., Gatter, K. C., and Carmichael, J. (1993) Association between expression of activated 72-kilodalton gelatinase and tumor spread in non-small-cell lung carcinoma. *J. Natl. Cancer Inst.* 85, 574–578.
140. Vaisanen, A., Tuominen, H., Kallioinen, M., and Turpeenniemi-Hujanen, T. (1996) Matrix metalloproteinase-2 (72 kd type IV collagenase) expression occurs in the early stage of human melanocytic tumour progression and may have prognostic value. *J. Pathol.* 180, 283–289.
141. Barille, S., Akhoundi, C., Collette, M., Mellerin, M. P., Rapp, M. J., Harousseau, J. L., et al. (1997) Metalloproteinases in multiple myeloma—production of matrix metalloproteinase-9 (MMP-9), activation of proMMP-2, and induction of MMP-1 by myeloma cells. *Blood* 90, 1649–1655.
142. Shima, I., Sasaguri, Y., Kusukawa, J., Yamana, H., Fujita, H., Kakegawa, T., et al. (1992) Production of matrix metalloproteinase-2 and metalloproteinase-3 related to malignant behavior of esophageal carcinoma: A clinicopathologic study. *Cancer* 70, 2747–2753.
143. Young, T. N., Rodriguez, G. C., Rinehart, A. R., Bast, R. C., Pizzo, S. V., and Stack, M. S. (1996) Characterization of gelatinases linked to extracellular matrix invasion in ovarian adenocarcinoma - purification of matrix metalloproteinase 2. *Gynecol. Oncol.* 62, 89–99.
144. Naylor, M. S., Stamp, G. W., Davies, B. D., and Balkwill, F. R. (1994) Expression and activity of MMPs and their regulators in ovarian cancer. *Int. J. Cancer* 58, 50–56.
145. Fishman, D. A., Bafetti, L. M., and Stack, M. S. (1996) Membrane-type matrix metalloproteinase expression and matrix metalloproteinase-2 activation in primary human ovarian epithelial carcinoma cells. *Invas. Metast.* 16, 150–159.
146. Koshiba, T., Hosotani, R., Wada, M., Fujimoto, K., Lee, J. U., Doi, R., et al. (1997) Detection of matrix metalloproteinase activity in human pancreatic cancer. *Surg. Today* 27, 302–304.
147. Bramhall, S. R., Stamp, G. W. H., Dunn, J., Lemoine, N. R., and Neoptolemos, J. P. (1996) Expression of collagenase (MMP2), stromelysin (MMP3) and tissue inhibitor of the metalloproteinases (TIMP1) in pancreatic and ampullary disease. *Brit. J. Cancer* 73, 972–978.
148. Stearns, M. E. and Stearns, M. (1996) Immunohistochemical studies of activated matrix metalloproteinase-2 (mmp-2a) expression in human prostate cancer. *Oncol. Res.* 8, 63–67.
149. Stearns, M. and Stearns, M. E. (1996) Evidence for increased activated metalloproteinase 2 (mmp-2a) expression associated with human prostate cancer progression. *Oncol. Res.* 8, 69–75.
150. Wood, M., Fudge, K., Mohler, J. L., Frost, A. R., Garcia, F., Wang, M., et al. (1997) In situ hybridization studies of metalloproteinases 2 and 9 and timp-1 and timp-2 expression in human prostate cancer. *Clin. Exp. Metastas.* 15, 246–258.
151. Gohji, K., Fujimoto, N., Hara, I., Fujii, A., Gotoh, A., Okada, H., et al. (1998) Serum matrix metalloproteinase-2 and its density in men with prostate cancer as a new predictor of disease extension. *Int. J. Cancer* 79, 96–101.
152. Pyke, C., Ralfkiaer, E., Huhtala, P., Hurskainen, T., and Tryggvason, K. (1992) Localization of messenger RNA for Mr 72,000 and 92,000 type IV collagenases in human skin cancers by in situ hybridization. *Cancer Res.* 52, 1336–1341.
153. Allgayer, H., Babic, R., Beyer, B., Grutzner, K., Tarabichi, A., Schildberg, F., et al. (1998) Prognostic relevance of MMP-2 (72-kD collagenase IV) in gastric cancer. *Oncol.* 55, 152–160.
154. Endo, K., Maehara, Y., Baba, H., Yamamoto, M., Tomisaki, S., Watanabe, A., et al. (1997) Elevated levels of serum and plasma metalloproteinases in patients with gastric cancer. *Anticancer Res.* 17, 2253–2258.
155. Nakagawa, T., Kubota, T., Kabuto, M., Sato, K., Kawano, H., Hayakawa, T., et al. (1994) Production of matrix metalloproteinases and tissue inhibitor of metalloproteinases-1 by human brain tumors. *J. Neurosurg.* 81, 69–77.
156. Nakano, A., Tani, E., Miyazaki, K., Furuyama, J., and Matsumoto, T. (1993) Expressions of matrilysin and stromelysin in human glioma cells. *Biochem. Biophys. Res. Commun.* 192, 999–1003.

157. Schonermark, M., Mester, B., Kempf, H. G., Blaser, J., Tschesche, H., and Lenarz, T. (1996) Expression of matrix-metalloproteinases and their inhibitors in human cholesteatomas. *Acta Oto-Laryngol.* 116, 451–456.

158. Kusukawa, J., Sasaguri, Y., Morimatsu, M., and Kameyama, T. (1995) Expression of matrix metalloproteinase-3 in stage I and II squamous cell carcinoma of the oral cavity. *J. Oral Maxill. Surg.* 53, 530–534.

159. Majmudar, G., Nelson, B. R., Jensen, T. C., and Johnson, T. M. (1994) Increased expression of matrix metalloproteinase-3 (stromelysin-1) in cultured fibroblasts and basal cell carcinomas of nevoid basal cell carcinoma syndrome. *Mol. Carcinogen.* 11, 29–33.

160. Yoshimoto, M., Itoh, F., Yamamoto, H., Hinoda, Y., Imai, K., and Yachi, A. (1993) Expression of MMP-7 (pump-1) mRNA in human colorectal cancers. *Int. J. Cancer* 54, 614–618.

161. McDonnell, S., Navre, M., Coffey, R. J., and Matrisian, L. M. (1991) Expression and localization of the matrix metalloproteinase pump-1 (MMP-7) in human gastric and colon carcinomas. *Mol. Carcinogen.* 4, 527–533.

162. Mori, M., Barnard, G. F., Mimori, K., Ueo, H., Akiyoshi, T., and Sugimachi, K. (1995) Overexpression of matrix metalloproteinase-7 mRNA in human colon carcinomas. *Cancer* 75, 1516–1519.

163. Bradl, M., Klein-Szanto, A., Porter, S., and Mintz, B. (1991) Malignant melanoma in transgenic mice. *Proc. Natl. Acad. Sci. USA* 88, 164–168.

164. Ichikawa, Y., Ishikawa, T., Momiyama, N., Yamaguchi, S., Masui, H., Hasegawa, T., et al. (1998) Detection of regional lymph node metastases in colon cancer by using RT-PCR for matrix metalloproteinase-7, matrilysin. *Clin. Exp. Metastas.* 16, 3–8.

165. Pajouh, M., Nagle, R., Breathnach, R., Finch, J., Brawer, M., and Bowden, G. (1991) Expression of metalloproteinase genes in human prostate cancer. *J. Cancer Res. Clin. Oncol.* 117, 144–150.

166. Honda, M., Mori, M., Ueo, H., Sugimachi, K., and Akiyoshi, T. (1996) Matrix metalloproteinase-7 expression in gastric carcinoma. *Gut* 39, 444–448.

167. Yamashita, K., Azumano, I., Mai, M., and Okada, Y. (1998) Expression and tissue localization of matrix metalloproteinase 7 (matrilysin) in human gastric carcinomas. Implications for vessel invasion and metastasis. *Int. J. Cancer* 79, 187–194.

168. Senota, A., Itoh, F., Yamamoto, H., Adachi, Y., Hinoda, Y., and Imai, K. (1998) Relation of matrilysin messenger RNA expression with invasive activity in human gastric cancer. *Clin. Exp. Metastas.* 16, 313–321.

169. Ueda, Y., Imai, K., Tsuchiya, H., Fujimoto, N., Nakanishi, I., Katsuda, S., et al. (1996) Matrix metalloproteinase 9 (gelatinase B) is expressed in multinucleated giant cells of human giant cell tumor of bone and is associated with vascular invasion. *Am. J. Path.* 148, 611–622.

170. Monteagudo, C., Merino, M. J., San-Juan, J., Liotta, L. A., and Stetler-Stevenson, W. G. (1990) Immunohistochemical distribution of type IV collagenase in normal, benign, and malignant breast tissue. *Am. J. Pathol.* 136, 585–592.

171. Zeng, Z. S. and Guillem, J. G. (1995) Distinct pattern of matrix metalloproteinase 9 and tissue inhibitor of metalloproteinase 1 mRNA expression in human colorectal cancer and liver metastases. *Brit. J. Cancer* 72, 575–582.

172. Zucker, S., Lysik, R. M., Zarrabi, M. H., and Moll, U. (1993) M_r 92,000 type IV collagenase is increased in plasma of patients with colon cancer and breast cancer. *Cancer Res.* 53, 140–146.

173. Zeng, Z. and Guillem, J. (1996) Colocalisation of matrix metalloproteinase-9 mRNA and protein in human colorectal cancer stromal cells. *Brit. J. Cancer* 74, 1161–1167.

174. Zeng, Z. and Guillem, J. (1998) Unique activation of matrix metalloproteinase-9 within human liver metastases from colorectal cancer. *Brit. J. Cancer* 78, 349–353.

175. Uemura, K., Takao, S., and Aikou, T. (1998) In vitro determination of basement membrane invasion predicts liver metastases in human gastrointestinal carcinoma. *Cancer Res.* 58, 3727–3731.

176. Zucker, S., Lysik, R. M., DiMassimo, B. I., Zarrabi, H. M., Moll, U. M., Grimson, R., et al. (1995) Plasma assay of gelatinase B: Tissue inhibitor of metalloproteinase complexes in cancer. *Cancer* 76, 700–708.

177. Hayasaka, A., Suzuki, N., Fujimoto, N., Iwama, S., Fukuyama, E., Kanda, Y., et al. (1996) Elevated plasma levels of matrix metalloproteinase-9 (92kd type IV collagenase/gelatinase B) in hepatocellular carcinoma. *Hepatology* 24, 1058–1062.

178. Tolnay, E., Wiethege, T., Kuhnen, C., Wulf, M., Voss, B., and Muller, K. (1997) Expression of type IV collagenase correlates with the ·xpression of vascular endothelial growth factor in primary non-small cell lung cancer. *J. Cancer Res. Clin. Oncol.* 123, 652–658.

179. Gress, T. M., Mueller-Pillasch, F., Lerch, M. M., Friess, H., Buechler, M., and Adler, G. (1995) Expression and in-situ localization of genes coding for extracellular matrix proteins and extracellular matrix degrading proteases in pancreatic cancer. *Int. J. Cancer* 62, 407–413.

180. Stahle-Backdahl, M. and Parks, W. (1993) 92Kd gelatinase is actively expressed by eosinophils and stored by neutrophils in squamous cell carcinoma. *Am. J. Pathol.* 142, 995–1000.

181. Van den Oord, J., Paemen, L., Opdenakker, G., and de Wolf-Peeters, C. (1997) Expression of gelatinase B and the extracellular matrix metalloproteinase inducer EMMPRIN in benign and malignant pigment cell lesions of the skin. *Am. J. Pathol.* 151, 665–670.

182. Muller, D., Wolf, C., Abecassis, J., Millon, R., Engelmann, A., Bronner, G., et al. (1993) Increased stromelysin 3 gene expression is associated with increased local invasiveness in head and neck squamous cell carcinomas. *Cancer Res.* 53, 165–169.

183. Kawami, H., Yoshida, K., Ohsaki, A., Kuroi, K., Nishiyama, M., and Toge, T. (1993) Stromelysin-3 mRNA expression and malignancy: Comparison with clinicopathological features and type IV collagenase mRNA expression in breast tumors. *Anticancer Res.* 13, 2319–2324.

184. Wolf, C., Rouyer, N., Lutz, Y., Adida, C., Loriot, M., Bellocq, J.-P., et al. (1993) Stromelysin 3 belongs to a subgroup of proteinases expressed in breast carcinoma fibroblastic cells and possibly implicated in tumor progression. *Proc. Natl. Acad. Sci. USA* 90, 1843–1847.

185. Johnson, L., Hunt, D., Kim, K., and Nachtigal, M. (1996) Amplification of stromelysin-3 transcripts from carcinomas of the colon. *Hum. Pathol.* 27, 964–968.

186. Urbanski, S., Edwards, D., Hershfield, N., Huchcroft, S., Shaffer, E., Sutherland, L., et al. (1993) Expression pattern of metalloproteinases and their inhibitors changes with the progression of human sporadic colorectal neoplasia. *Diagn. Mol. Pathol.* 2, 81–89.

187. Mueller, J., Mueller, E., Arras, E., Bethke, B., Stolte, M., and Hofler, H. (1997) Stromelysin-3 expression in early (pt1) carcinomas and pseudoinvasive lesions of the colorectum. *Virchows Arch.* 430, 213–219.

188. Thewes, M., Pohlmann, G., Atkinson, M., Mueller, J., Putz, B., and Hofler, H. (1996) Stromelysin-3 (st-3) mRNA expression in colorectal carcinomas—localization and clinicopathologic correlations. *Diagn. Mol. Pathol.* 5, 284–290.

189. Porte, H., Triboulet, J., Kotelevets, L., Carrat, F., Prevot, S., Nordlinger, B., et al. (1998) Overexpression of stromelysin-3, BM40/SPARC, and MET genes in human esophageal carcinoma: implications for prognosis. *Clin. Cancer Res.* 4, 1375–1382.

190. Wagner, S., Ruhri, C., Kunth, K., Holocek, B., Goos, M., Hofler, H., et al. (1992) Expression of stromelysin-3 in the stromal elements of human basal cell carcinoma. *Diagn. Mol. Pathol.* 1, 200–205.

191. Unden, A., Sandstedt, B., Bruce, K., Hedblad, M., and Stahle-Backdahl, M. (1996) Stromelysin-3 mRNA associated with myofibroblasts is overexpressed in aggressive basal cell carcinoma and in dermatofibroma but not in dermatofibrosarcoma. *J. Invest. Dermatol.* 107, 147–153.

192. Majmudar, G., Nelson, B. R., Jensen, T. C., Voorhees, J. J., and Johnson, T. M. (1994) Increased expression of stromelysin-3 in basal cell carcinomas. *Mol. Carcinogen.* 9, 17–23.

193. Wolf, C., Chenard, M.-P., De Grossouvre, P. D., Bellocq, J.-P., Chambon, P., and Basset, P. (1992) Breast-cancer-associated stromelysin-3 gene is expressed in basal cell carcinoma and during cutaneous wound healing. *J. Invest. Dermatol.* 99, 870–872.

194. Freije, J. M. P., Diez-Itza, I., Balbín, M., Sanchez, L. M., Blasco, R., Tolivia, J., et al. (1994) Molecular cloning and expression of collagenase-3, a novel human matrix metalloproteinase produced by breast carcinomas. *J. Biol. Chem.* 269, 16766–16773.

195. Johansson, N., Airola, K., Grenman, R., Kariniemi, A. L., Saarialho-Kere, U., and Kahari, V. M. (1997) Expression of collagenase-3 (matrix metalloproteinase-13) in squamous cell carcinomas of the head and neck. *Am. J. Path.* 151, 499–508.

196. Airola, K., Johansson, N., Kariniemi, A. L., Kahari, V. M., and Saarialho-Kere, U. K. (1997) Human collagenase-3 is expressed in malignant squamous epithelium of the skin. *J. Invest. Dermatol.* 109, 225–231.

197. Ueno, H., Nakamura, H., Inoue, M., Imai, K., Noguchi, M., Sato, H., et al. (1997) Expression and tissue localization of membrane-types 1,2, and 3 matrix metalloproteinases in human invasive breast carcinomas. *Cancer Res.* 57, 2055–2060.

198. Polette, M., Nawrocki, B., Gilles, C., Sato, H., Seiki, M., Tournier, J. M., et al. (1996) MT-MMP expression and localisation in human lung and breast cancers. *Virchows Arch.* 428, 29–35.

199. Gilles, C., Polette, M., Piette, J., Munaut, C., Thompson, E. W., Birembaut, P., et al. (1996) High level of MT-MMP expression is associated with invasiveness of cervical cancer cells. *Int. J. Cancer* 65, 209–213.

200. Harada, T., Arii, S., Mise, M., Imamura, T., Higashitsuji, H., Furutani, M., et al. (1998) Membrane-type matrix metalloproteinase-1 (MT1-MMP) gene is overexpressed in highly invasive hepatocellular carcinomas. *J. Hepatol.* 28, 231–239.

201. Imamura, T., Ohshio, G., Mise, M., Harada, T., Suwa, H., Okada, N., et al. (1998) Expression of membrane-type matrix metalloproteinase-1 in human pancreatic adenocarcinomas. *J. Cancer Res. Clin. Oncol.* 124, 65–72.

202. Nomura, H., Sato, H., Seiki, M., Mai, M., and Okada, Y. (1995) Expression of membrane-type matrix metalloproteinase in human gastric carcinomas. *Cancer Res.* 55, 3263–3266.

203. Shipley, J. M., Wesselschmidt, R. L., Kobayashi, D. K., Ley, T. J., and Shapiro, S. D. (1996) Metalloelastase is required for macrophage-mediated proteolysis and matrix invasion in mice. *Proc. Natl. Acad. Sci. USA* 93, 3942–3946.

204. D'Armiento, J., Dalal, S. S., Okada, Y., Berg, R. A., and Chada, K. (1992) Collagenase expression in the lungs of transgenic mice causes pulmonary emphysema. *Cell* 71, 955–961.

205. Witty, J. P., Wright, J., and Matrisian, L. M. (1995) Matrix metalloproteinases are expressed during ductal and alveolar mammary morphogenesis, and misregulation of stromelysin-1 in transgenic mice induces unscheduled alveolar development. *Mol. Biol. Cell* 6, 1287–1303.

206. Rudolph-Owen, L. A., Cannon, P., and Matrisian, L. M. (1998) Overexpression of the matrix metalloproteinase matrilysin results in premature mammary gland differentiation and male infertility. *Mol. Biol. Cell* 9, 421–435.

5 Hydroxamic Acid Matrix Metalloproteinase Inhibitors

Peter D. Brown, DPhil,
Alan H. Davidson, MA, PhD,
Alan H. Drummond, PhD,
Andrew Gearing, PhD, and
Mark Whittaker, DPhil

CONTENTS

INTRODUCTION
MEDICINAL CHEMISTRY
PHARMACOLOGICAL EFFECTS IN DISEASE MODELS
CLINICAL DEVELOPMENT
CONCLUSION

1. INTRODUCTION

It is now apparent that the matrix metalloproteinases (MMPs) play a key role in the remodeling of basement membrane that is associated with tumor metastasis, growth, and angiogenesis. Thus there is considerable interest in the design of MMP inhibitors (MMPIs) *(1–6)* as they promise to provide a novel noncytotoxic means of treating human cancer. Furthermore, pharmacological studies of MMPIs in animal models of human disease suggest that the potential therapeutic applications will encompass other endpoints such as arthritis and multiple-sclerosis. Recently, evidence has shown that MMP inhibitors can also reduce the production of TNF-α by inhibiting a TNF-α converting enzyme (TACE) *(7–9)*. As a consequence, this "dual activity" may be of benefit in diseases which involve both inflammation and matrix remodeling. In this chapter we review the hydroxamic acid class of MMPIs with specific reference to the re-

From: *Cancer Drug Discovery and Development:*
Matrix Metalloproteinase Inhibitors in Cancer Therapy
Edited by: Neil J. Clendeninn and Krzysztof Appelt © Humana Press Inc., Totowa, NJ

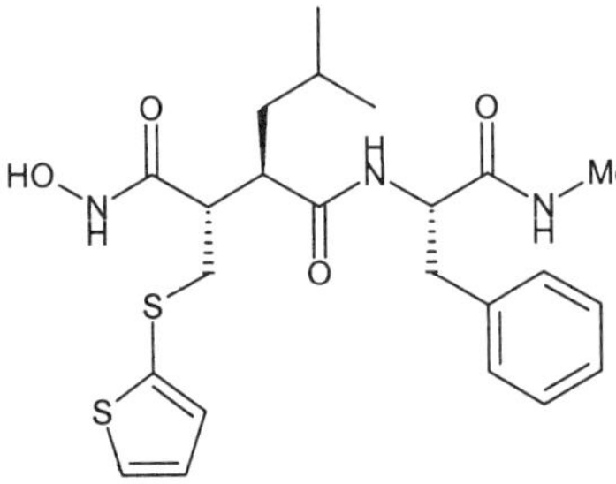

Batimastat (1)

IC_{50}	Fibroblast collagenase	3 n*M*
	Neutrophil collagenase	10 n*M*
	Gelatinase A	4 n*M*
	Gelatinase B	1 n*M*
	Stromelysin-1	20 n*M*

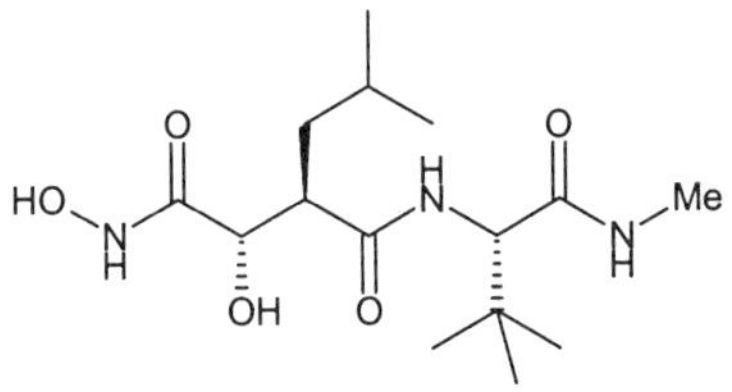

Marimastat (2)

IC_{50}	Fibroblast collagenase	5 n*M*
	Neutrophil collagenase	2 n*M*
	Gelatinase A	6 n*M*
	Gelatinase B	3 n*M*
	Stromelysin-1	200 n*M*
	Matrilysin	20 n*M*
	Cellular TACE	3,800 n*M*

Fig. 1. Structures and in vitro activities of batimastat (BB-94) and marimastat (BB-2516).

search program at British Biotech and the compounds batimastat 1 (BB-94) and marimastat 2 (BB-2516) (Fig. 1). Batimastat was the first MMPI to enter human clinical trials in cancer patients. This compound has been superseded by the orally active MMPI marimastat which is now under Phase III clinical evaluation in late-stage cancer patients. Here we present an overview of the medicinal chemistry relating to batimastat and marimastat, discuss the preclinical evaluation of compounds of this class in animal models of cancer and other human diseases and review the current clinical status for marimastat.

2. MEDICINAL CHEMISTRY

The requirement for a molecule to be an effective inhibitor of the MMP class of enzymes is a functional group (e.g., carboxylic acid, hydroxamic acid, and sulfhydryl, etc.) capable of chelating the active site zinc(II) ion (this will be referred to as zinc binding group or ZBG), at least one functional group which provides a hydrogen bond interaction with the enzyme back-bone and one or more side chains which undergo effective Van der Waals interactions with the enzyme subsites. It is now apparent that this requirement can be satisfied by a variety of different structural classes of MMPIs which have been discovered by a number of methods including structure-based design *(10)* and combinatorial chemistry *(11)*. The discovery of batimastat predated these methods and followed a substrate-based approach to inhibitor design which had been pioneered by early workers in the field *(12–16)*. The earliest MMP inhibitors were designed from a knowledge of the amino acid sequence of human triple helical collagen at the site of cleavage by collagenase-1 (MMP-1) (Fig. 2). In this

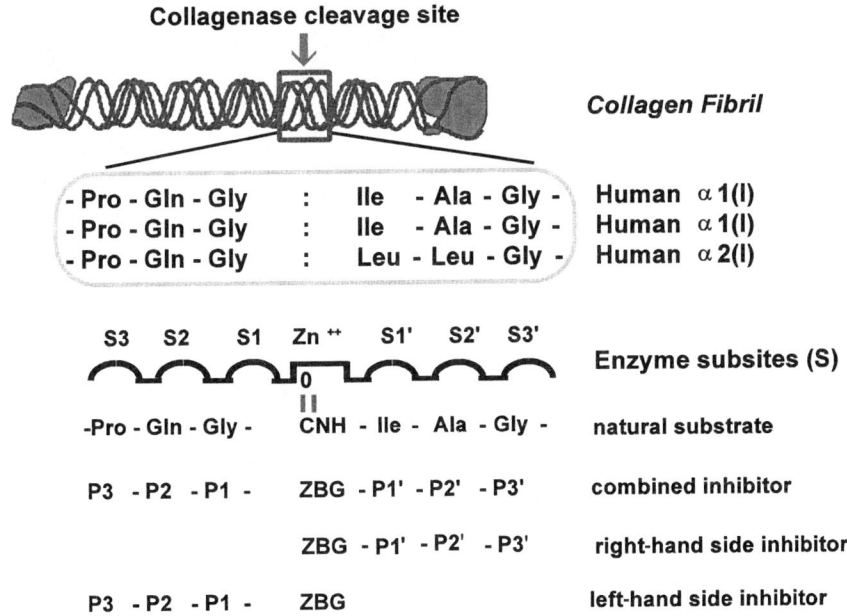

Fig. 2. Design of matrix metalloproteinase inhibitors based on the sequence of the collagen substrate cleavage site.

approach, a ZBG was attached to peptide derivatives which mimicked part of this sequence. Three classes of compounds were developed; those in which the ZBG is flanked on both sides by amino acid residues and those in which the amino acid residues are present on either the left-hand side or the right-hand side of the ZBG. The variety of different MMPIs that have been identified following this approach incorporate a range of different ZBG functionality and have been summarized in a number of early reviews *(12–16)*. It was generally found that compounds which mimic the sequence to the "right-hand side" of the active site (P1′ and P2′) and incorporate a hydroxamic acid ZBG exhibited particularly potent inhibition. In contrast, the corresponding "left-hand side" inhibitors were reported to possess only modest inhibitory potency. At British Biotech, we have investigated both the "left-hand side" and "right-hand side" approaches to MMP inhibition and have also identified nonpeptidic inhibitors.

2.1. "Left-Hand Side" Inhibitors

The "left-hand side" hydroxamate MMPIs are compounds which feature side chains that bind to the unprimed (S1, S2, and S3) enzyme subsites. Compounds of this class were first described in 1986 *(17–18)* but have not received as much attention *(19–21)* as "right-hand side" MMPIs. Early investigations resulted in the identification of "left-hand side" hydroxamates with micromolar inhibitory activity such as Z-Pro-Leu-Ala-NHOH 3 *(17–18)*. Although the major focus of our MMPI program has been on the "right-hand side" inhibitors, we were interested to discover whether the activity of "left-hand side" inhibitors could be improved by investigating a larger range of tripeptide derivatives. We have developed a series of O-hydroxylamine presenting resins for the preparation of hydroxamic acid derivatives by solid phase synthesis methods *(22–25)*. Similar resins have been subsequently reported by others *(26–33)*. We employed a modified Wang resin for the preparation of combinatorial libraries of "left-hand side" hydroxamates both by "split-pool" and parallel synthesis strategies *(22–25)*. The aim of this study was to identify optimal amino acids for each subsite and so improve the inhibitory potency over that reported for the literature lead compound Z-Pro-Leu-Ala-NHOH 3. The "split-pool" method was examined first and involved the generation of a 500 member library (Fig. 3) as 10 mixtures each of 50 compounds in which the identity of the amino acid at P1 was defined but varied at the P2 and P3 positions. The tripeptide library mixtures were prepared using standard Fmoc protocols and the product hydroxamic acids were obtained following cleavage from the resin with trifluoroacetic acid. Assay of the mixtures against MMP-1, MMP-2, and MMP-3 suggested that D-leucine at P1 would give selectivity for MMP-2 whereas L-isoleucine at this position would provide potent broad-spectrum activity (Fig. 4). Iterative deconvolution of the mixtures with P1 D-leucine and P1 L-isoleucine in each case did not lead to the identification of compounds with improved activity over the literature lead compound Z-Pro-Leu-Ala-NHOH 3. This disappointing result may reflect insufficient diversity within the library or cooperative effects between the mixture components on assay. With this experience, we decided to concentrate on producing single compounds by parallel synthesis methods and we undertook a systematic variation of the amino acid residues at P3, P2, and P1. From the synthesis of over 200 individual tripeptides it was found that substitution of L-proline by L-thioproline at P3 and L-leucine by L-homophenylalanine at P2 gave a significant improvement in the inhibition of MMP-2 and MMP-3 (Table 1: Compound 4). For modification of the P1 side-chain it was found that D-stereochemistry tended to give selective inhibition of MMP-2 over MMP-1 and MMP-3 whereas L-stereochemistry and an extended side-chain gave nanomolar inhibition of the three enzymes evaluated (Table 1: Compounds 5 and 6). Although, there is a literature X-ray crystal structure of a tripeptide (Pro-Leu-Ala-NHOH) bound into the "left-hand side" (unprimed region) of the active site of human neutrophil collagenase (MMP-8) *(34)* it does not necessarily follow that the more potent analogs adopt a similar binding mode. Whereas this study provided useful structure-activity relationships (SARs) and demonstrated the ability to optimize inhibitory activity by combinatorial methods, the peptidic nature of the compounds limits their utility as pharmaceutical agents.

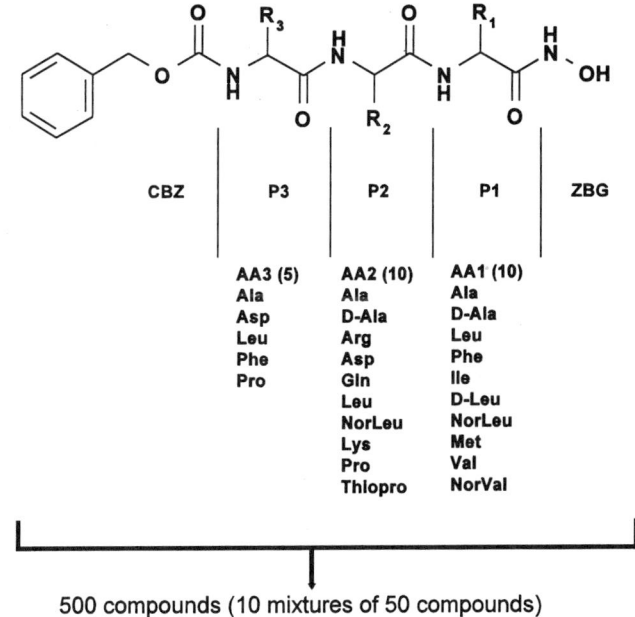

Fig. 3. "Left-hand side" matrix metalloproteinase inhibitor library.

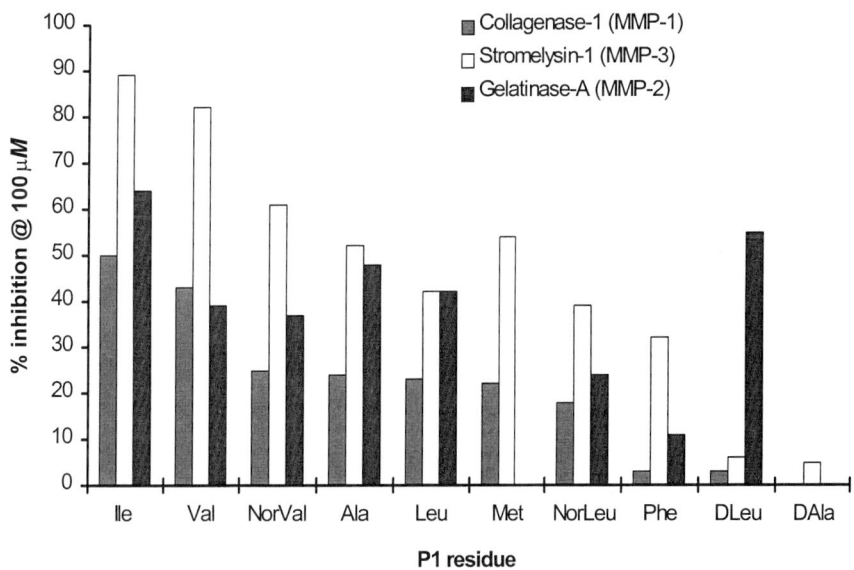

Fig. 4. 1st Level Assay of "left-hand side" matrix metalloproteinase inhibitor library.

Table 1
In Vitro Results for Selected "Left-Hand Side" MMP Inhibitors

Compound	Structure	IC_{50} (or % inhibition) nM		
		MMP-1	MMP-2	MMP-3
3		8,000	8,000	3,500
4		6,000	200	100
5		50% @ 100,000	5	10% @ 1,000
6		40	0.4	8

2.2. *"Right-Hand Side" Inhibitors*

The main focus of the British Biotech MMPI program has been a series of hydroxamic acid based pseudopeptide "right-hand side" inhibitors. This series of pseudopeptide derivatives, of the general formula shown in Figure 5, feature a hydroxamate ZBG, and side chains that bind to the S1′ and S2′ enzyme subsites.

2.2.1. IN VITRO SAR FOR "RIGHT-HAND SIDE" INHIBITORS

In contrast to the "left-hand side" inhibitors described above the literature lead compound SC-44463 7 *(35)* already possessed potent inhibitory activity in vitro. Thus, the focus of the program was to understand the SAR and to obtain a molecule that was effective in animal models of human disease and which had suitable pharmacokinetics for clinical evaluation in man.

Within this series, we and others have investigated the effect of the substituents Ra, R1, R2, and R3 on inhibitory potency and selectivity of the inhibitors. Structure-activity relationships within this series are summarized in Figure 6. In particular, we found that a lipophilic α-substituent (Ra) confers the property of broad spectrum activity against a variety of MMP enzymes. This led to the discovery of batimastat 1 (BB-94) *(36,37)* and later BB-1101 8 *(38)*. The former possesses a thienylthiomethylene α-substituent (Ra) whereas the latter features the smaller allyl α-substituent. Both batimastat 1 (BB-94) and BB-1101 8 are broad spectrum inhibitors that have displayed efficacy in animal models of human disease following intraperitoneal (ip) administration *(vide infra)*. We later found the presence of certain α-substituents had a beneficial effect on the inhibition of TACE.

There has been considerable debate as to whether selective inhibitors would be equally effective for particular diseases. At British Biotech we have focused on broad spectrum inhibitors since MMPs are rarely, if ever, expressed singly in human diseases, but are usually produced as "gangs" of several enzymes at a time. In addition, different tumor types express different patterns of MMPs. In reality, with over sixteen known MMP enzymes it is difficult to obtain MMPIs which are uniquely selective for a particular enzyme. Rather it has been possible to obtain compounds with different spectra of activity against the members of the MMP family. Seminal work from the Celltech group showed that a degree of enzyme selectivity could be obtained: The introduction of larger P1′ substituents (e.g., 3-phenylpropyl as in 9) enhances inhibition of the gelatinases (MMP-2 and MMP-9) and neutrophil collagenase (MMP-8) at the expense of activity against fibroblast collagenase (MMP-1) and matrilysin (MMP-7) *(39)*.

The advent of high resolution X-ray crystal structures of MMP inhibitor-enzyme complexes has confirmed the presumed binding mode for inhibitors such as batimastat and, very importantly, provided insight into differences in the active site for the different MMPs *(10)*. The most significant difference is in

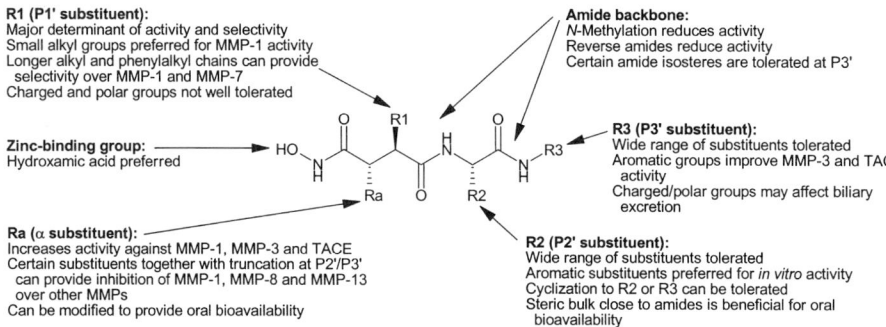

Fig. 5. General formula for hydroxamic acid MMP inhibitors. Ra is referred to as the α-substituent and may interact with the S1 subsite of the enzyme. R1, R2, and R3 are referred to respectively as the P1′, P2′, and P3′ substituents which interact respectively with the S1′, S2′, and S3′ enzyme subsites.

R1 (P1′ substituent):
Major determinant of activity and selectivity
Small alkyl groups preferred for MMP-1 activity
Longer alkyl and phenylalkyl chains can provide
 selectivity over MMP-1 and MMP-7
Charged and polar groups not well tolerated

Amide backbone:
N-Methylation reduces activity
Reverse amides reduce activity
Certain amide isosteres are tolerated at P3′

Zinc-binding group:
Hydroxamic acid preferred

R3 (P3′ substituent):
Wide range of substituents tolerated
Aromatic groups improve MMP-3 and TACE
 activity
Charged/polar groups may affect biliary
 excretion

Ra (α substituent):
Increases activity against MMP-1, MMP-3 and TACE
Certain substituents together with truncation at P2′/P3′
 can provide inhibition of MMP-1, MMP-8 and MMP-13
 over other MMPs
Can be modified to provide oral bioavailability

R2 (P2′ substituent):
Wide range of substituents tolerated
Aromatic substituents preferred for *in vitro* activity
Cyclization to R2 or R3 can be tolerated
Steric bulk close to amides is beneficial for oral
 bioavailability

Fig. 6. Summary of structure-activity relationships for "right-hand side" MMP inhibitors.

the size and shape of the S1′ pocket for the various MMPs. The S1′ subsite is a deep pocket that penetrates into the core of all MMPs, with the exception of MMP-1 and MMP-7, for which the S1′ subsite is relatively shallow. The observation of the difference in the size of the S1′ pocket between the MMPs explains the selectivity that the researchers at Celltech obtained by the incorporation of large P1′ groups. This has been exploited by other workers, notably the Sterling Winthrop (*40–42*) and Agouron (*10*) groups which have identified other compounds with more extended P1′ substituents. We have investigated the effect of extended alkyl P1′ substituents and have shown that a C_8 substituent provides potent inhibition of MMP-2 for compound 10 but that effective inhibition is still observed upon extending the side chain to C_{16} as in compound 11 (*43,44*). Recently, we identified a series of "deep-pocket" selective compounds that feature a rigid arylalkylmethylene P1′ substituent such as compound 12 (*45*).

SAR studies, later confirmed by X-ray crystal structures, indicated substituents in the P2′ position point away from the active site of the enzyme and hence a large number of groups can be accommodated. Tryptophan at P2′ is reported to yield more potent inhibitors than other amino acid side chains (*46,47*). To date, there is no evidence that selectivity can be achieved by modifications at this position.

We have found that a wide range of groups can be accommodated at P3' but that methyl, or heteroaryl amides are often preferred. Heterocyclic and aromatic groups appear to enhance MMP-3 and TACE activity. Disubstitution of the P2'-P3' amide leads to a loss of activity. The P1'-P2' central amide bond also picks up key backbone interactions and either removal of, or substitution on, the secondary amide leads to greatly reduced potency. Although these hydrogen bond interactions between the enzyme and inhibitor are important for the pseudopeptide inhibitors it has been possible, by increasing the interactions at the other subsites (e.g. S1 and S1'), to produce potent inhibitors where either or both of the amide bonds have been replaced.

Hydroxamate MMPIs with good in vitro and in vivo potency have been known for a considerable period of time, and the structural features which determine potency are now reasonably well understood. The main reason it has taken so long to progress such compounds into and through the clinic has been the lack of acceptable oral bioavailability. The major indications for these agents (e.g., cancer and arthritis), will require chronic dosing and hence the need for compounds which can be given by mouth. Over the last few years, considerable advances have been made and several compounds are now in clinical development as oral agents. Unfortunately, pseudopeptide molecules often have inherent difficulties in terms of oral bioavailabilty—rapid metabolism, poor absorption, high first pass metabolism *(48)*. There difficulties have been overcome either by modifying the pseudopeptide structure to circumvent these problems or by developing nonpeptide like molecules.

The "right-hand side" hydroxamic acid MMPIs possess two secondary amide groups and might therefore be expected to exhibit poor oral bioavailability. Indeed, batimastat has poor oral availability. Drug metabolism and pharmacokinetic (DMPK) studies have shown that 97% of a radiolabeled sample of orally administered batimastat was excreted intact in the feces. Batimastat is not degraded in the gastrointestinal tract, and the low oral bioavailability is therefore due to low absorbtion and/or high first pass metabolism. Workers at Sterling-Winthrop have shown that a related hydroxamate MMPI undergoes rapid first pass metabolism by glucuronidation and biliary excretion *(49)*. This could be reduced by placing basic or thioether groups at P3'. Even with such improvements, bioavailabilty was still less than 10% suggesting that oral absorption was still low *(49)*. We considered that the low aqueous solubility and high log P of batimastat were the principal factors contributing to poor absorption of batimastat. Accordingly, a program of work was undertaken to modify the physicochemical properties of batimastat. Over 50 compounds were produced in which solubilizing groups were introduced at the P3', P2', and/or α-position without adverse effect on in vitro potency *(50–53)*. The aqueous solubilities of the resulting compounds ranged from 0.003 to 30 mg/mL and the log P values from −2 to 4, but the blood levels of active species seen in the rat ex vivo bioassay following oral administration were not significantly improved. It was known from the literature that molecular weight also has an important effect on absorption and the route and rate of metabolism *(54)*. Thus compounds with molecular weight above a certain threshold are rapidly cleared via the liver, whereas compounds with lower molecular weight are cleared more slowly via the kidneys. In rats this molecular weight cut-off is at around 500, and the molecular weight of batimastat (478) is close to this limit. Furthermore, the more soluble analogs of batimastat described above, which were weakly absorbed, generally possessed higher molecular weights than batimastat itself.

Analysis of structure activity data suggested that the size of the α-substituent, and hence the molecular weight, could be reduced without adversely affecting the in vitro activity of the compounds. We thought that replacement of the α-thienylthiomethylene group of batimastat by a hydroxy substituent would produce active compounds with lower molecular weight and increased aqueous solubility. The first compound to be produced, BB-1090 13 with a P2′ phenylalanine residue *(55)*, was indeed more soluble than batimastat and possessed comparable in vitro activity although the activity against stromelysin was somewhat reduced. We have routinely used an ex vivo bioassay in the rat to provide an indication of oral absorption (Table 2). Following oral administration of batimastat (10 mg/kg p.o.) the concentration of active inhibitor in the blood remained below the limit of sensitivity of the assay. On changing the thienylthiomethylene α-substituent of batimastat to an α-hydroxy substituent, providing BB-1090 13, a substantial increase in the systemic exposure was observed (Table 2).

We hypothesized that the replacement of the P2′ phenylalanine residue of BB-1090 13 with an unnatural amino acid residue might reduce proteolytic metabolism and hence increase oral activity and duration of action. From the series of analogs, BB-1433 14 stood out as possessing potent broad spectrum activity with enhanced inhibition of stromelysin-1 in comparison to BB-1090 13, but disappointingly, the oral absorption of this compound 14 was no better than that of BB-1090 13 (Table 2) *(56)*.

Workers at Upjohn have demonstrated that a major problem in transporting peptides and pseudopeptides across membranes is the presence of secondary amide bonds *(57)*. These can form strong hydrogen bonds to water and this solvation energy is lost on entering a lipid membrane. Evidence has been presented showing that this effect is not only dependent on the hydrogen bond number but as expected, on hydrogen bond strength. Thus it appeared to be desirable to introduce specific groups that lead to a reduction in intermolecular hydrogen bond potential. Indeed, the beneficial effect of a hydroxyl α-substituent may in part be due to intramolecular hydrogen bonds being formed at the expense of intermolecular hydrogen bonds.

However, N-methylation of either the P1′-P2′ amide or the P2′-P3′ amide was inappropriate since structure-activity studies had previously shown that this caused a reduction in potency. This observation can be rationalized by analysis of X-ray

Table 2
Results from the Ex Vivo Bioassay Following Oral Dosing of Compounds to Rats and Marmosets

	Rat ex vivo bioassay (10 mg/kg p.o.)		Marmoset ex vivo bioassay (30 mg/kg p.o.)	
Compound	Peak Conc (ng/mL)	AUC (0.5–6h) (ng/mL.h)	Peak Conc (ng/mL)	AUC (0.5–24h) ng/mL.h
BB-1090 (13)	143 @ 0.5h	540	nd	nd
BB-1433 (14)	102 @ 0.5h	297	320 @ 0.5h	1550
Marimastat (2)	278 @ 0.5h	686	4050 @ 1h	16300
(17)	336 @ 1h	2087	38,110 @ 1h	246,440

crystal structure of batimastat bound to human neutrophil collagenase *(58)*, which shows that the carbonyl and N-H groups of the two amides are intimately involved in hydrogen bonding to the enzyme. As an alternative to alkylation of the amides we considered that the introduction of steric bulk in the vicinity of the two amides might reduce intermolecular hydrogen bond potential. Indeed, it has been shown using solution infra-red spectroscopy that in a series of alkyl amides the t-butyl group greatly reduces intermolecular hydrogen bonding *(59)*.

We considered that a bulky t-butyl P2′ group might shield these amide bonds from intermolecular hydrogen bonding without affecting enzyme inhibitory activity since it was clear from structure-activity studies, and subsequently from structural studies, that the P2′ substituent points away from the enzyme. Indeed, we found that combination of the P2′ *tert*-leucine modification with the favorable α-hydroxy substituent identified earlier had a synergistic effect on oral absorption for the compound marimastat (BB-2516) 2 *(56)*. Following oral administration of marimastat to the marmoset, both C_{max} and AUC were greater than those seen in rats (Table 2). By comparison of the AUC following oral and intravenous administration using liquid chromatography mass spectroscopy (LCMS) assay (data not shown), the oral bioavailability of marimastat was found to be 18% in the rat and 50% in the marmoset.

The greater oral bioavailability of marimastat as compared with batimastat is likely to be due to a combination of its reduced molecular weight, a lower log P, good aqueous solubility and the effect of the α-hydroxy group and P2′ *tert*-butyl group. These two groups may lower the desolvation energy penalty for oral absorption by participating in internal hydrogen bonding (α-hydroxy group) and shielding the amide backbone (P2′ *tert*-butyl group). Marimastat is a broad spectrum inhibitor of MMP enzymes (Table 1) although it is less active against stromelysin-1 than batimastat. In addition, marimastat is a selective

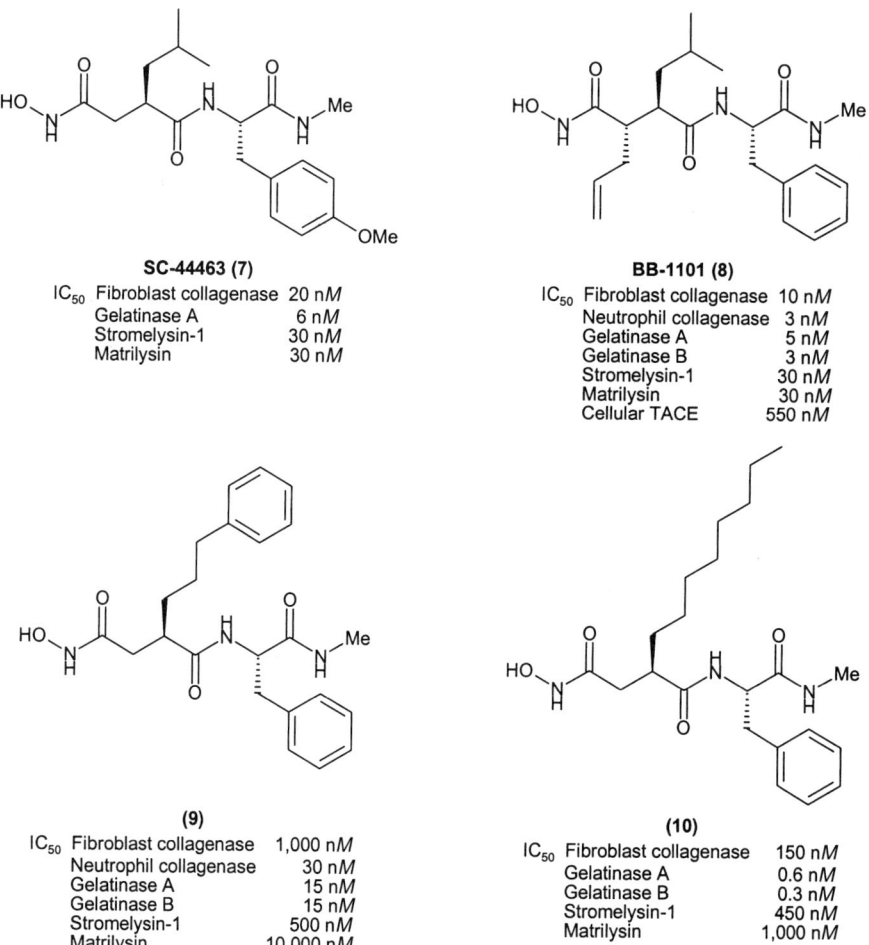

Fig. 7. Structures and in vitro activities of selected "right-hand side" matrix metalloproteinase inhibitors.

inhibitor of the MMP enzymes over vascular metalloproteinases such as angiotensin converting enzyme (30% inhibition at 100 μM) and enkephalinase (IC$_{50}$ 4 μM).

Since the first reports of the discovery of marimastat, there has been considerable interest in the synthesis of analogs. The DuPont Merck group introduced an α-methyl in addition to the α-hydroxy group (e.g., 15; Fig. 7) *(60)*. There is a strong preference for S-stereochemistry at this position (i.e., α-hydroxy group orientation is opposite to that for marimastat). Furthermore, phenylpropyl is reported to be the optimal substituent at P1′ in the DuPont Merck series and, rather surprisingly, compound 15 potently inhibits not only MMP-3 and MMP-9 which

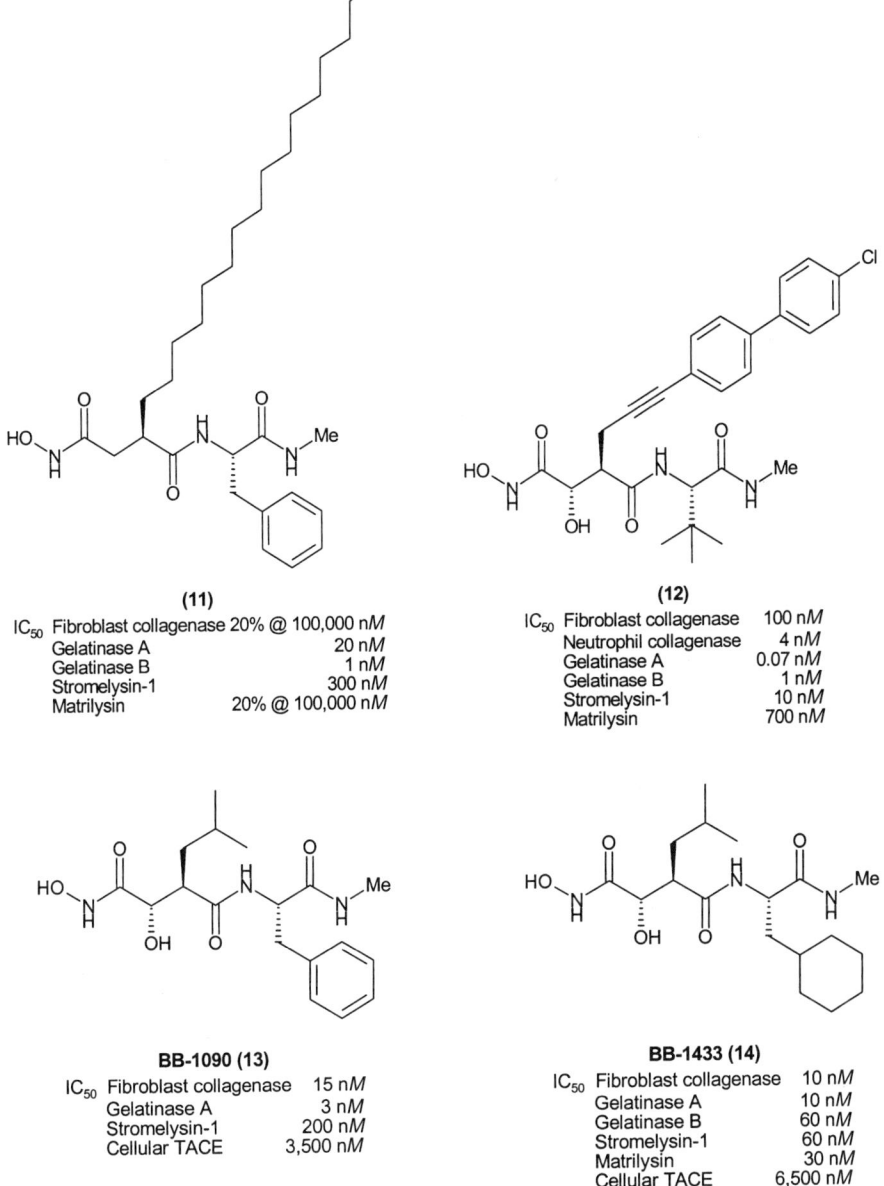

(11)

IC$_{50}$ Fibroblast collagenase 20% @ 100,000 nM
Gelatinase A 20 nM
Gelatinase B 1 nM
Stromelysin-1 300 nM
Matrilysin 20% @ 100,000 nM

(12)

IC$_{50}$ Fibroblast collagenase 100 nM
Neutrophil collagenase 4 nM
Gelatinase A 0.07 nM
Gelatinase B 1 nM
Stromelysin-1 10 nM
Matrilysin 700 nM

BB-1090 (13)

IC$_{50}$ Fibroblast collagenase 15 nM
Gelatinase A 3 nM
Stromelysin-1 200 nM
Cellular TACE 3,500 nM

BB-1433 (14)

IC$_{50}$ Fibroblast collagenase 10 nM
Gelatinase A 10 nM
Gelatinase B 60 nM
Stromelysin-1 60 nM
Matrilysin 30 nM
Cellular TACE 6,500 nM

Fig. 7. *(continued on next page)*

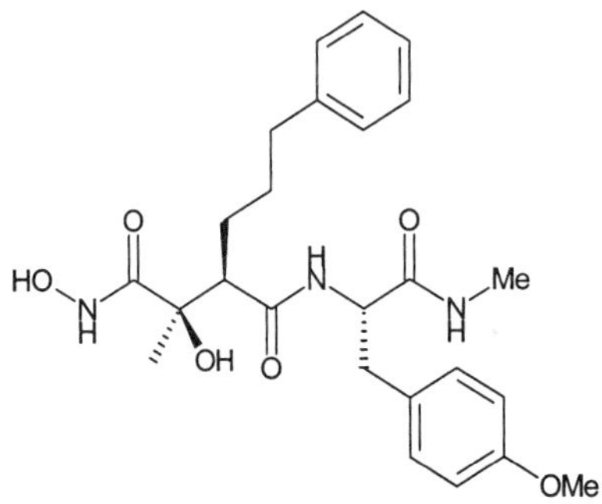

DuPont Merck (15)

IC$_{50}$ Fibroblast collagenase 2 nM
      Gelatinase B   < 1 nM
      Stromelysin-1   3 nM

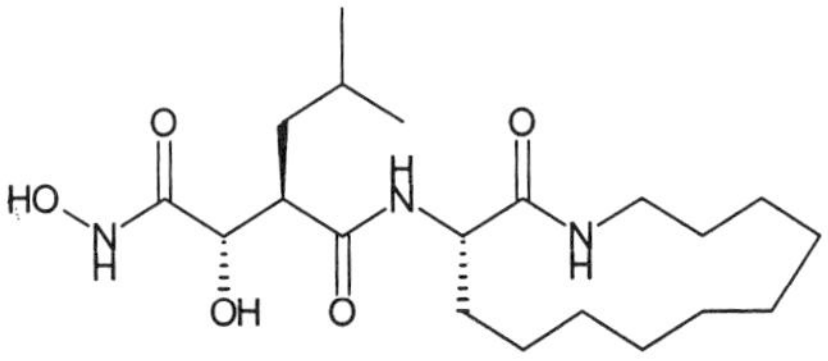

BB-1909 (16)

IC$_{50}$ Fibroblast collagenase   30 nM
      Neutrophil collagenase 20 nM
      Gelatinase A   20 nM
      Stromelysin-1   500 nM
      Matrilysin   200 nM
      Cellular TACE   2,250 nM

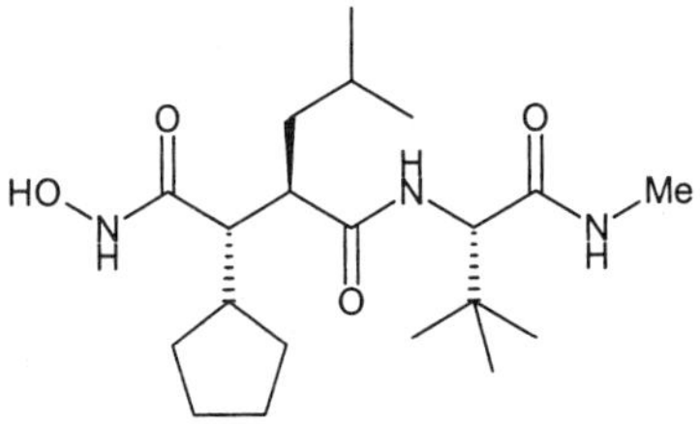

(17)

IC$_{50}$ Fibroblast collagenase   4 nM
      Neutrophil collagenase 20 nM
      Gelatinase A   3 nM
      Gelatinase B   9 nM
      Stromelysin-1   30 nM
      Matrilysin   20 nM
      Cellular TACE   900 nM

Fig. 7. *(continued)*

both have a deep extended S1′ pocket, but also MMP-1 which has a shorter S1′ pocket. An X-ray crystal structure of 15 complexed to the catalytic domain of MMP-3 indicates the presence of a hydrogen bond between the α-hydroxy group and the backbone of Ala[165], as predicted by modeling, and a Van-der-Waals (VDW) interaction between the P1′ aryl group and His[201] *(60)*. An X-ray crystal structure of BB-1909 16, an analog of marimastat, complexed to the catalytic domain of human neutrophil collagenase reveals that the hydroxyl is directed away from the protein surface and is hydrogen-bonded to a solvent molecule *(61)*. In BB-1909, the P2′ and P3′ groups are cyclized via a lactam. The ring size has to be such that it allows the P2′-P3′ amide bond to exist in the *trans* conformation since both the carbonyl and NH hydrogen bond to the enzyme backbone.

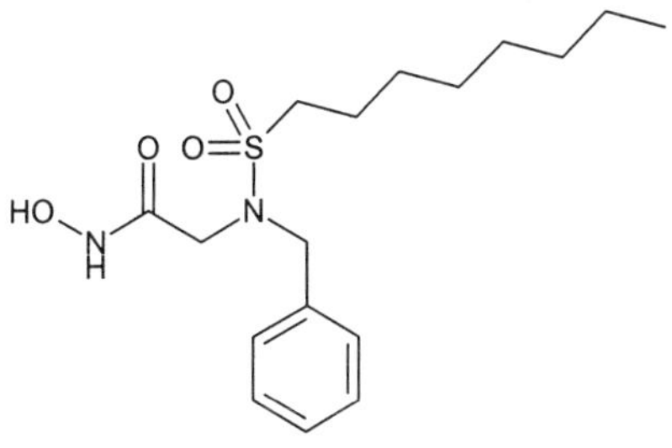

(18)

IC$_{50}$	Fibroblast collagenase 50% @ 100,000 nM
	Gelatinase A	200 nM
	Stromelysin-1	700 nM

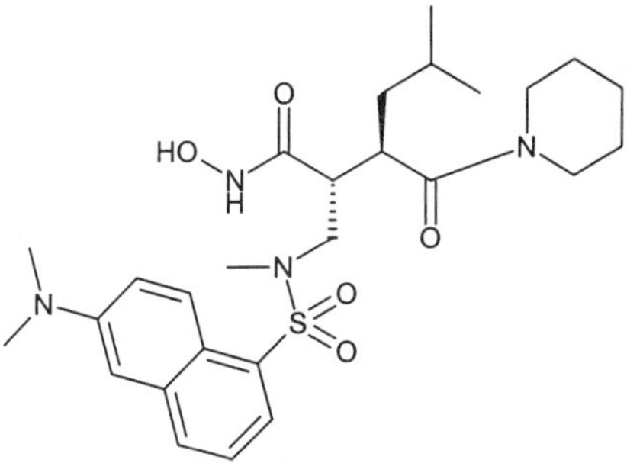

(19)

IC$_{50}$	Fibroblast collagenase	6 nM
	Neutrophil collagenase	4 nM
	Collagenase-3	6 nM
	Gelatinase A	40 nM
	Stromelysin-1	30 nM

Fig. 8. Structures and in vitro activities of selected nonpeptidic matrix metalloproteinase inhibitors.

Others have prepared cyclic BB-1101 analogs by linking the α- and P2′ substituents *(62,63)*. We have investigated compounds in which an α-cycloalkyl group is introduced as possible backup to marimastat. In the case of the α-cyclopentyl derivative (17; Fig 7), a high level of oral availability was observed in rat and marmoset MMP-1 ex vivo bioassays (Table 2) *(64)*.

2.3. Nonpeptidic Inhibitors

Independently of workers at Ciba-Geigy (now Novartis) *(65,66)*, we identified a series of sulfonamide hydroxamic acid derivatives (e.g., 18; Fig. 8) *(67,68)*. We have been able to prepare a large number of analogs using solid-phase methods for array synthesis of hydroxamic acids *(22,23)*.

Truncation of the P2′–P3′ group of pseudo-peptide succinyl hydroxamic acid derivatives has been shown by the Roche group to lead to orally active compounds which tend to be selective for the collagenases *(69)*. The Roche compounds feature a cyclic imide group at P1. We have shown that a sulfonamide moiety can be incorporated at P1 (e.g., 19; Fig. 8) and different substituents can be used to vary the enzyme selectivity *(70)*.

3. PHARMACOLOGICAL EFFECTS IN DISEASE MODELS

The MMPs are produced by tumor cells, activated leucocytes, and connective tissue cells in a wide range of malignant or inflammatory diseases *(71,72)*. In any diseased tissue, multiple MMPs are over-expressed or activated when compared to normal tissues. The presence of active MMPs in local excess over the levels of their natural inhibitors, the TIMPs, is thought to mediate pathology in many of these conditions *(73)*. It is only by testing MMP inhibitors in models of these disorders that their pathological significance can be confirmed. MMPs may be involved in at least three aspects of cancer progression *(74)*. First, MMPs are implicated in facilitating tumor metastasis, which is the process whereby tumor cells enter neighboring blood vessels and lymphatics where they are transported to different organs and establish secondary tumors. Secondly, the growth at secondary tumor sites requires MMPs to aid breakdown and remodeling of the surrounding tissue. Thirdly, tumors need a blood supply in order to grow above a certain size and it has been hypothesized that MMP activity aids the invasive ingrowth of new blood vessels (angiogenesis). Opdenakker has proposed that MMPs function in analogous ways in inflammation, mediating migration of inflammatory leucocytes through connective tissues, contributing to the tissue destruction and remodeling seen in many inflammatory diseases and even to the angiogenesis observed in chronic arthritis *(75)*. The effects of MMP inhibitors in animal models of cancer, inflammatory and infectious diseases are now reviewed.

3.1. Cancer Models

Experimental models of cancer usually involve the transfer of human tumor cell lines into immunocompromized nude or severe combined immunodeficiency (SCID) mice, although some models involve the transfer of mouse or rat tumor cells into immunologically intact rodents. Endpoints for these models can include survival, extent of tumor spread, or tumor burden. MMP inhibitors have been tested in models of almost all forms of human cancer including lymphoma, colorectal, pancreatic, lung, prostate, hemangioma, melanoma, ovarian, and breast.

In a model of human breast carcinoma regrowth of tumor at the site of primary tumor resection was significantly inhibited by batimastat *(76)*, as could the number and size of lung metastases. Batimastat has also been shown to enhance survival and inhibit the growth of secondary lesions and lymphatic metastases from a rat mammary carcinoma *(77)*. CT-1746, a hydroxamate inhibitor with selectivity for gelatinases, enhanced survival and caused a marked inhibition in the growth and metastatic spread of human colon carcinomas implanted orthotopically in the colon wall *(78)*. Batimastat was also shown to increase survival and decrease tumor growth in a model using transplanted tumor fragments *(79)*, and to decrease in vivo growth of two tumor lines *(80)*. In a peritoneal ascites model of ovarian cancer, batimastat when given alone increased survival and reduced tumor burden *(81)* and when given in combination with cisplatin had a synergistic effect on survival *(82)*. Batimastat also prolonged survival and decreased tumor burden in models of pancreatic *(83)* and prostate cancers *(84)*. Batimastat has also been shown to reduce the growth of a murine hemangioma caused by subcutaneous injection of a transformed endothelioma cell line *(85)*, but was ineffective in controlling the spread or growth of a Burkitt lymphoma cell line in SCID mice *(86)*. Santos and coworkers have shown that AG3340 and related compounds could reduce the growth of a Lewis Lung carcinoma in mice *(87)*. They also showed that the growth of a B-16 mouse melanoma could be reduced by AG3287 and AG3296.

3.2. Autoimmune Inflammation

MMP inhibitors have been tested in models of rheumatoid arthritis, multiple sclerosis, uveitis, and Guillain-Barre syndrome.

Rheumatoid arthritis is a chronic inflammatory disease which predominantly involves the joints, resulting in pain, swelling and eventual destruction of the normal joint architecture. Affected joints are infiltrated with activated leucocytes. An arthritis-like syndrome can be induced in rodents following injection with complete Freunds adjuvant. In the rat adjuvant arthritis model, batimastat given intraperitoneally from onset of symptoms significantly reduced paw swelling, bone degradation, and cartilage breakdown *(88)*. BB-1101 and BB-1433 given orally were similarly effective on paw swelling and bone degradation *(89)*. Connolly and coworkers also showed that GI168 administered by minipump commencing prior to symptom onset significantly reduced ankle swelling, bone and cartilage destruction and also reduced the deposition of new bone and pannus *(90)*.

Multiple sclerosis (MS) is a chronic disabling condition in which activated leucocytes accumulate at local sites within the brain or spinal cord, where they are associated with edema and damage to the insulating myelin sheath around nerves. The majority of animal models of MS involve the generation of an autoimmune response to components of the myelin sheath which leads to a T cell-dependent inflammation of the spinal cord or brain. In classical experimental autoimmune encephalomyelitis (EAE), animals are immunized with myelin or one of its protein components in adjuvant, resulting in a progressive paralytic disease that resolves over a period of 1 to 2 wk. Transfer of activated T cells can also result in a chronic disease with recurrent episodes of paralysis or relapse. An alternative model of MS has been described in which a demyelinated inflammatory lesion is induced as a consequence of a delayed-type hypersensitivity response (DTH) generated locally in the brain. MMP inhibitors have shown efficacy in models of MS. Gijbels and coworkers have shown that GM-6001 given continuously or from disease onset can ameliorate symptoms of EAE *(91)*. Hewson and coworkers using Ro 31-9790 showed a reduction in disease severity in both EAE and in an adoptive transfer EAE model when compound was given from disease induction *(92)*. BB-1101 was shown to reduce the severity of disease in EAE when given prior to symptom onset *(93)*, and to reduce both the severity and incidence of relapse in chronic relapsing EAE *(94)*. Matyszak and Perry have also shown that BB-1101 inhibits the inflammation and demyelination associated with the DTH model of MS *(95)*.

Guillain Barré syndrome (GBS) is an acute inflammatory paralytic disease of the peripheral nervous system in which leucocytes infiltrate nerves causing demyelination and edema. Experimental autoimmune neuritis (EAN), the animal model of GBS, results from immunization with peripheral nerve myelin which leads to a T cell-dependent inflammation in peripheral nerves. BB-1101 given from initial immunization could prevent the development of symptoms and reduced the inflammation, demyelination, and weight loss in EAN *(96)*. When given from onset of symptoms, the compound significantly reduced disease severity.

Uveoretinitis is an autoimmune inflammatory disease of the eye. Animal models of uveitis involve immunization with retinal antigens in adjuvant. Treatment with BB-1101 was shown to reduce retinal damage in experimental autoimmune uveitis *(97)*.

3.3. Other Inflammatory Diseases

In stroke, a blood vessel in the brain becomes blocked either by a blood clot or by a local hemorrhage. The lack of oxygen in the infarcted area of brain supplied by the blocked vessel causes loss of neurons resulting in disability. The infarcted area becomes the focus for an inflammatory response which may be exacerbated during reperfusion of the tissue. Animal models of stroke usually involve clipping or blocking the midcerebral artery to give either permanent or temporary occlusion and reperfusion. Alternatively, injection of blood or bacterial collagenase into the brain can cause a local hemorrhage. Rosenberg has shown that BB-1101 reduces the early phases of blood brain barrier leakage in an ischemia reperfusion model in the rat *(98)*, and the secondary brain edema which occurs following hemorrhage *(99)*.

Restenosis of vessels is a common complication of balloon catheter angioplasty, which is used to treat atherosclerosis. Similar thickening of the vessel wall can be seen in rats following balloon angioplasty. Batimastat given for 7–14 d post angioplasty was shown to reduce thickening of the carotid artery significantly *(100)*. In similar studies, treatment with GM6001 only resulted in a transient effect on vessel thickening *(101)*, but significantly reduced collagen deposition in the vessel wall *(102)*.

Glomerulonephritis is an inflammatory disease which can result in destruction and fibrosis of the kidney. A nephritic syndrome can be generated in rats by injection of an antibody against Thy-1.1. BB-1101 given prior to disease induction significantly reduced the inflammatory response and kidney damage, but was less effective given after disease induction *(103)*.

3.4. Infectious Diseases

Bacterial meningitis is an acute life-threatening disease of the central nervous system. Rodents can develop meningitis following infection with particular bacteria. Batimastat was shown to be effective in reducing intracranial pressure and blood brain barrier breakdown in a model of meningococcal meningitis *(104)*.

4. CLINICAL DEVELOPMENT

British Biotech has taken four MMPIs into clinical development starting with batimastat which was subsequently superseded by the orally active compound marimastat. More recently BB-2983 and BB-3644 have been evaluated in the clinic, the former in collaboration with Glaxo Wellcome.

4.1. Clinical Trials with Batimastat

Batimastat was the first MMP inhibitor to be administered systemically to humans. The initial study with this compound was conducted in April 1992 in six patients with advanced breast cancer. The compound was given as a capsule to be taken by mouth and patients received single doses ranging from 50 to 1000 mg. Unfortunately, little or no batimastat was detected in plasma samples taken following administration. Attempts were made to improve oral bioavailability through different formulations but these were largely unsuccessful. In a comparative bioavailability study, a single dose of 250 mg of batimastat given to healthy male volunteers only resulted in low plasma exposure (AUC 0–24 of 70–120 μg/L.hr). Although batimastat was tested as a repeated oral treatment in a second study in patients with advanced breast cancer, the low oral bioavailability led to the exploration of other routes of delivery. Further development of batimastat took the form of a suspension to be administered intra-peritoneally or intra-pleurally in patients with malignant effusions. This indication was supported by promising results from a xenograft model of human ovarian malignant ascites in which intraperitoneal batimastat was shown to resolve the ascites and significantly prolong survival *(81)*.

A phase I study of intraperitoneal batimastat was conducted in patients with symptomatic malignant ascites. Patients with any form of malignancy who required paracentesis for symptomatic relief were eligible for the study. Sixteen of the 23 patients in the study had ascites secondary to an ovarian carcinoma. Patients received a single intraperitoneal dose of batimastat ($150–1350$ mg/m^2) in 500 mL 5% dextrose after paracentesis. In this study batimastat was generally well tolerated and there were early signs of efficacy with several patients requiring no further paracentesis for over 3 mo. Surprisingly, high plasma concentrations of batimastat were demonstrated 1 h after dosing, the mean Cmax ranging from 595 μg/L following 150 mg/m^2 to 1436 μg/L following 1350 mg/m^2. Batimastat was still present in plasma at day 28 at concentrations ranging from mean 20 μg/L after 150 mg/m^2 to 226 μg/L after 1350 mg/m^2. Blood concentrations fell with a long half-life of 19 d and this was attributed to the slow dissolution of batimastat within the peritoneum, where the suspension effectively formed a depot. The total AUC (0–28 d) following a dose of 150 mg/m^2 (approx 240 mg) was 80,112 μg/L.h. Vomiting, fatigue, fever, and abdominal pain were the most common events recorded during the study but were not considered unusual for this patient group. No significant acute peritoneal reactions were seen *(105)*.

A second phase I study in patients with malignant ascites secondary to a gastrointestinal malignancy gave similar results with signs of efficacy in some patients and a reasonable safety profile *(106)*. Batimastat was also administered intra-peritoneally to patients with advanced malignancy without ascites. In this setting, abdominal discomfort appeared to limit the dose of batimastat that could be administered.

A phase I study was also conducted in patients with malignant pleural effusion. Patients with symptomatic malignant pleural effusion received lower doses of batimastat (15–135 mg/m^2), given intrapleurally in 50 mL 5% dextrose after aspiration of the effusion. Batimastat was well tolerated and again there were early signs that the drug might be effective in palliation of this condition, with patients receiving the higher doses showing a significant improvement in dyspnoea scores *(107)*.

Although initial clinical results gave signs of efficacy with batimastat, larger Phase III studies indicated issues with tolerability and the clinical program was discontinued in favor of the orally available drug marimastat.

4.2. Clinical Trials with Marimastat

As a result of the experience with batimastat and other early compounds, improved oral bioavailability became an important milestone in the design and development of MMP inhibitors. Marimastat can be classed as a "second generation" inhibitor, and distinguished from earlier compounds on this basis. Like batimastat, it is a broad spectrum inhibitor with low nanomolar activity against the principal members of the MMP family except stromelysin-1 (IC$_{50}$ 200 n*M*). In single and repeat dose studies in healthy volunteers, oral marimastat gave good plasma exposure in a dose proportional manner (Fig. 9). A dose of 200 mg (the highest dose used in the repeat dose study) gave an AUC$_{0-12\,hrs}$ of 5461 μg/l.h following the initial dose, rising to 8009 μg/l.h on the final day of a seven day study of twice daily administration *(108)*. This increase in plasma exposure can be attributed to the attainment of steady-state. Accumulation has not been observed during longer treatment periods. The terminal elimination half-life measured in healthy subjects ranged from 7–10 h. Marimastat was well tolerated in both of these studies and significant findings were confined to a serial rise in serum alanine aminotransferase (ALT) in one subject receiving 200 mg twice daily. The levels in this subject reached 2.5 times the upper limit of the normal range 5 d after the end of the study but returned to normal in the following 2 wk. More modest increases in transaminase levels were recorded in the three remaining subjects at this dose level. There were no accompanying changes in γGT or bilirubin *(108)*.

Early studies in cancer patients with marimastat have followed both conventional and nonconventional routes. The former is represented by a phase I study, of standard dose-escalating design, in patients with advanced lung cancer *(109)*. The primary objective of this study was to establish a maximum tolerated dose on the basis of toxicity and side effect profile. Twelve patients received doses of 25, 50, or 100 mg twice daily over the study period of 12 wk. As expected, there were no objective cytoreductive responses to marimastat although two patients showed stable disease for a period of at least 8 wk. The study was successful in identifying the principal treatment-related side effect for marimastat, namely musculoskeletal pain and joint stiffness. At the lower doses of 25 and 50 mg these effects were generally mild and patients continued treatment. However, at a dose of 100 mg twice daily, musculoskeletal side effects were severe and led to an interruption in treatment in 5 of 6 patients within 18–58 d. The most commonly affected region was the shoulder girdle although in some patients multiple joints in the arms and legs were also affected. The condition has been described variously as tenosynovitis, tendinitis, or polyarthralgia. It was not found to be responsive to prophylactic treatment with either nonsteroidal antiinflammatory drugs or low dose prednisone (10–20 mg/d). However, the effects were generally reversible within a period of approx 2 wk of stopping treatment.

The plasma concentrations of marimastat in these patients were higher than predicted from the healthy volunteer studies with 12 h trough levels ranging from 173 μg/L at a dose of 25 mg to 540 μg/L at 100 mg. By comparison trough levels in healthy subjects receiving 100 mg twice daily would be expected to be in the range of 80–100 μg/l. The conclusion from this study was that a dose of 50 mg twice daily should be reasonably well tolerated over a period of 8 wk but that, in view of the higher than expected plasma levels, lower doses of marimastat should also be explored.

Marimastat was expected to be tumorostatic rather than cytotoxic and hence for Phase II the conventional approach of measuring reduction in tumor size could not be used. Two approaches were therefore utilized; the first was to monitor cancer antigen levels and the second was to look at changes in histology of accessible tumors.

For the first approach a series of similarly designed studies that recorded the rate of rise of serum cancer antigens in cancer patients, both in the month prior to receiving marimastat and in a one month treatment period were designed. The antigens measured (CEA, PSA, CA125, and CA19-9) have been used clinically to follow the course of malignant disease, with a fall in levels accompanying a response to cytotoxic therapy and a rise often preceding a clinical manifestation of relapse *(110,111)*. The intention was to use changes in the rate of rise of these antigens as a pharmacodynamic marker of the activity of the drug, where a fall or slower rate of rise might reflect a slowing in the rate of disease progression, and to relate this to the side effect profile observed.

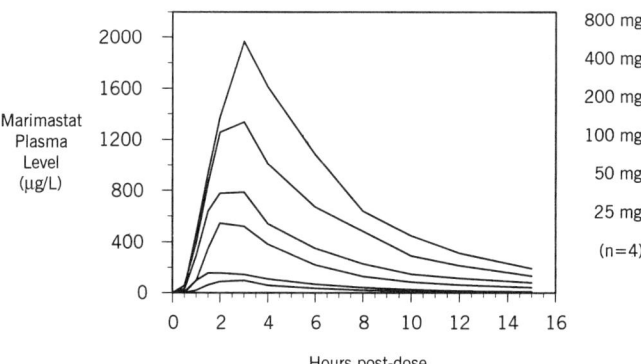

Fig. 9. Plasma concentrations of BB-2516 in human volunteers after a single oral dose.

In total six "cancer antigen" studies were performed, two each in patients with ovarian and colorectal cancer, and one each in patients with pancreatic and prostatic cancer. Patients were recruited in dose groups, with doses ranging from 5 mg once daily to 50 mg twice daily. The inherent variability in cancer antigen levels meant that it was difficult to draw conclusions from the individual studies but a combined analysis did reveal a significant relationship between dose and a reduction in the rate of rise of cancer antigens *(112–114)* (Fig. 10). From these results, it appeared that a biological activity might exist at doses equal to or greater than 10 mg twice daily. Analysis of adverse events during these studies, and during a continuation treatment period, showed musculoskeletal pain and inflammation to be the predominant treatment/dose-related effect. On the basis of the effects on cancer antigens and the side effect profile a dose range of 10–25 mg twice daily was recommended for further study *(112)*.

The second approach of looking for indications of the intended activity of marimastat involved the examination of samples of tumor tissue for evidence of increased fibrosis. In some of the animal cancer models in which MMP inhibitors have been tested there appeared to be an encapsulation of the tumor in fibrotic tissue *(81)*. This approach was explored in the clinic in a phase I study in which patients with advanced gastric or gastro-oesophageal adenocarcinoma were examined endoscopically before and after a one month treatment period with marimastat (50 mg twice daily or 25 mg once daily). Treatment at both doses was shown to be associated with changes in the macroscopic and histological appearance of the tumors consistent with an increase in the quantity of fibrotic stromal tissue *(115)*.

The safety and tolerability of marimastat has also been studied clinically in combination with cytotoxic chemotherapies. Results from a trial of marimastat and carboplatin in patients with advanced ovarian cancer showed that the two agents

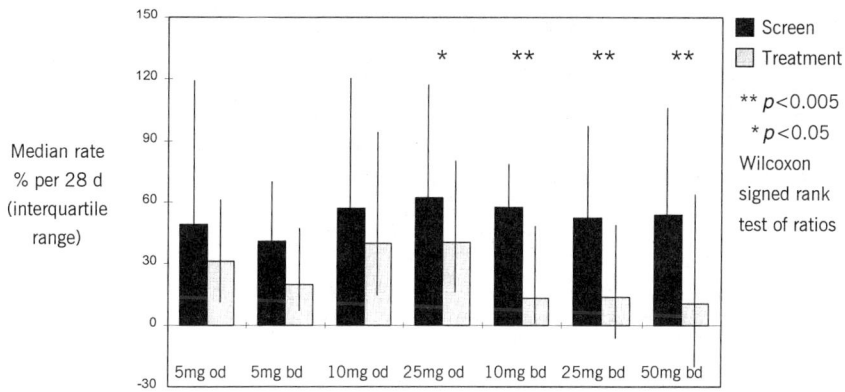

Fig. 10. Rate of rise of serum cancer antigens in patients with advanced cancer before (screen) and during treatment with different doses of marimastat.

could be administered in combination without apparent potentiation of the side effects of either drug *(116)*. Similarly, marimastat and gemcitabine appear to be well tolerated in combination in patients with pancreatic cancer *(117)*. The combinations of marimastat and 5-fluorouracil or marimastat and doxorubicin/cyclophosphamide have also been explored in Phase I studies. Preliminary results indicate that these combinations are well tolerated *(118,119)*. These results are important since animal cancer model data indicate that it is likely that MMP inhibitors will be most effective if used early in combination with chemotherapy *(82,120,121)*.

Marimastat is currently being tested in a range of randomized placebo-controlled studies in patients with advanced pancreatic, gastric, lung, breast, and ovarian cancers, as well as in patients with glioblastoma. Although advanced cancer may not be the ideal setting for a tumorostatic agent, these trials may show a survival advantage for patients receiving marimastat, and should also provide the sort of controlled safety data that will be required to conduct studies in the adjuvant setting, where from a theoretical basis one might expect the effects of these inhibitors to be greatest.

5. CONCLUSION

MMP inhibitors such as marimastat may be an important new class of therapeutic agents for the treatment of diseases characterized by excessive extracellular matrix degradation and/or remodeling, such as cancer. However, rather than treating the primary cause of the disease, they will serve as disease-modifying agents which should stabilize the condition. Results from randomized clinical trials which will become available in the next few years will define the true utility of MMP inhibitors.

ACKNOWLEDGMENTS

The authors wish to thank the many scientists at British Biotech who have been involved in the MMP inhibitor research and development program. Thanks are due also to Jenny Edge for assistance in the preparation of this review and Dr. Paul Beckett for helpful discussions.

REFERENCES

1. Beckett, R.P., Davidson, A.H., Drummond, A.H., Huxley, P., and Whittaker, M. (1996) Recent advances in matrix metalloproteinase inhibitor research. *Drug Discovery Today,* 1, 16–26.
2. Beckett, R.P. (1996) Recent advances in the field of matrix metalloproteinase inhibitors. *Exp. Opin. Ther. Patents,* 6, 1305–1315.
3. Davidson, A.H., Drummond, A.H., Galloway, W.A., and Whittaker, M. (1997) The inhibition of matrix metalloproteinase enzymes. *Chem. Ind.,* 258–261.
4. Brown, P., and Whittaker, M. (1998) Matrix metalloproteinase inhibitors; design, development and early clinical trials. *Biotech. Med.,* 9, 11–16.
5. Whittaker, M., and Brown, P. (1998) Recent advances in matrix metalloproteinase inhibitor research and development. *Curr. Opin. Drug Disc. Dev.,* 1, 157–164.
6. Beckett, R.P., and Whittaker, M. (1998) Matrix metalloproteinase inhibitors 1998. *Exp. Opin. Ther. Patents,* 8, 259–282.
7. Mohler, K.M., Sleath, P.R., Fitzner, J.N., Cerretti, D.P., Alderson, M., Kerwar, S.S., Torrance, D.S., Otten-Evans, C., Greenstreet, T., Weerawarna, K., Kronheim, S.R., Petersen, M., Gerhart, M., Kozlosky, C.J., March, C.J., and Black, R.A. (1994) Protection against a lethal dose of endotoxin by an inhibitor of tumor necrosis factor processing. *Nature,* 370, 218–220.
8. Gearing, A.J.H., Beckett, P., Christodoulou, M., Churchill, M., Clements, J., Davidson, A.H., Drummond, A.H., Galloway, W.A., Gilbert, R., Gordon, J.L., Leber, T.M., Mangan, M., Miller, K., Nayee, P., Owen, K., Patel, S., Thomas, W., Wells, G., Wood, L.M., and Woolley K. (1994) Processing of tumor necrosis factor-α by metalloproteinases. *Nature,* 370, 555–557.
9. McGeehan, G.M., Becherer, J.D., Bast, R.C., Boyer, C.M., Champion, B., Connolly, K.M., Conway, J.G., Furdon, P., Karp, S., Kidao, S., McElroy, A.B., Nichols, J., Pryzwansky, K.M., Schoenen, F., Sekut, L., Truesdale, A., Verghese, M., Warner, J., and Ways, J.P. (1994) Regulation of Tumor Necrosis Factor-α Processing by a Metalloproteinase Inhibitor. *Nature,* 370, 558–561.
10. Babine, R.E., and Bender, S.L. (1997) Molecular recognition of protein-ligand complexes: Applications to drug design. *Chem. Rev.,* 97, 1359–1472.
11. Whittaker, M. (1998) Discovery of protease inhibitors using targeted libraries. *Curr. Opin. Chemical Biology,* 2, 386–396.
12. Johnson, W.H., Roberts, N.A., and Borkakoti, N. (1987) Collagenase inhibitors: Their design and potential therapeutic use. *J. Enzyme Inhibition,* 2, 1–22.
13. Wahl, R.C., Dunlap, R.P., and Morgan, B.A. (1989) Biochemistry and inhibition of Collagenase and Stromelysin. *Ann. Rep. Med. Chem.,* 25, 177–184.
14. Johnson, W.H. (1990) A new class of disease-modifying antirheumatic drugs. *Drug News and Perspectives,* 3, 453–458.
15. Henderson, B., Docherty, A.J.P., and Beeley, N.R.A. (1990) Design of Inhibitors of Articular Cartilage Destruction. *Drugs of the future,* 15, 495–508.
16. Schwartz, M.A. and van Wart, H. (1992) Synthetic Inhibitors of Bacterial and Mammalian Interstitial Collagenases, in *Progress in Medicinal Chemistry;* Ellis G.P., Luscombe D.K., Eds., Elsevier Science Publishers BV.: The Netherlands, 29, 271–334.

17. Moore, W.M. and Spilburg, C.A. (1986) Peptide hydroxamic acids inhibit skin collagenase. *Biochem. Biophys. Res. Comm.,* 136, 390–395.

18. Moore, W.M. and Spilburg, C.A. (1986) Purification of human collagenases with a hydroxamic acid affinity column. *Biochem.,* 25, 5189–5195.

19. Odake, S., Okayama, T., Obata, M., Morikawa, T., Hattori, S., Hori, S., and Nagai, Y. (1990) Vertebrate collagenase inhibitor I. Tripeptidyl hydroxamic acids. *Chem. Pharm. Bull.,* 38, 1007–1011.

20. Odake, S., Okayama, T., Obata, M., Morikawa, T., Hattori, S., Hori, H., and Nagi, Y. (1991) Vertebrate collagenase inhibitor II. Tetrapeptidyl hydroxamic acids. *Chem. Pharm. Bull.,* 39, 1489–1494.

21. Odake, S., Morita, Y., Morikawa, T., Yoshida, N., Hori, H. and Nagai Y. (1994) Inhibition of matrix metalloproteinases by peptidyl hydroxamic acids. *Biochem. Biophys. Res. Comm.,* 199, 1442–1446.

22. Floyd, C.D. and Lewis, C.N. (1996) Synthesis of hydroxamic acid derivatives. PCT Patent WO9626223.

23. Floyd, C.D., Lewis, C.N., Patel, S.R., and Whittaker, M. (1996) A method for the synthesis of hydroxamic acids on solid phase. *Tetrahedron Lett.,* 37, 8045–8048.

24. Floyd, C.D., Lewis, C., Patel, S., and Whittaker, M. (1996) The automated synthesis of organic compounds—some newcomers have some success. *ISLAR '96 Proc.,* pp 51–76.

25. Floyd, C.D., Lewis, C.N., Patel, S.R., and Whittaker, M. (1996) Automated synthesis of organic compounds—A success story. *Screening Forum,* 4, 3–6.

26. Richter, L.S., and Desai, M.C. (1997) A TFA-cleavable linkage for solid-phase synthesis of hydroxamic acids. *Tetrahedron Lett.,* 38, 321–322.

27. Bauer, U., Ho, W-B., and Koskinen, A.M.P. (1997) A novel linkage for the solid-phase synthesis of hydroxamic acids. *Tetrahedron Lett.,* 38, 7233–7236.

28. Gordeev, M.F., Hui, H.C., Gordon, E.M., and Patel, D.V. (1997) A general and efficient solid phase synthesis of quinazoline-2,4-diones. *Tetrahedron Lett.,* 38, 1729–1732.

29. Mellor, S.L., McGuire, C., and Chan, W.C. (1997) N-Fmoc-aminooxy-2-chlorotrityl polystyrene resin: A facile solid-phase methodology for the synthesis of hydroxamic acids. *Tetrahedron Lett.,* 38, 3311–3314.

30. Ngu, K. and Patel, D.V. (1997) A new and efficient solid phase synthesis of hydroxamic acids. *J. Org. Chem.,* 62, 7088–7089.

31. Groneberg, R.G., Neuenschwander, K.W., Djuric, S.W., McGeehan, G.M., Burns, C.J., London, S.M., Morrissette, M.M., Salvino, J.M., Scotese, A.C., and Ullrich, J.W. (1997) Substituted (aryl, heteroaryl, arylmethyl or heteroarylmethyl) hydroxamic acid compounds. PCT Patent, WO9724117.

32. Patel, D. and Ngu, K. (1998) PCT Patent Application, WO 9818754.

33. Salvino, J.M., Morton, G.L., Mason, H.J., and Labaudiniere. (1998) PCT Patent Application, WO9829376.

34. Bode, W., Reinemer, P., Huber, R., Kleine, T., Schnierer, S., and Tschesche, H. (1994) The X-ray crystal structure of the catalytic domain of human neutrophil collagenase inhibited by a substrate analogue reveals the essentials for catalysis and specificity. *EMBO J.,* 13, 1263–1269.

35. Dickens, J.P., Donald, D.K., Kneen, G., and McKay, W.R. (1986), European Patent Application, EP-214,639-A.

36. Campion, C., Davidson, A.H., Dickens, J.P., and Crimmin, M.J. (1990) PCT Patent Application, WO9005719.

37. Ngo, J., Graul, A., and Castaner, J. (1996) Batimastat. *Drugs Future,* 21, 1215–1220.

38. Crimmin, M.J., Ayscough, A.P., and Beckett, R.P. (1994) PCT Patent Application, WO9424140.

39. Porter, J.R., Beeley, N.R.A., Boyce, B.A., Mason, B., Millican, A., Millar, K., Leonard, J., Morphy, J.R., and O'Connell, J.P. (1994) Potent and selective inhibitors of gelatinase-A 1. Hydroxamic acid derivatives. *Bioorg. Med. Chem. Lett.,* 4, 2741–2746.

40. Tomczuk, B.E., Gowravaram, M.R., Johnson, J.S., Delecki, D., Cook, E.R., Ghose, A.K., Mathiowetz, A.M., Spurlino, J.C., Rubin, B., Smith, D.L., Pulvino, T., and Wahl, R.C. (1995) Hydroxamate inhibitors of the matrix metallo-proteinases (MMPs) containing novel P1' heteroatom based modifications. *Bioorg. Med. Chem. Lett.*, 5, 343–348.

41. Wahl, R.C., Pulvino, T.A., Mathiowetz, A.M., Ghose, A.K., Johnson, J.S., Delecki, D., Cook, E.R., Gainor, J.A., Gowravaram, M.R., and Tomczuk, B.E. (1995) Hydroxamate inhibitors of human gelatinase B (92 kDa), *Bioorg. Med. Chem. Lett.*, 5, 349–352.

42. Gowravaram, M.R., Tomczuk, B.E., Johnson, J.S., Delecki, D., Cook, E.R., Ghose, A.K., Mathiowetz, A.M., Spurlino, J.C., Rubin, B., Smith, D.L., Pulvino, T., and Wahl, R.C. (1995) Inhibition of matrix metalloproteinases by hydroxamates containing heteroatom-based modifications of the P1' group, *J. Med. Chem.*, 38, 2570–2581.

43. Miller, A., Beckett, P.R., Martin, F.M., and Whittaker, M. (1995) PCT Patent Application, WO9532944.

44. Miller, A., Askew, M., Beckett, R.P., Bellamy, C.L., Bone, E.A., Coates, R.E., Davidson, A.H., Drummond, A.H., Huxley, P., Martin, F.M., Saroglou, L., Thompson, A.J., van Dijk, S.E., and Whittaker, M. (1997) Inhibition of matrix metalloproteinases: An examination of the S1' pocket. *Bioorg. Med. Chem. Lett.*, 7, 193–198.

45. Whittaker, M., Beckett, R.P., Spavold, Z.M., and Martin, F.M. (1998) PCT Patent Application, WO9824759.

46. Galardy, R.E. (1993) Galardin™, *Drugs of the Future*, 18, 1109–1111.

47. Levy, D.E., Lapierre, F., Liang, W., Ye, W., Lange, C.W., Li, X., Brobelny, D., Casabonne, M., Tyrrell, D., Holme, K., Nadzan, A., and Galardy, R.E. (1998) Matrix metalloproteinase inhibitors: A structure-activity study. *J. Med. Chem.*, 41, 199–223.

48. Plattner, J.J., and Norbeck, D.W. (1990) In Drug Discovery Technologies, eds. Clark, C.R. & Moos, W.H., (Ellis Horwood Ltd, Chichester, U.K.), pp. 92–126.

49. Singh, J., Conzentino, P., Cundy, K., Gainor, J.A., Gilliam, C.L., Gordon, T.D., Johnson, J.A., Morgan, B.A., Schneider, E.D., Wahl, R.C., and Whipple, D.A. (1995) Relationship between structure and bioavailability in a series of hydroxamate based metalloproteinase inhibitors. *Bioorg. Med. Chem. Lett.*, 5, 337–342.

50. Davidson, A.H., Dickens, J.P., and Crimmin, M.J. (1990) PCT Patent Application, WO9005716.

51. Campion, C., Davidson, A.H., Dickens, J.P., and Crimmin, M.J. (1991) PCT Patent Application, WO9102716.

52. Crimmin, M.J., Beckett, P.R., and Davis, M.H. (1994) PCT Patent Application, WO9421625.

53. Crimmin, M.J., and Beckett, R.P. (1995) PCT Patent Application, WO9509841.

54. Klaassen, C.D., and Watkins, J.B. (1984) Mechanisms of bile formation, hepatic uptake, and biliary excretion. *Pharmacol. Rev.*, 36, 1–67.

55. Dickens, S.P., Crimmin, M.S., and Beckett, R.P. (1994) PCT Patent Application, WO9402446.

56. Dickens, J.P., Crimmin, M.J., and Beckett, R.P. (1994) PCT Patent Application, WO9402447.

57. Conradi, R.A., Hilgers, A.R., Ho, N.F.H., and Burton, P.S. (1992) The influence of peptide structure on transport across Caco-2 cells. II. Peptide bond modification which results in improved permeability. *Pharm. Res.*, 9, 435–439.

58. Grams, F., Crimmin, M., Hinnes, L., Huxley, P., Pieper, M., Tschesche, H., and Bode, W. (1995) Structure determination and analysis of human neutrophil collagenase complexed with a hyroxamate inhibitor. *Biochemistry*, 34, 14012–14020.

59. Jones, R.L. (1964) Steric inhibition of hydrogen-bonding in a secondary amide. *Spectrochimica Acta*, 20, 1879–1882.

60. Jacobson, I.C., Reddy, P.G., Wasserman, Z.R., Harman, K.D., Covington, M.B., Arner, E.C., Copeland, R.A., Decicco, C.P., and Magolda, R.L. (1998) Structure-based design and synthesis of a series of hydroxamic acids with a quaternary-hydroxy group in P1 as inhibitors of matrix metalloproteinases. *Bioorg. Med. Chem. Lett.*, 8, 837–842.

61. Betz, M., Huxley, P., Davies, S.J., Mushtaq, Y., Pieper, M., Tschesche, H., Bode, W., and Gomis-ruth, F.X. (1997) 1.9-Å crystal structure of the catalytic domain of human neutrophil collagenase (matrix metalloproteinase-8) complexed with a peptidomimetic hydroxamate primed-side inhibitor with a distinct selectivity profile. *Eur. J. Biochem.,* 247, 356–363.

62. Xue, C-B., He, X., Roderick, J., DeGrado, W.F., Cherney, R.J., Hardman, K.D., Nelson, D.J., Copeland, R.A., Jaffee, B.D., and Decicco, C.P. (1998) Design and synthesis of cyclic inhibitors of matrix metalloproteinases and TNF-α production. *J. Med. Chem.,* 41, 1745–1748.

63. Steinman, D.H., Curtin, M.L., Garland, R.B., Davidson, S.K., Heyman, H.R., Holms, J.H., Albert, D.H., Magoc, T.J., Nagy, I.B., Marcotte, P.A., Li, J., Morgan, D.W., Hutchins, C., and Summers, J.B. (1998) The design, synthesis, and structure-activity relationships of a series of macrocyclic MMP inhibitors. *Bioorg. Med. Chem. Lett.,* 8, 2087–2092.

64. Pratt, L.M., Beckett, R.P., Bellamy, C.L., Corkill, D.J., Cossins, J., Courtney, P.F., Davies, S.J., Davidson, A.H., Drummond, A.H., Helfrich, K., Lewis, C.N., Mangan, M., Martin, F., Miller, K., Nayee, P., Ricketts, M.L., Thomas W., Todd, R.S., and Whittaker, M. (1998) The synthesis of novel matrix metalloproteinase inhibitors employing the Ireland-Claisen rearrangement. *Bioorg. Med. Chem. Lett.,* 8, 1359–1364.

65. MacPherson, L.J. and Parker, D.T. (1994), European Patent Application, EP-606,046A.

66. MacPherson, L.J., Bayburt, E.K., Capparelli, M.P., Carroll, B.J., Goldstein, R., Justice, M.R., Zhu, L., Hu, S., Melton, R.A., Fryer, L., Goldberg, R.L., Doughty, J.R., Spirito, S., Blancuzzi, V., Wilson, D., O'Byrne, E.M., Ganu, V., and Parker, D.T. (1997) Discovery of CGS 27023A, a non-peptidic, potent, and orally active stromelysin inhibitor that blocks cartilage degradation in rabbits. *J. Med. Chem.,* 40, 2525–2532.

67. Miller, A., Beckett, R.P., and Whittaker, M. (1995) PCT Patent Application, WO9535275.

68. Miller, A., Beckett, R.P., and Whittaker, M. (1995) PCT Patent Application, WO9535276.

69. Broadhurst, M.J., Brown, P.A., Lawton, G., Ballantyne, N., Borkakoti, N., Bottomley, K.M.K., Cooper, M.I., Eatherton, A.J., Kilford, I.R., Malsher, P.J., Nixon, J.S., Lewis, E.J., Sutton, B.M., and Johnson, W.H. (1997) Design and synthesis of the cartilage protective agent (CPA, Ro 32-3555). *Bioorg. Med. Chem. Lett.,* 7, 2299–2302.

70. Beckett. R.P., Martin, F.M., Miller, A., Todd, R.S., and Whittaker, M. (1998) PCT Patent Application, WO 9817655.

71. Nagase, H. (1996) Matrix metalloproteinases in zinc metalloproteases in health and disease (ed Hooper, N.M.). Taylor and Francis, London.

72. Chandler, S., Miller, K.M., Clements, J.M., Lury, J., Corkill, D., Anthony, D.C.C., Adams, S.E., and Gearing, A.J.H. (1997) Matrix metalloproteinases, tumor necrosis factor and multiple sclerosis: an overview. *J. Neuroimmun.,* 72, 155–161.

73. Greenwald, R.A. and Golub, L.M. (1994) Inhibition of matrix metalloproteinases: Therapeutic potential. *Ann. N.Y. Acad Sci.,* 732.

74. Wojtowiczpraga, S.M., Dickson, R.B., and Hawkins, M.J. (1997) Matrix metalloproteinase inhibitors. *Investigational New Drugs,* 15, 61–75.

75. Opdenakker, G. and Van Damme, J. (1992) Cytokines and proteases in invasive processes: molecular similarities between inflammation and cancer. *Cytokine,* 4, 251–258.

76. Sledge, G.W., Qulali, M., Goulet, R., Bone, E.A., and Fife, R. (1995) Effect of matrix metalloproteinase inhibitor batimastat on breast cancer regrowth and metastasis in athymic mice. *J. Natl. Cancer Inst.,* 87, 1546–1550.

77. Eccles, S.A., Box, G.M., Court, W.J., Bone, E.A., Thomas, W., and Brown, P.D. (1996) Control of lymphatic and hematogenous metastasis of a rat mammary carcinoma by the matrix metalloproteinase inhibitor batimastat (BB-94). *Cancer Res.,* 56, 2815–2822.

78. An, Z., Wang, X., Willmott, N., Chander, S.K., Tickle, S., Docherty, A.J.P., Mountain, A., Millican, A.T., Morphy, R., Porter, J.R., Epemolu, R.O., Kubota, T., Moossa, A.R., and Hoffman, R.M. (1997) Conversion of a highly malignant colon cancer from an aggressive to a controlled disease by oral administration of a metalloproteinase inhibitor. *Clin. Exp. Metastasis.,* 15, 184–195.

79. Wang, X., Fu, X., Brown, P.D., Crimmin, M.J., and Hoffman, R.M. (1994) Matrix metallo-proteinase inhibitor BB-94 (Batimastat) inhibits human colon tumor growth and spread in a patient-like orthotopic model in nude mice. *Cancer Res.,* 54, 4726–4728.

80. Watson, S.A., Morris, T.M., Robinson, G., Crimmin, M.J., Brown, P.D., and Hardcastle, J.D. (1995) Inhibition of organ invasion by the matrix metalloproteinase inhibitor batimastat (BB-94) in two human colon carcinoma metastasis models. *Cancer Res.,* 55, 3629–3633.

81. Davies, B., Brown, P.D., East, N., Crimmin, M.J., and Balkwill, F.R. (1993) A synthetic Matrix Metalloproteinase Inhibitor Decreases Tumor Burden and Prolongs Survival of Mice Bearing Human Ovarian Carcinoma Xenografts. *Cancer Res.,* 53, 2087–2091.

82. Giavazzi, R., Garofalo, A., Ferri, C., Lucchini, V., Bone, E.A., Chiari, S., Brown, P.D., Nicoletti, M.I., and Taraboletti, G. (1998) Batimastat, a synthetic inhibitor of matrix metal-loproteinases, potentiates the antitumor activity of cisplatin in ovarian carcinoma xenografts. *Clin. Cancer Res.,* 4, 985–992.

83. Zervos, E.E., Norman, J.G., Gower, W.R., Franz, M.G., and Rosemurgy, A.S. (1997) Matrix metalloproteinase inhibition attenuates human pancreatic cancer growth in vitro and de-creases mortality and tumorgenesis in vivo. *J. Surgical Res.,* 69, 367–371.

84. Knox, J.D., Bretton, L., Lynch, T., Bowden, G.T., and Nagle, R.B. (1998) Synthetic matrix metalloproteinase inhibitor, BB-94, inhibits the invasion of neoplastic human prostate cells in a mouse model. *Prostate,* 35, 248–254.

85. Taraboletti, G., Garofalo, A., Belotti, D., Drudis, T., Borsotti, P., Scanziani, E., Brown, P.D., and Giavazzi, R. (1995) Inhibition of angiogenesis and murine hemangioma growth by Batimastat, a synthetic inhibitor of matrix metalloproteinases. *J. Natl. Cancer Inst.,* 87, 293–298.

86. Zubair, A.C., Ali, S.A., Rees, R.C., Goepel, J.R., and Goyns, M. H. (1996) Investigation of the effect of BB-94 (Batimastat) on the colonization potential of human lymphoma cells in scid mice. *Cancer Lett.,* 107, 91–95.

87. Santos, O., McDermott, C.D., Daniels, R.G., and Appelt, K. (1997) Rodent pharmacoki-netic and anti-tumor efficacy studies with a series of synthetic inhibitors of matrix metallo-proteinases. *Clin. Exp. Metastasis,* 15, 499–508.

88. Di Martino, M.J., High, W., Galloway, W.A., and Crimmin, M.J. (1994) Preclinical Antiarthritic Activity of Matrix Metalloproteinase Inhibitors. *Ann. N. Y. Acad. Sci.,* 732, 411–413.

89. Di Martino, M., Wolff, C., High, W., Stoup, G., Hoffman, S., Laydon, J., Lee, J.C., Bertolini, D., Galloway, W.A., Crimmin, M.J., Davis, M., and Davies, S. (1997) Anti-arthritic activity of hydroxamic acid-based pseudopeptide inhibitors of matrix metallopro-teinases and TNF-α processing. *Inflamm. Rev.,* 46, 211–215.

90. Conway, J.G., Wakefield, J.A., Brown, R.H., Marron, B.E., Sekut, L., Stimpson, S.A., McElroy, A., Menius, J.A., Jeffreys, J.J., Clark, R.L., McGeehan, G.M., and Connolly, K.M. (1995) Inhibition of cartilage and bone destruction in adjuvant arthritis in the rat by a matrix metalloproteinase inhibitor. *J. Exp. Med.,* 182, 449–457.

91. Gijbels, K., Galardy, R.E., and Steinman, L. (1994) Reversal of experimental autoimmune encephalomyelitis with a hydroxamate inhibitor of matrix metalloproteinases. *J. Clin. Invest.,* 94, 2177–2182.

92. Hewson, A.K., Smith, T., Leonard, J.P., and Cuzner, M.L. (1995) Suppression of experi-mental allergic encephalomyelitis in the Lewis rat by the matrix metalloproteinase inhibitor Ro31-9790. *Inflamm. Res.,* 44, 345–349.

93. Clements, J.M., Cossins, J.A., Wells, G.M.A., Corkill, D.J., Helfrich, K., Wood, L.M., Pigott, R., Stabler, G., Ward, G.A., Gearing, A.J.H., and Miller, K. M. (1997) Matrix me-talloproteinase expression during experimental autoimmune encephalomyelitis and effects of a combined matrix metalloproteinase and tumor necrosis factor-α inhibitor. *J. Neuroimmunol.* 74, 85–94.

94. Liedtke, W., Cannella, B., Mazzaccaro, R.J., Clements, J.M., Miller, K.M., Wucherpfenning, K.W., Gearing, A.J.H., and Raine, C.S. (1998) Effective treatment of models of multiple sclerosis by matrix metalloproteinase inhibitors. *Annals. Neurology,* 44, 35–46.

95. Matyszak, M.K. and Perry, V.H. (1996) Delayed-type hypersensitivity lesions in the central nervous system are prevented by inhibitors of matrix metalloproteinases. *J. Neuroimun.,* 69, 141–149.
96. Redford, E.J., Smith, K.J., Gregson, N.A., Davies, M., Hughes, P., Gearing, A.J.H., Miller, K., and Hughes, R.A.C. (1997) A combined inhibitor of matrix metalloproteinase activity and tumor necrosis factor-alpha processing attenuates experimental autoimmune neuritis. *Brain,* 120, 1895–1905.
97. Wallace, G., Stansford, M.R., Whiston, R.A., and Clements, J. (1996) The MMP inhibitor BB-1101 is effective in reducing the incidence of EAN. *Immunology,* 89, Suppl. 1, 53.
98. Rosenberg, G.A., Estrada, E.Y., and Dencoff, J.E. (1998) Matrix metalloproteinases and TIMPS are associated with blood-brain barrier opening after reperfusion in rat brain. *Stroke,* 29, 2189–2195.
99. Rosenberg, G.A., and Navratil, M. (1997) Metalloproteinase inhibition blocks edema in intracerebral hemorrhage in the rat. *Neurology,* 48, 921–926.
100. Zempo, N., Koyama, N., Kenagy, R.D., Lea, H.J., and Clowes, A.W. (1996) Regulation of vascular smooth muscle cell migration and proliferation in vitro and in injured rat arteries by a synthetic matrix metalloproteinase inhibitor. *Arteriosclerosis Thrombosis & Vascular Biology,* 16, 28–33.
101. Bendeck, M.P., Irvin, C., and Reidy, M.A. (1996) Inhibition of matrix metalloproteinase activity inhibits smooth muscle cell migration but not neointimal thickening after arterial injury. *Circ. Res.,* 78, 38–43.
102. Strauss, B.H., Robinson, R., Batchelor, W.B., Chisholm, R.J., Ravi, G., Natarajan, M.K., Logan, R.A., Mehta, S.R., Levy, D.E., Ezrin, A.M., and Keeley, F.W. (1996) In vivo collagen turnover following experimental balloon angioplasty injury and the role of matrix metalloproteinases. *Circulation Research,* 79, 541–550.
103. Steinmann-Niggli, K., Ziswiler, R., Kung, M., and Marti, H.P. (1998) Inhibition of matrix metalloproteinases attenuates anti-thyl.l nephritis. *J. Am. Soc. Nephrology,* 9, 397–407.
104. Paul, R., Lorenzyl, S., Koedel, U., Vogel, U., and Pfister, H.W. (1997) Involvement of matrix metalloproteinases in the disruption of the blood-brain barrier in bacterial meningitis Poster Presentation at 37th ICAAC Toronto Ontario Canada Sept 28–Oct 1 1997.
105. Beattie, G.J. and Smyth, J.F. (1998) Phase I study intraperitoneal metalloproteinase inhibitor BB94 in patients with malignant ascites. *Clin. Cancer Res.,* 4, 1899–1902.
106. Parsons, S.L., Watson, S.A., and Steele, R.J.C. (1997) Phase I/II trial of batimastat, a matrix metalloproteinase inhibitor, in patients with malignant ascites. *Eur. J. Surg. Oncol.,* 23, 526–531.
107. Macaulay, V.M., O'Byrne, K.J., Saunders, M.P., Long, L., Gleeson, F., Mason, C.S., Harris, A.L., Brown, P., and Talbot, D.C. (1998) Phase I study of the matrix metalloproteinase inhibitor batimastat in patients with malignant pleural effusion. *Clin. Cancer Res.,* In Press.
108. Millar, A.W., Brown, P.D., Moore, J., Galloway, W.A., Cornish, A.G., Lenehan, T.J., and Lynch, K.P. (1998) Results of single and repeat dose studies of the oral matrix metalloproteinase inhibitor marimastat in healthy male volunteers. *Br. J. Clin. Pharm.,* 45, 21–26.
109. Wojtowiczpraga, S., Torri, J., Johnson, M., Steen, V., Marshall, J., Ness, E., Dickson, R., Sale, M., Rasmussen, H.S., Chiodo, T.A., and Hawkins, M.J. (1998) Phase I trial of marimastat, a novel matrix metalloproteinase inhibitor, administered orally to patients with advanced lung cancer. *J. Clin. Oncol.,* 16, 2150–2156.
110. Rubin, S.C., Hoskins, W.J., and Hakes, T.B. CA 125 levels and surgical findings in patients undergoing secondary operations for epithelial ovarian cancer. *Am. J. Obstet. Gynecol.,* 160, 667–671, 1989.
111. Ward, U., Primrose, J.N., Finan, P.J., Perren, T.J., Selby, P., Purves, D.A., and Cooper, E.H. (1993) The use of tumor markers CEA, CA-195 and CA-242 in evaluating the response to chemotherapy in patients with advanced colorectal cancer. *Br. J. Cancer,* 67, 1132–1135.

112. Nemunaitis, J., Poole, C., Primrose, J., Rosemurgy, A., Malfetano, J., Brown, P., Berrington, A., Cornish, A., Rasmussen, H., Kerr, D., Cox, D., and Millar, A. (1998) Combined analysis of studies of the effects of the matrix metalloproteinase inhibitor marimastat on serum tumor markers in advanced cancer: Selection of a biologically active and tolerable dose for longer-term studies. *Clin. Cancer Res.,* 4, 1101–1111.

113. Primrose, J.N., Bleiberg, H., Daniel, F., Van Belle, S., Mansi, J.L., Seymour, M., Johnson, P.W., Neoptolemos, J.P., Baillet, M., Barker, K., Berrington, A., Brown, P.D., Millar, A.W., and Lynch, K.P. Pilot study of oral marimastat in recurrent colorectal cancer: an evaluation of biological activity by measurement of carcinoembryonic antigen. *Br. J. Cancer,* In Press.

114. Rosemurgy, A., Harris, J., Langleben, A., Casper, E., and Rasmussen, H.S. Marimastat in patients with advanced pancreatic cancer—a dose finding study. *Am. J. Clin. Oncol.,* In Press.

115. Tierney, G., Steele, R., Griffin, N., Stuart, R., Kasem, H., Lynch, K.P., Lury, J.T., Brown, P.D., Millar, A.W., and Parsons, S. A pilot study of the effects of the matrix metalloproteinase inhibitor marimastat in gastric cancer. Submitted.

116. Adams, M., and Thomas, H. (1998) A phase I study of the matrix metalloproteinase inhibitor, marimastat, administered concurrently with carboplatin, to patients with relapsed ovarian cancer. *Proc. Am. Soc. Clin. Oncol.,* 17, 217a.

117. Carmichael, J., Ledermann, J., Woll, P.J., Gulliford, T., and Russell, R.C. (1998) Phase IB study of concurrent administration of marimastat and gemcitabine in non-resectable pancreatic cancer. *Proc. Am. Soc. Clin. Oncol.,* 17, 232a.

118. O'Reilly, S., Mani, S., Ratain, M.J., Elza Brown, K., Johnson, S., Vogelzang, N.J., Kennedy, M.J., Donehower, R.C., and Rugg, T. (1998) Schedules of 5FU and the matrix metalloproteinase inhibitor marimastat (MAR): a phase I study. *Proc. Am. Soc. Clin. Oncol.,* 17, 217a.

119. Gradishar, W., Sparano, J., Cobleigh, M., Kennedy, M.J., Schuchter, L., Wicks, J., and Rasmussen, H. (1998) A phase I study of marimastat in combination with doxorubicin and cyclophosphamide in patients with metastatic breast cancer. *Proc. Am. Soc. Clin. Oncol.,* 17, 144a.

120. Anderson, I.C., Shipp, M.A., Docherty, A.J.P., and Teicher, B.A. (1996) Combination therapy including a gelatinase inhibitor and cytotoxic agent reduces local invasion and metastasis of murine Lewis lung carcinoma. *Cancer Res.,* 56, 715–718.

121. Neri, A., Goggin, B., Kolis, S., Brekken, J., Khelemskaya, N., and Gabriel, L. (1998) Pharmacokinetics and efficacy of a novel matrix metalloproteinase inhibitor, AG3340, in single agent and combination therapy against B16-F10 melanoma tumors developing in the lung after Iv tail vein implantation in C57BL/6 mice. *Proc. Am. Assoc. Cancer Res.,* 39, 302.

6

Prinomastat

A Potent and Selective Matrix Metalloprotease Inhibitor—Preclinical and Clinical Development for Oncology

David R. Shalinsky, PhD, Bhasker Shetty, PhD, Yazdi Pithavala, PhD, Steve Bender, PhD, Anthony Neri, PhD, Stephanie Webber, PhD Krzysztof Appelt, PhD, and Mary Collier, BS

CONTENTS

1. INTRODUCTION

Several members of the matrix metalloprotease (MMP) enzyme family expressed by tumors and surrounding stromal components participate in the growth and spread of cancer *(1–4)*. Accumulating data indicate that MMP-2 (gelatinase A), MMP-9 (gelatinase B), and MMP-14 (MT-MMP-1, a membrane bound enzyme) are commonly associated with growing and invasive tumors and with neovascularization *(5–9, 9a, 9b)*. Other MMPs commonly found in the vicinity of invasive tumors include MMP-1 (collagenase-1), MMP-3 (stromelysin-1), MMP-11 (stromelysin-3), MMP-13 (collagenase-3), and

From: *Cancer Drug Discovery and Development:*
Matrix Metalloproteinase Inhibitors in Cancer Therapy
Edited by: Neil J. Clendeninn and Krzysztof Appelt © Humana Press Inc., Totowa, NJ

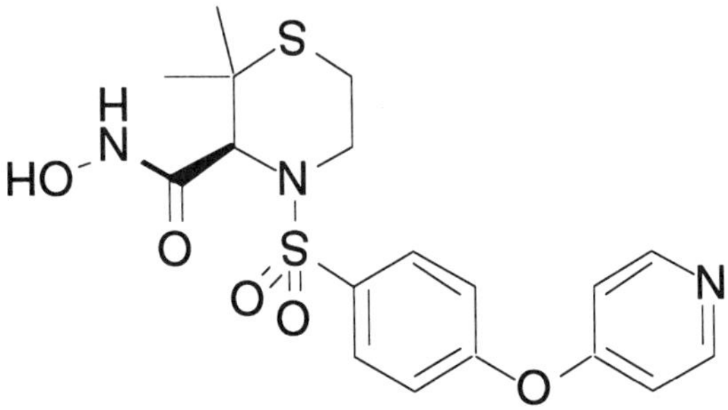

Fig. 1. Structure of prinomastat.

MMP-7 *(10–11)*. MMP-1 and MMP-7 have also been associated with carcinogenic processes *(12,13)*.

Broad inhibition of MMP activities may result in undesirable side effects whereas inhibition of a subset of MMPs may produce a positive therapeutic index for inhibiting tumor growth. Some synthetic MMP inhibitors have been associated with reversible joint complaints, most often observed as arthralgias but also progressing in some patients to contractures of the fingers and limited range of motion in shoulders with prolonged exposure. The inhibition of MMP-1, which functions to remodel triple-helical collagens, may be responsible for this side effect *(14,15)*. The hypothesis pursued by Agouron Pharmaceuticals, Inc. is that selective inhibition of the MMPs most closely associated with invasive tumors, with less potent inhibition of MMP-1, will result in inhibition of tumor growth and angiogenesis although limiting the potential for side effects.

In 1993, Agouron Pharmaceuticals, Inc. undertook a research program to design MMP inhibitors. The structures of human MMPs -1, -3, -7, and -13 were solved*. X-ray crystallographic methods were applied to recombinant human proteins to describe the active site pocket of each enzyme. Models of other members of the MMP family were constructed using knowledge of the sequence homology. Prinomastat (also known as AG3340) is the lead development candidate to emerge from this discovery program. Prinomastat is a small molecule (molecular weight 423), nonpeptidic, hydroxamate inhibitor of selected MMPs (Fig. 1). It is a potent inhibitor of MMPs -2, -3, -9, -13, and -14 but is less potent for inhibiting the activities of MMP-1 and MMP-7. The K_i values for enzyme inhibition by prinomastat against a series of MMPs are summarized in Table 1. The results of preclinical investigations, phase I clinical trials and our approach to design of pivotal oncology efficacy studies will now be discussed.

*Dr. K. Appelt and coworkers, Agouron Pharmaceuticals, Inc., in collaboration with Dr. M. Browner and coworkers, Syntex Corporation/Roche Bioscience (unpublished data).

Table 1
K_i Values for Inhibition of Selected MMPs by Prinomastat

Enzyme		K_i (nM)
Collagenase-3	MMP-13	0.03
Gelatinase A	MMP-2	0.05
Gelatinase B	MMP-9	0.26
Stromelysin-1	MMP-3	0.30
MT-MMP-1	MMP-14	0.33
Collagenase-1	MMP-1	8.3
Matrilysin	MMP-7	54.0

2. PRECLINICAL PHARMACOLOGY

2.1. Preclinical Pharmacokinetics, Distribution, and Metabolism

The pharmacokinetics of prinomastat were studied in the rat, dog, and monkey after intravenous and oral administration. In mice, pharmacokinetics were studied after intraperitoneal and oral administration. Plasma concentrations of prinomastat were assessed by high-performance liquid chromatography (HPLC) coupled with detection by ultraviolet light absorbance (240 λ) or by mass spectrometry. In the rat, dog, and monkey, evidence of enterohepatic recycling was observed, complicating the determination of the plasma half-life. Half-life values across all species studied were in the range of 0.6 to 2.6 h. Systemic clearance ranged from 0.76 (monkey) to 3.2 L/h*kg (rat); the volume of distribution exceeded that of total body water in most species.

Significant oral bioavailability (20–40%) was recorded in all animal species tested. Oral bioavailability was generally higher in the fasted state; this was linked to rapid absorption and high C_{max} values in the fasted state. In monkeys in particular, administration to fed animals led to more consistent, sustained blood levels. Pharmacokinetics in rodents and monkeys were dose proportional within the range employed for toxicity studies. The plasma vs time curve for prinomastat in mice is shown in Figure 2. This curve illustrates the rapidity with which prinomastat enters the bloodstream after oral and intraperitoneal administration. It also illustrates that the pharmacokinetic curves are virtually superimposable after either intraperitoneal or oral dosing with the main difference being a higher C_{max} after intraperitoneal dosing.

The potential for accumulation of prinomastat or metabolic induction during daily oral dosing was evaluated in the rat. Animals received 200 mg/kg prinomastat once daily for 5 d. Pharmacokinetic profiles through 7 h post-dose were obtained on days 1 and 5, and trough levels were obtained prior to dosing on days 2, 3, and 4. The pharmacokinetic profiles were similar on days 1 and 5. No

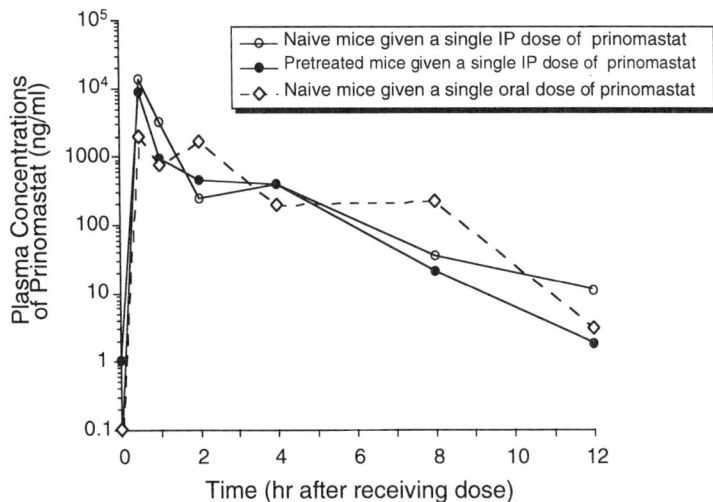

Fig. 2. Plasma concentrations of prinomastat after dosing with 100 mg/kg prinomastat, given as a single dose in naive and in pretreated mice. One hundred mg/kg prinomastat was administered IP, BID to C57BL/6 mice over a 15 d period. On day 15, these mice were given a single IP dose of 100 mg/kg prinomastat 17 h after the previous dose. Naive mice were also given a single IP dose. Naive nude mice were given a single PO dose. Values are mean of 3 mice/point.

prinomastat accumulation or metabolic induction were observed. Similarly, no change in prinomastat accumulation has been observed in nude mice when they were given a single oral dose after 4 wk of twice daily pretreatment *(16)*, or when a single intraperitoneal dose was given to C57BL/6 mice after 2 wk of twice daily intraperitoneal dosing (Fig. 2).

Tissue distribution and excretion of ^{14}C-prinomastat was evaluated after a single oral dose of 50 mg/kg in rats (Table 2). Concentrations exceeding those in plasma 30 min after dosing were found in the gastrointestinal tract, kidneys, liver, lung, pancreas, lymph nodes, spleen, and heart. High levels of prinomastat equivalents (^{14}C-labeled species) were transient and declined rapidly to less than 1 μg/g by 48 h in all tissues except the gastrointestinal tract and liver, likely related to an apparent biliary excretion of prinomastat. Excretion of prinomastat equivalence was approx equal in feces (38%) and urine (35%).

In vitro metabolism studies with prinomastat were conducted in human and nonhuman liver microsomes from both sexes and cDNA-derived human cytochrome P450. Human microsomes metabolized prinomastat to a lesser extent than did microsomes from the other species investigated. Glucuronide conjugation accounted for the majority of metabolism, with the cytochrome P450 system contributing to a lesser extent. Both the extent of metabolism and its

Table 2
Tissue Distribution of ^{14}C-Prinomastat After a Single 50 mg/kg Oral Dose in the Rat

Tissues	\multicolumn{4}{c}{Concentration of prinomastat equivalent (μg/g)[a]}			
	0.5h	4h	24h	48h
Blood (RBC)	5.49 ± 2.74	1.45 ± 0.18	0.86 ± 0.29	0.70 ± 0.53
Bone	3.70 ± 2.31	1.32 ± 0.24	0.54 ± 0.12	0.42 ± 0.23
Bone Marrow	0.20 ± 0.12	0.24 ± 0.07	0.28 ± 0.18	0.27 ± 0.38
Brain	0.95 ± 0.76	0.69 ± 0.44	0.16 ± 0.12	0.18 ± 0.13
Eyes	3.08 ± (31.65)[b]	1.52 ± 0.54	1.23 ± 0.31	0.36 ± 0.29
Fat	0.07 ± 0.05	0.07 ± 0.04	ND[c]	ND
Heart	7.92 ± 3.86	1.64 ± 0.18	0.73 (5.81)[b]	0.30 ± 0.08
Kidneys	29.79 ± 13.78	10.17 ± 6.99	2.51 ± 0.41	0.88 ± 0.14
Large Intestine	10.27 ± 3.22	407.45 ± 79.30	127.08 ± 24.86	60.67 ± 28.87
Large Intestine Content	4.27 ± 2.63	1036.04 ± 211.25	719.58 ± 252.94	207.43 ± 98.04
Liver	90.71 ± 31.83	32.56 ± 7.47	18.34 ± 2.29	5.30 ± 0.42
Lungs	8.73 ± 4.06	2.18 ± 0.26	1.00 ± 0.17	0.48 ± 0.11
Mesenteric Lymph Node	8.39 ± 7.01	3.58 ± 1.23	1.94 ± 0.40	0.81 ± 0.03
Muscle	4.48 ± 2.97	1.23 ± 0.27	0.82 ± 0.22	0.21 ± 0.07
Oesophagus	86.72 ± 59.67	5.17 ± 2.24	3.21 ± 1.73	1.82 ± 0.78
Pancreas	49.92 ± 20.50	4.23 ± 0.61	1.27 ± 0.33	0.58 ± 0.19
Plasma	6.58 ± 2.85	1.65 ± 0.33	1.31 ± 0.29	0.76 ± 0.18
Prostate	6.22 ± 2.78	4.70 ± 4.16	1.02 ± 0.21	0.81 ± 0.62
Seminal vesicles	3.09 ± 1.61	0.86 ± 0.12	0.86 ± 0.07	0.53 ± 0.25
Skin	3.99 ± 1.65	0.95 ± 0.17	1.12 ± 0.56	0.27 ± 0.14
Small Intestine	949.58 ± 419.27	605.25 ± 196.51	215.65 ± 69.95	86.11 ± 34.76
Small Intestine Content	428.44 ± 151.14	422.23 ± 161.65	289.15 ± 85.13	51.88 ± 19.24
Spinal cord	1.31 ± 0.94	0.80 ± 0.66	0.41 ± 0.25	0.17 ± 0.11
Spleen	7.91 ± 2.71	1.57 ± 0.56	1.11 ± 0.42	0.36 ± 0.13
Stomach	586.15 ± 470.86	230.48 ± 218.86	3.68 ± 1.47	1.60 ± 1.09
Stomach Content	3437.92 ± 1916.73	649.37 ± 350.16	63.70 ± 46.22	30.03 ± 12.71
Submaxillary Glands	9.14 ± 4.93	1.29 ± 0.86	0.89 ± 0.44	0.37 ± 0.44
Testes	1.72 ± 1.07	0.85 ± 0.10	0.35 ± 0.11	0.16 ± 0.04
Thymus	6.05 ± 3.21	1.27 ± 0.24	0.56 ± 0.11	0.49 ± 0.03
Thyroid Glands	0.55 ± 0.24	0.28 ± 0.06	0.14 ± 0.03	0.15 ± 0.06

[a]Values presented are mean ± SD of data from 3 rats; [b]Mean of two rats (outlier); [c]ND = Not detected

147

complexity, as seen in the HPLC chromatogram traces, suggested that monkeys may exhibit a pattern of prinomastat metabolism more similar to humans than dogs or rodents.

Protein binding determinations were conducted using equilibrium dialysis and ^{14}C-prinomastat to evaluate the free fraction in mouse, rat, monkey, and human serum. The results showed a percent unbound in the range of 20% (rat) to 38% (monkey) with 31% free in human serum*. Binding to both α_1-acid glycoprotein and human serum albumin was documented. The mean in vitro blood to plasma ratio was 1.0 in monkey and 0.65 in human.

2.2. Toxicology

Acute toxicity studies with prinomastat have been conducted in the rat and mouse by oral gavage administration. In both species, the no observable effect level was $\geq$2000 mg/kg, the highest dose level administered.

Long-term good laboratory practice (GLP) toxicology studies with prinomastat have been conducted to date for 26 wk in rats and cynomolgus monkeys. Findings of these studies were consistent with the pharmacological activity of prinomastat as an MMP inhibitor and included joint-related effects that diminished in severity upon cessation of prinomastat treatment. In monkeys, joint-related effects were observed only at very high exposure levels compared to those expected to be therapeutic in patients. In rats, joint effects were noted at lower exposures. The rat is believed to represent a particularly sensitive test system for collagen-related effects due to its postulated dependence on a single MMP (MMP-13) for remodeling of collagen in the joints in comparison to humans who express both MMP-1 and MMP-13 *(17,18)*. Prinomastat is a potent inhibitor of MMP-13 (K_i = 0.03 nM) as compared to MMP-1 (K_i = 8.3 nM). By comparison, humans, and presumably monkeys, possess both MMP-1 and MMP-13. Much higher plasma concentrations were required in monkeys to produce similar joint effects to those observed in rats. In non-GLP tumor efficacy studies in mice, prinomastat has been well-tolerated at doses up to 400 mg/kg/day (on a twice daily dosing regimen) given for up to 12 wk.

2.3. Preclinical Efficacy Studies

The efficacy of prinomastat in preclinical model systems was investigated primarily in in vivo models due to the mechanism of action of the agent requiring interaction between tumor cells and the surrounding stromal matrix.

2.3.1. Single Agent Prinomastat in Murine and Human Xenograft Tumor Models

The anticancer effects of prinomastat were tested in the B16-F10 melanoma model *(16,19)*. Tumor cells were injected intravenously into the tail vein of

*Dr. Mark Zorbas, Agouron Pharmaceuticals, Inc., unpublished data.

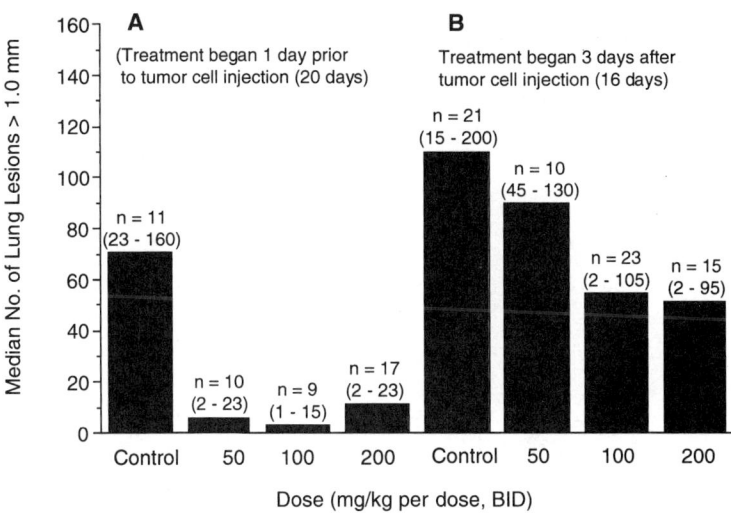

Fig. 3. Inhibition of the number of B16-F10 lesions developing in the lung after IV tail implantation of tumor cells. Prinomastat was administered IP, BID either 1 d before or 3 d after tumor cell implantation. The number of lung lesions in all prinomastat-treated groups was significantly decreased from control ($p < 0.01$) with the exception of the low dose of prinomastat in **B**.

mice. Treatment with prinomastat (administered by intraperitoneal injection twice daily at doses between 50 and 200 mg/kg/dose) was initiated 1 d prior to tumor implantation or 3 or 7 d following tumor implantation. Efficacy was assessed by counting tumors (> 1.0 mm) in the lung 16 to 20 d following injection. Results of these experiments are shown in Figures 3 and 4. Prinomastat efficacy was greatest (90% tumor inhibition) when treatment was begun prior to tumor injection.

Prinomastat was less effective when treatment was begun 1 or 3 d after tumor injection ($\cong 50\%$ inhibition) and ineffective when begun 7 d after implantation (data not shown). These results are consistent with the hypothesized role of MMPs in a sequence of tumor growth-related events. MMP inhibition, particularly MMP-9 inhibition *(20)*, could be expected to reduce extravasation of tumors from the circulation into the lung. MMP inhibitors may also have a prominent role in disrupting the extracellular matrix to prevent the growth of tumors shortly after seeding into the lung has occurred *(21)*. MMP inhibition following extravasation but early in the neovascularization process would be expected to reduce the number of lesions reaching a critical size. Treatment of established, vascularized tumors with an MMP inhibitor alone would be expected to be least effective.

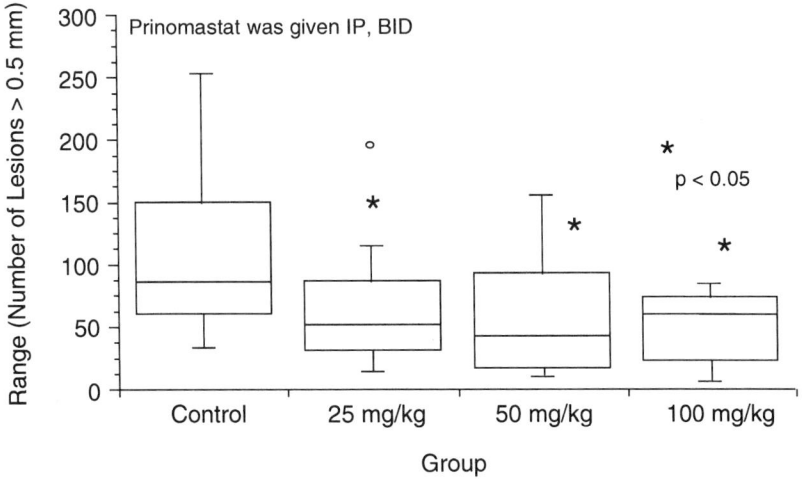

Fig. 4. Dose-dependent inhibition of the number and range of B16-F10 lesions developing in the lung after IV tail implantation of tumor cells. The box plot shows the 10th, 25th, 50th (median), 75th, and 90th percentile for lesion number (from bottom to top of box). Prinomastat was administered IP, BID beginning 1 day after tumor cell implantation. Lesion number in all treated-groups was significantly decreased from control ($p < 0.05$)(n = 12 mice/group). The circle over the 25 mg/kg box represents the number of lesions in an animal that had an outlying number of lesions.

The efficacy of single agent prinomastat has been tested in eight xenograft models involving human tumor cell lines implanted into immunocompromised mice *(16)*. In five models (COLO-320DM colon adenocarcinoma *[16]*, PC-3 prostate cancer *[16]*, MV522 nonsmall cell lung cancer *[16,22]*, U87 glioma *[23]*, and KKLS gastric cancer *[16]*), tumors were implanted subcutaneously into the flank of the animals. In two models (MB-MDA-435 breast cancer *[16]*, and NCI-H460 large cell lung cancer *[24]*, tumors were implanted orthotopically. In most experiments, prinomastat was administered orally, twice daily. In mice bearing U87 glioma tumors, prinomastat was given intraperitoneally, once daily. Prinomastat was well-tolerated in all models and was even beneficial in protecting mice from ill health induced in some of the models (PC-3) *(16)*. Among the models studied, prinomastat was effective in all except the KKLS gastric cancer model.

COLO-320DM is a colorectal adenocarcinoma xenograft model. Mice with tumors implanted into the flank were treated with prinomastat twice daily beginning 5 d after tumor implantation. The role of treatment schedule was investigated by treating animals 4 (Mon–Thur), 5 (Mon–Fri) or 7 (Mon–Sun) days each week. Significant reduction in tumor growth (approx 75%) was observed 14 d after the start of treatment (Fig. 5A). The 5 and 7 d regimens produced sim-

A   **B**

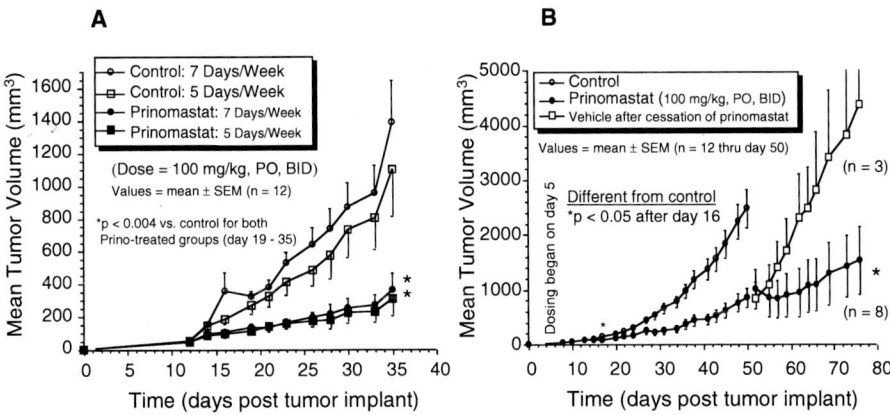

Fig. 5. Inhibition of the growth of human colon COLO-320DM tumors by prinomastat. One hundred mg/kg prinomastat was given orally, BID, 5 or 7 per week (**A**). Prinomastat inhibited tumor growth equivalently in both regimens. In a separate study, dosing with prinomastat was stopped on day 50 (**B**). Tumor volumes rapidly increased after cessation of dosing.

ilar efficacy. Prinomastat was substantially less effective when administered 4 d each week (data not shown). During treatment, tumor growth was markedly decreased relative to vehicle controls. To observe the effect of treatment cessation, prinomastat dosing was stopped on day 50 in a subset of treated animals. Cessation of treatment resulted in rapid increase in tumor volume similar to the rate of increase observed in control tumors (Fig. 5B). However, histological examination of tumors after hematoxylin and eosin staining indicated that the increase in tumor volume was artifactual. Tumors from mice sacrificed two weeks following the cessation of treatment had a remarkable degree of necrosis and hemorrhage (Fig. 6C) compared to control tumors (Fig. 6A). Importantly, the rate of proliferation in the peripheral viable tumor regions, assessed by bromodeoxyuridine staining, remained suppressed at a level similar to that recorded in tumors from animals continuing prinomastat treatment (Fig. 6F). Thus, increased fluid retention and necrosis, greater than that observed in continually-treated tumors, rather than tumor proliferation, accounted for the increasing tumor volume following cessation of prinomastat treatment.

PC-3 is an androgen-independent prostate cancer xenograft model. Mice with tumors implanted into the flank were treated with prinomastat beginning 5 d after tumor implantation. Results of the growth inhibition assay are presented in Figure 7A. Statistically significant reduction of the rate of tumor growth was observed in the prinomastat-treated group by d 28 of the experiment *(16)*. Differences in tumor size between the control and prinomastat treated groups became more pronounced late in the study. The PC-3 model is

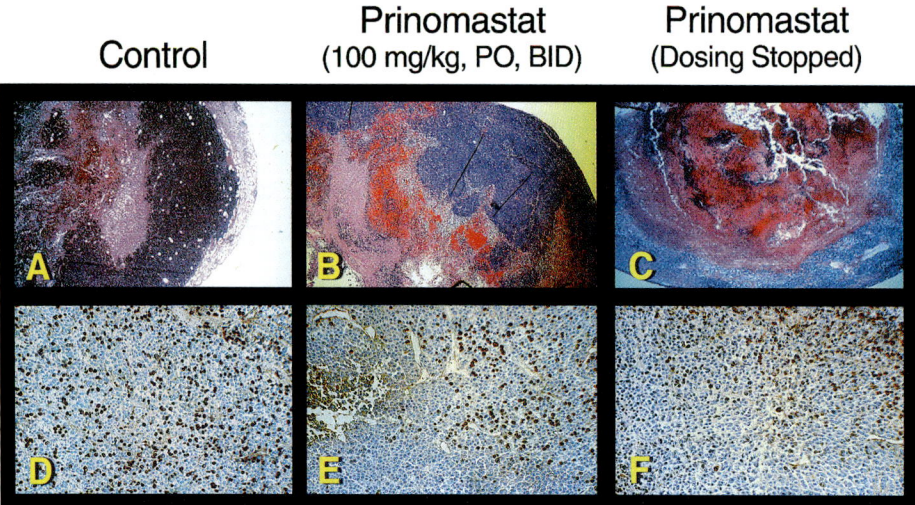

Fig. 6. Morphologies and BrdU staining of COLO-320DM tumors in the presence and absence of prinomastat treatment. Hematoxylin and eosin-stained tumors are shown in **A–C.** The morphologies of control and prinomastat-treated tumors (>5 wk of treatment) were similar (**A** and **B**). There was a marked increase in tumor necrosis and hemhorrage 2 wk after cessation of prinomastat treatment (**C**). Control tumors had extensive BrdU staining in the area of viable tumor cells (**D**). Prinomastat decreased the staining by >90% (**E**). Staining remained inhibited 2 wk after cessation of dosing (**F**).

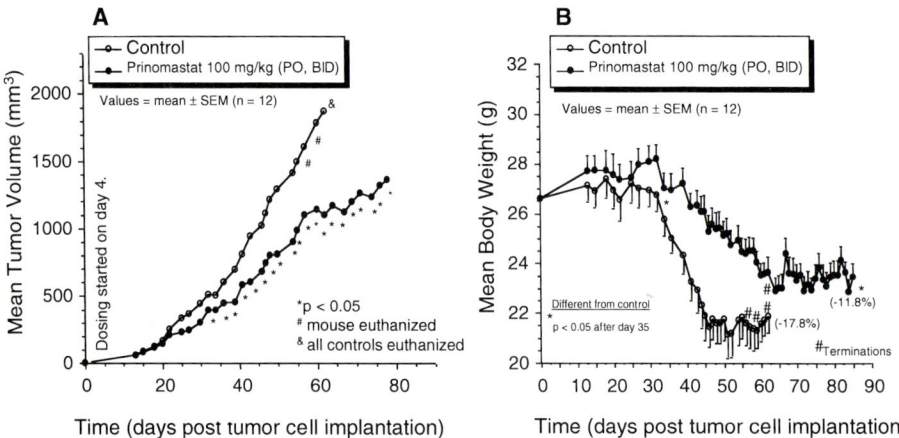

Fig. 7. Prinomastat inhibited the growth of human androgen-independent PC-3 prostate tumors (**A**). Control mice became moribund and were euthanized as indicated in the figure. In comparison, prinomastat attenuated body weight losses, ill health, and morbidity observed in control tumor-bearing mice (**B**). Panel A is reprinted with the permission of the *New York Academy of Sciences* (*16*).

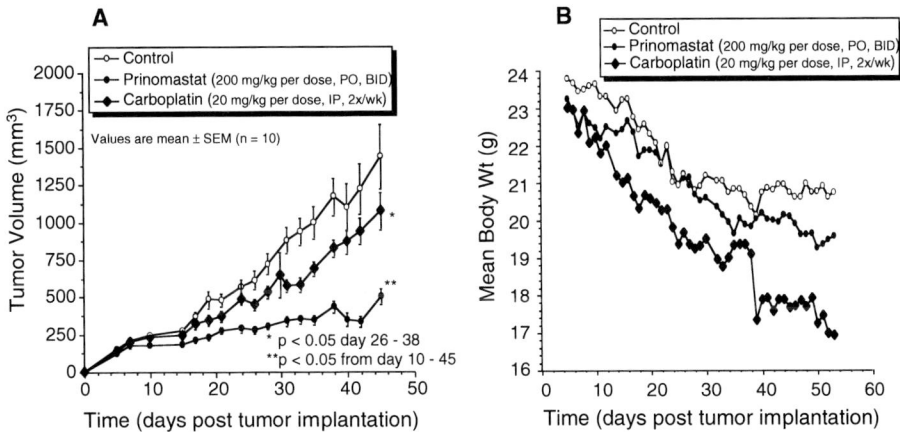

Fig. 8. Prinomastat has a superior therapeutic index to carboplatin as shown by marked inhibition of the growth of NSCLC MV522 tumors (compared to inhibitions produced by carboplatin; (**A**) and tolerance to these agents (**B**). Prinomastat did not affect body weights or animal health at a dose that markedly decreased tumor growth; carboplatin modestly decreased tumor growth at a dose that significantly decreased the body weights of mice. Data in this figure printed with permission of *Clinical Cancer Research* (*22*).

associated with progressive body weight loss as tumor size increases. Treatment with prinomastat attenuated body weight loss, preventing the onset of a moribund condition. Individual control animals were sacrificed on d 58 and 60 of the experiment due to a moribund condition coupled with unacceptable tumor burden. All remaining control animals were sacrificed on d 62 of the study due to morbidity. In contrast, prinomastat-treated animals did not become moribund in this study. A group of prinomastat-treated animals was sacrificed on day 62 to allow comparison of histological findings with control samples. The remaining treated animals had a clearly-suppressed tumor growth rate and a stabilized attenuation of weight loss relative to control animals when the experiment was terminated on day 84. Thus, prinomastat contributed to increased survival in this subcutaneous tumor model.

MV522 is a xenograft model of nonsmall cell lung cancer that is known to be particularly resistant to treatment with chemotherapy agents (*25*). Treatment with prinomastat at 50 or 200 mg/kg per dose, twice daily, resulted in dose-dependent inhibition of tumor growth (Fig. 8A). After 45 d of treatment, tumor volumes were decreased by 31.8 ± 2.7 and $65.1 \pm 7.1\%$, respectively, compared to controls ($p < 0.05$) (22). In this model, prinomastat was more efficacious and better tolerated than standard chemotherapy agents, such as carboplatin (Fig. 8) or paclitaxel (*22*), demonstrating a superior therapeutic index for prinomastat compared to these cytotoxic agents.

U87 is a human malignant glioma cell line that was grown subcutaneously in the flank of severe combined immunodeficiency (SCID) mice. Prinomastat (100 mg/kg administered intraperitoneally once daily) or vehicle was administered to animals beginning approx 3 wk after implantation when tumors measured 0.25 cm^2 *(23)*. After 31 d of treatment, tumors in control animals had grown to a size requiring euthanasia. Tumor size in the prinomastat-treated group was reduced by 78% compared to controls ($p < 0.01$). A group of treated animals, allowed to continue on study beyond day 31, required sacrifice after 71 d of treatment, a greater than twofold increase in survival.

2.3.2. EFFECTS OF PRINOMASTAT ON CELLULAR PROLIFERATION AND APOPTOSIS

The effect of prinomastat treatment on the rate of tumor cell proliferation and apoptosis was investigated in tumor samples obtained from in vivo treatment experiments. Tumor cell proliferation rate was assessed using bromodeoxyuridine (BrdU) staining of fixed paraffin-embedded tissues and apoptosis was investigated using the terminal deoxynucleotidyl transferase-mediated deoxyuridine triphosphate nick end labeling (TUNEL) assay, as previously described *(16)*. Figure 6 illustrates the outcome of a typical experiment conducted in mice bearing human COLO-320DM tumors. In brief, mice implanted in the flank with the COLO-320DM cell line were treated with vehicle or prinomastat for over 7 wk. Sacrifice of the control animals became necessary due to tumor burden. Tumors from some prinomastat-treated animals were also collected simultaneously for BrdU analyses. BrdU incorporation in vehicle-treated tumors was extensive with 238 ± 38 positive-staining tumor cells/200X field *(16)* (Fig. 6D). In contrast, tumors from animals receiving continuous prinomastat treatment (100 mg/kg, twice daily) showed a >90% reduction in BrdU staining *(16)* (Fig. 6E). Most of the treated animals continued to receive prinomastat for an additional two weeks while a subset of three animals was discontinued from treatment. Tumor samples from this subset were harvested two weeks after cessation of treatment. The suppression of proliferation rate was sustained in the tumors (Fig. 6F). Cellular proliferation was also markedly decreased in U87 glioma tumors concomitant with decreased invasiveness and tumor growth in vivo *(23)*. The rate of apoptosis in the viable regions of COLO-

---

Fig. 10. (Opposite page) Inhibition of angiogenesis and induction of tumor necrosis by prinomastat in human nonsmall cell lung cancer MV522 (**D** vs **C**) and colon cancer COLO-320DM (**B** vs **A**) xenograft tumors in nude mice. After dosing with 200 mg/kg prinomastat PO, BID, angiogenesis was decreased by 77% as assessed by inhibition of CD-31 staining ($p < 0.002$)(**D**) compared to control tumors (**C**). Prinomastat increased tumor necrosis as well (panel **D** vs **C**). After dosing with 100 mg/kg prinomastat PO, BID, prinomastat also decreased CD-31 staining in COLO-320DM tumors (**B** vs **A**). This figure reprinted with the permission of the *New York Academy of Sciences (16)*.

Prinomastat
Control
(100 mg/kg, PO, BID)

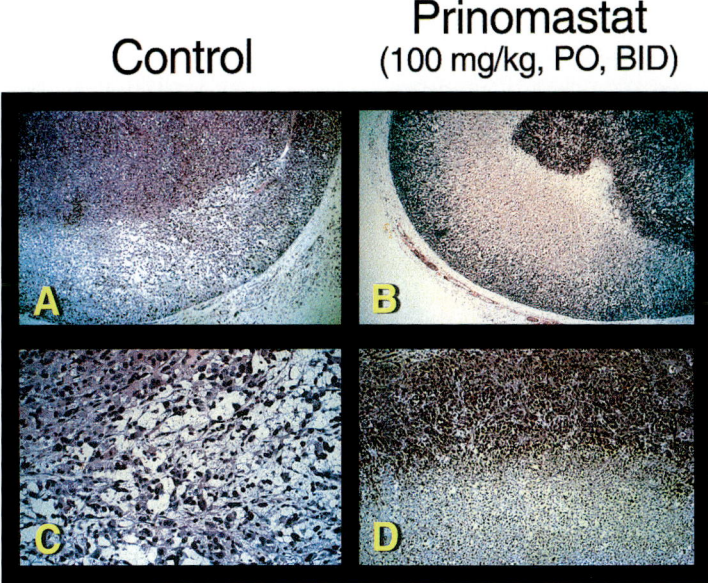

Fig. 9. Morphologies of PC-3 tumors in the presence and absence of prinomastat treatment. Tumors were collected on d 62 of the study shown in Figure 7A. Control tumors were stained with H & E (**A**, X40). Part of **A** is shown at higher magnification in **C** (X200). Prinomastat (**B** and **D**) markedly increased tumor necrosis compared to controls. The sharp border between viable (upper) and necrotic (lower) cells is shown in **B**, and at higher magnification in **D**. Portions of this figure are reprinted with the permission of the *New York Academy of Sciences* (*16*).

Control   Prinomastat

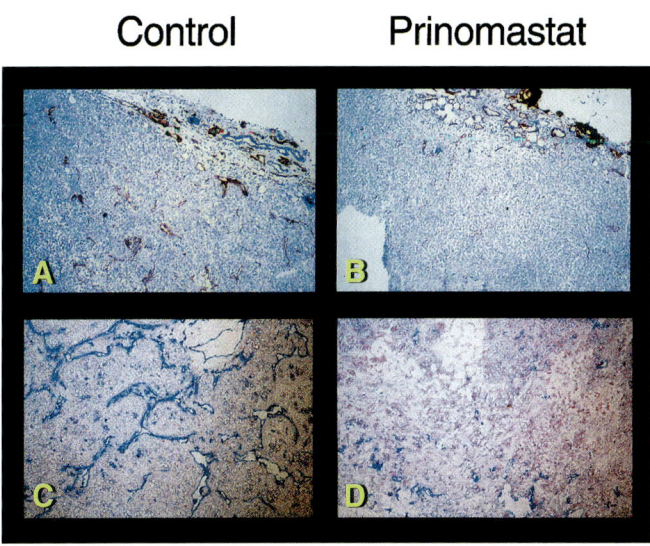

320DM tumors was increased by ≅ 2.9-fold in the prinomastat-treated group as compared to controls *(16)*.

Studies on the effect of prinomastat on cellular proliferation and apoptosis were also conducted in mice bearing the PC-3 human prostate cancer xenograft *(16)*. PC-3 tumors had a neglible fraction of cells incorporating BrdU and decreases in proliferation could not be reliably quantified due to the low basal staining *(16)*. Shown in Figure 9 are tumors from animals treated with vehicle or prinomastat for 62 d prior to sacrifice. Tumors were stained with hematoxylin and eosin. Control tumors were comprised primarily of viable, undifferentiated cells (Fig. 9A; Fig. 9C shows the same area at higher magnification); viable cells are interspersed with dead or dying cells in the periphery of the control tumors (Fig. 9C). In contrast, treatment with prinomastat markedly increased tumor necrosis in the periphery (Fig. 9B; and Fig. 9D shows a similar area at higher magnification), resulting in a sharp border between viable and nonviable zones. The amount of necrosis in the treated tumors increased by twofold, an effect that could not be observed by physical caliper measurements. In this experiment, treatment with prinomastat increased the rate of apoptosis within the viable region of the tumor by 2.4-fold ($p < 0.04$) *(16)*. Marked increases in tumor necrosis have also been observed in MV522 nonsmall cell lung tumors after exposure to prinomastat *(22)* but the mechanism for this effect has not yet been investigated.

2.3.3. INHIBITION OF ANGIOGENESIS BY PRINOMASTAT

Antiangiogenic affects of prinomastat were investigated in four human tumor xenograft models: MV522 nonsmall cell lung cancer, PC-3 prostate cancer, COLO-320DM colon adenocarcinoma, and U87 glioma. Animals bearing tumors were treated with prinomastat by oral administration beginning 5 d following tumor implantation. U87-tumor bearing animals were treated with prinomastat intraperitoneally beginning approx 30 d after tumor implantation. The formation of new blood vessels in mice was assessed by staining tumors with an antibody to CD-31, an endothelial cell marker that is expressed on new vessels *(26,27)*. In four tumor model systems, prinomastat treatment resulted in a significant inhibition of angiogenesis coupled with inhibition of tumor growth. In the MV522 lung cancer model, administration of prinomastat at doses of 50 and 200 mg/kg per dose twice daily for 52 d resulted in dose-dependent reduction in vessel counts of 45% and 77% per 200X field compared to controls *(22)*. Representative CD-31 staining of control and prinomastat-treated tumors is shown in Figure 10. In MV522 tumors, only remnants of CD-31 positive vessels were evident at the high dose (Fig. 10D) compared to the highly vascular control tumors (Fig. 10C). In COLO-320DM tumors, prinomastat also decreased CD-31 staining significantly, by about 50%, but without inducing necrosis to the extent produced in MV522 tumors (Fig. 10A vs

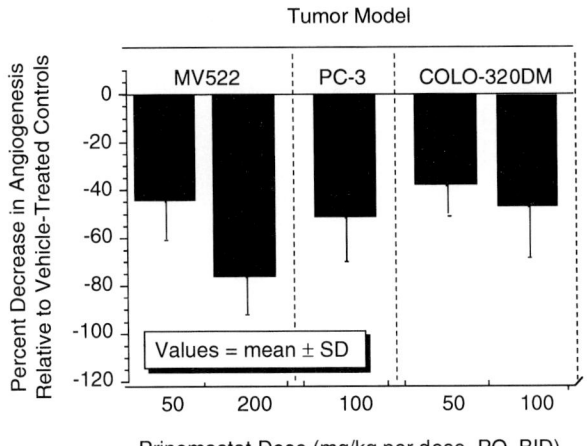

Fig. 11. Inhibition of angiogenesis, as assessed by CD-31 staining of tumors, by prinomastat across preclinical tumor models. Dose-dependent inhibitions were observed. The range of inhibition was 37–77%.

10B). Similarly, reductions in vessel count were observed in the PC-3 prostate cancer model, with 100 mg/kg prinomastat twice daily resulting in approx 50% inhibition compared to controls (Fig. 11) *(16)*. Inhibition of the invasiveness of PC-3 tumor cells and angiogenesis (by Factor VIII staining) was also demonstrated in a SCID mouse model in which tumor cells were placed onto human foreskin and grafted into mouse dermis *(28)*. Reduction (> 60%) in CD-31 staining was also observed in the human U87 glioma model *(38)*, in which prinomastat produced a remarkable tumor growth inhibition, decreased invasiveness, and a survival advantage *(23)*. The inhibition of angiogenesis in U87 tumors is a recent finding obtained after optimization of the process for tissue collection. We have previously reported inadequate baseline staining for CD-31 to definitively quantify changes in vessel densities in these tumors *(23)*.

2.3.4. CORRELATION BETWEEN PLASMA TROUGH CONCENTRATIONS AND EFFICACY

The correlation between various pharmacokinetic parameters and efficacy was addressed using the COLO-320DM colon tumor model. Groups of tumor-bearing mice received a total daily prinomastat dose of 25 mg/kg as one, or two or four equally divided doses (25 mg/kg once daily, 12.5 mg/kg twice daily, or 6.25 mg/kg four times daily) *(29)*. In addition, a group of animals received an eightfold higher total daily dose, 200 mg/kg/d (100 mg/kg twice daily). Tumors were measured over time and pharmacokinetic parameters including peak and trough plasma prinomastat concentrations and total exposure (area-under-the-curve) were calculated. The results of the study are presented in Table 3.

Table 3

Independence of the Antitumor Efficacy of Prinomastat from Total Dose and Total Plasma Exposure in Nude Mice

Total daily dose (mg/kg)	Prinomastat given per dose (mg/kg)	Dosing regimen	Daily AUC value (0–24h) (ng/mL*h)	Trough concentrations (ng/mL)	Percent tumor growth inhibition (day 38)
25	6.25	Four times daily	672[a]	2.3[c]	74.4*,#
25	12.5	Twice daily	ND[b]	0.12[c]	40.5
25	25	Once daily	684	0.0003[c]	19.9
200	100	Twice daily	10882	1.0 ± 0.2^d	82.0*

[a]Value calculated by multiplying single dose AUC by number of doses/day as described.
[b]Value not determined (plasma samples collected only over 4 h).
[c]Value estimated at 24 h based on log-linear extrapolation of mean 0 to 4 or 0 to 12 h concentrations after repeated dosing.
[d]Value determined experimentally 17 h after second of the daily BID doses after repeated dosing (n = 3) (ref. 29).
*$p < 0.05$ vs control; #$p < 0.05$ vs 50 mg/kg/day (given 25 mg/kg, BID).
This table is reprinted with permission of *Investigational New Drugs*.

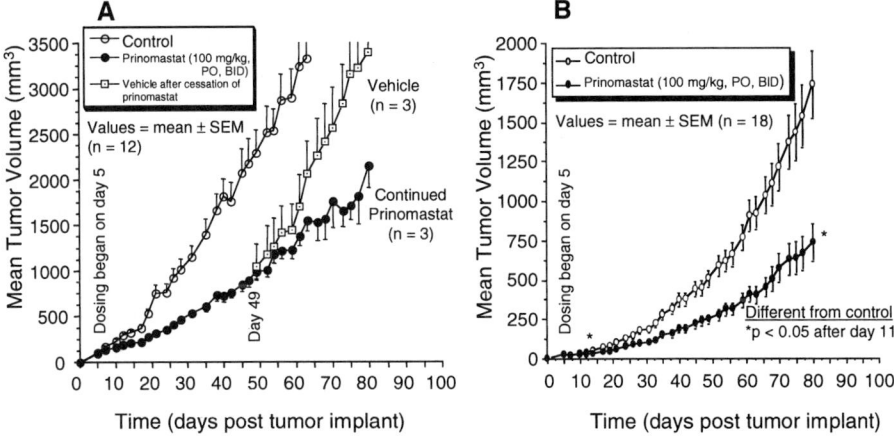

Fig. 12. Prinomastat significantly delayed the growth of NSCLC MV522 tumors with continued dosing. When dosing was stopped, tumors regrew (**A**). In a subsequent study, growth-inhibited tumors were serially passaged into naive mice. Pretreated tumors retained their sensitivity to prinomastat after serial passage and extended treatment (**B**).

Efficacy correlated with trough concentration as opposed to peak concentration or AUC. The trough prinomastat concentrations observed after administration of 6.25 mg/kg four times daily or 100 mg/kg twice daily were similar as were inhibitions of tumor growth. The target trough concentration for future study was identified as 1–2 ng/mL. The rate of elimination of prinomastat in mice is substantially more rapid than in humans. As will be discussed below, the target concentration of 1 ng/mL is easily exceeded in patients when prinomastat is administered in low doses twice daily.

2.3.5. INVESTIGATIONS OF TUMOR RESISTANCE TO PRINOMASTAT

Questions concerning treatment-induced tumor resistance were addressed using serial passage and treatment of various tumor models. In the experiment shown in Figure 12A, MV522 tumors were implanted into the flank of mice and were treated with prinomastat or vehicle twice daily beginning 5 d after implantation and continuing for at least 50 d. Animals were then sacrificed and viable tumor pieces from prinomastat-treated animals were transferred to new animals. Treatment with prinomastat or vehicle began again 5 d after implantation. The results of this experiment are shown in Figure 12B. No evidence of change in sensitivity to treatment was observed after passage of previously-treated MV522 tumors. Similar data have been generated in other tumor models after months of extended treatment *(30)*. The basis of these observations is under continuing investigation. However, these findings are consistent with the expectation that many of the tumor growth-promoting MMP enzymes secreted by surrounding stromal cells, a normal cell population, would not be susceptible to selective pressure due to low mutation rate.

2.3.6. PRINOMASTAT IN COMBINATION WITH CYTOTOXIC CHEMOTHERAPIES IN MURINE AND HUMAN XENOGRAFT TUMOR MODELS

The efficacy of prinomastat in combination with cytotoxic chemotherapies was investigated using the murine B16-F10 model, the human MV522 lung cancer model implanted subcutaneously into nude mice, and the NCI-H460 lung cancer model implanted orthotopically in nude rats. In the B16-F10 model, treatment with prinomastat (100 mg/kg twice daily orally), with or without carboplatin or paclitaxel (by intraperitonal injection two to three doses each week), began one day after tumor cell implantation. In this experiment, after 15 d of study, prinomastat administration resulted in 33% reduction in the number of lung lesions. Single agent carboplatin (25 mg/kg/dose) was inactive but paclitaxel (7.5 or 15 mg/kg/dose, given 3 times weekly) resulted in a dose dependent reduction in lesion number (47 and 77% inhibition, respectively, $p < 0.05$ for 15 mg/kg only). In combination, prinomastat plus carboplatin produced 72% fewer lung lesions ($p < 0.02$). Prinomastat in combination with 7.5 mg/kg paclitaxel resulted in 68% fewer lesions relative to controls ($p < 0.05$). Prinomastat in combination with both carboplatin and paclitaxel was well-tolerated without evidence of additional toxicity over that produced by the cytotoxic agents alone. In summary, prinomastat enhanced antitumor efficacy when used in combination with the cytotoxic agents, carboplatin or paclitaxel, in the B16-F10 intravenous tumor metastasis model.

The MV522 lung cancer model is well characterized as being resistant to chemotherapy *(25)*. As discussed previously, single agent prinomastat administration resulted in substantial inhibition of the growth of subcutaneous tumors. For the purposes of investigating combination regimens, it was necessary to reduce the dose of prinomastat from 200 mg/kg to 50 mg/kg twice daily to allow observation of a potential increase in efficacy. The chemotherapy regimens were used at or close to their maximum tolerated doses. After extended treatment, a 40 mg/kg per week dose of carboplatin exceeded its maximum tolerated dose (MTD) (Fig. 8B). Combinations of prinomastat and carboplatin, prinomastat and paclitaxel, and prinomastat and gemcitabine were investigated in this model. In the prinomastat/carboplatin experiment, single agent prinomastat resulted in 32% inhibition of tumor growth, single agent carboplatin (20 mg/kg twice weekly) produced 25% inhibition of tumor growth and the combination resulted in 60% reduction (Table 4) *(16)*. The high degree of necrosis noted in the combination-treated tumors during histological examination provided evidence of an interaction that was not appreciated by caliper assessments alone *(16,22)*. In the prinomastat/paclitaxel experiment, single agent prinomastat resulted in 32% inhibition of tumor growth, single agent paclitaxel (3.75 mg/kg twice weekly) produced no inhibition of tumor growth, and the combination resulted in a 48% reduction (Table 4). In the prinomastat/gemcitabine experiment, single agent prinomastat resulted in 67% inhibition of tumor growth, single agent gemcitabine (60 mg/kg d 7, 10, and 13) produced 52% inhibition of tumor growth and the combination resulted in 83% reduction (Fig. 13). Volumes in the combination groups were significantly different from the single agent groups in all studies except for the B16-F10 study, in which the prinomastat/paclitaxel combination was different only from prinomastat and not paclitaxel.

The KKLS gastric xenograft model was also used to study prinomastat in combination with paclitaxel *(16)*. In this model prinomastat was ineffective as a single agent (no inhibition of tumor growth), treatment with single agent paclitaxel resulted in 27% inhibition of tumor growth, and the combination produced a 67% reduction (Table 4).

In an orthotopic model of lung cancer, NCI-H460 tumor fragments were implanted into the nude rat lung to investigate the effect of prinomastat with and without carboplatin on the growth of primary tumors, metastasis, and animal survival *(24)*. As single agents, neither prinomastat (100 mg twice daily by oral administration) nor carboplatin (10 mg/kg twice weekly by intraperitoneal administration) enhanced survival over control. In combination, prinomastat plus carboplatin produced a mean survival of 41.6 ± 2.5 d as compared to 33.0 ± 0.8 d for controls ($p < 0.03$). The combination regimen was well-tolerated.

2.4. Summary of Preclinical Investigations

Preclinical pharmacology studies indicated that the free fraction of prinomastat in blood plasma is relatively high, that the agent distributes well to tissues and that the potential for drug interactions with chemotherapeutic agents on the basis of metabolism is low. Toxicology studies have demonstrated that prinomastat is well-tolerated in the species studied. Dose-dependent, reversible joint effects were the primary toxicity observed. The animal tumor models systems used to investigate the potential of prinomastat as a cancer therapy provided several guidelines for design of the clinical trials. Evidence of activity was demonstrated in many tumor models. The combination of prinomastat and cytotoxic chemotherapy produced enhanced antitumor efficacy in these models. Several biological effects were observed in different systems, including prinomastat-induced decreases in tumor cell proliferation, increases in tumor necrosis and apoptosis, and inhibition of tumor angiogenesis. A relationship between trough concentrations and efficacy was also observed. Resistance to prinomastat did not develop after extended treatment in in vivo experiments. All of these observations were taken into consideration in the clinical development plan.

Table 4
Tumor Growth Inhibition by Combination Chemotherapy of Prinomastat and Cytotoxic Agents

Tumor model	Agent	Dose (mg/kg)	Mean tumor volume (mm^3) after 5 to 7 wks[a]	Percent decrease in tumor volume	Statistical significance relative to monotherapy
Human Models					
MV522 (NSCLC)	Control	Vehicle	1440	—	
	prinomastat	50, PO, BID	982	32	
	carboplatin	20 (IP, 2X/wk)	1073	25	
	prinomastat + carboplatin	50 + 20	571	60	$p < 0.01$
	Control	Vehicle	860	—	
	prinomastat	50, PO, BID	581	32	
	paclitaxel	3.75 (IP, 3X/wk)	917	0	
	prinomastat + paclitaxel	50 + 3.75	365	48	$p < 0.04$
	Control	Vehicle	3165	—	
	prinomastat	100, PO, BID	1043	67	
	gemcitabine	60 × 3 doses, IP	1484	52	
	prinomastat + gemcitabine	100 + 60	555	83	$p < 0.01$

162

Model	Treatment	Dose			p
KKLS[b] (gastric)	Control	Vehicle	2349	—	
	prinomastat	100, PO, BID	2372	0	
	paclitaxel	3.75 (IP, 3X/wk)	1720	27	
	prinomastat + paclitaxel	100 + 3.75	865	67	$p < 0.01$
Murine Model			Number of Lung Lesions > 1 mm		
B16-F10[c]	Control	Vehicle	32.8	—	
	prinomastat	100, PO, BID	22.2	32	
	carboplatin	25, (IP, 2X/wk)	35.6	0	
	prinomastat + carboplatin	100 + 25	9.1	72	$p < 0.02$
	Control	Vehicle	21.8	—	
	prinomastat	100, PO, BID	14.3	34	
	paclitaxel	7.5 mg (IP, 3X/wk)	11.6	47	
	prinomastat + paclitaxel	100 + 7.5	7.5	68	$p < 0.05$[d]

[a]Except for the B16-F10 model when lung metastases were scored after 15 d.
[b,c]Portions of data are reprinted by permission of the *New York Academy of Sciences*.
[d]Significantly different from prinomastat and control only.

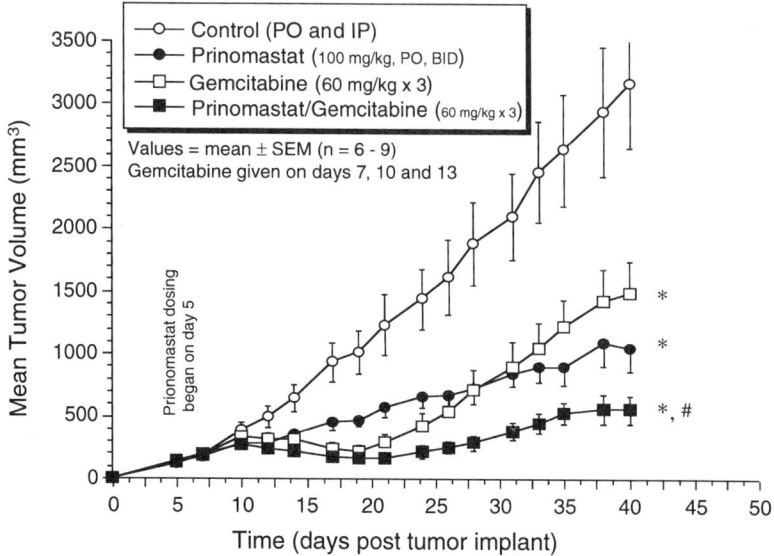

Fig. 13. Enhanced inhibition of the growth of NSCLC MV522 tumors by prinomastat and gemcitabine. Prinomastat was administered orally at 100 mg/kg BID. Gemcitabine was administered IP at 60 mg/kg on d 7, 10, and 13. The combination inhibited growth to a greater degree than either agent alone. *$p < 0.05$ vs control after d 14; #$p < 0.01$ vs prinomastat after d 18, and gemcitabine after d 24.

3. PRINOMASTAT CLINICAL DEVELOPMENT

3.1. Phase I Studies

3.1.1. SAFETY AND PHARMACOKINETIC STUDIES IN VOLUNTEERS

The safety and pharmacokinetics of prinomastat were first investigated in a single dose study conducted in healthy male volunteers. Groups of 7 volunteers (5 treated and 2 placebo) received prinomastat at 10, 25, 50, 100, or 200 mg or placebo with a light breakfast *(31)*. Prinomastat was well-tolerated; no treatment related adverse experiences were identified. Plasma pharmacokinetic parameters for prinomastat were estimated by noncompartmental of concentrations determined by a validated LC-MS-MS assay analysis. Absorption of prinomastat was rapid with peak concentrations generally observed by 1 to 2 h after dosing (data not shown). Mean peak concentrations were 114 ± 53 ng/mL in the 10 mg group and 2794 ± 484 ng/mL in the 200 mg group. The AUC$_\infty$ increased linearly between 10 and 100 mg (208 ± 67 and 2869 ± 444 ng*h/mL, respectively) with slightly higher exposure at 200 mg than projected. The plasma half-life was typically between 2 and 4 h. The plasma concentration-vs-time curves for some patients included a secondary peak between 8 and 12 h after dosing, consistent with preclinical observations, which may indicate enterohepatic recirculation.

The safety and steady-state pharmacokinetics of repeat prinomastat dosing were studied in volunteers administered prinomastat tablets twice daily for 6.5 d. Groups of 9 volunteers (6 treated and 3 placebo) received prinomastat 25 or 100 mg or placebo twice daily, for a total of 13 doses in the fed state. No treatment related adverse experiences were identified. Steady-state prinomastat pharmacokinetics were consistent with results of the single dose study. No evidence of accumulation or hepatic induction was found.

3.1.2. Dose Escalation Study in Patients having Advanced Cancer

A phase I dose escalation study in patients having advanced cancer was conducted at Vanderbilt University and the University of Wisconsin at Madison *(32,33)*. The safety and pharmacokinetics of prinomastat were evaluated in cohorts of at least 6 patients and as many as 12 patients at each dose level. Patients enrolled in this study had advanced solid tumors for which no potentially curative therapy was available. Patients had World Health Organization (WHO) Performance Status 0 or 1 at the time of entry and adequate renal, hepatic, and bone marrow function. Prinomastat was administered by oral tablet at doses of 1, 2, 5, 10, 25, 50, or 100 mg twice daily in the fasted state (i.e., 2 h prior to or 1 h following a meal). The MTD was defined as the dose associated with dose-limiting toxicity in at least 2 patients among as many as 6 during the first 4 weeks of treatment. Enrollment into this study included 75 patients. Demographics are presented in Table 5. No serious or acute drug-related adverse experiences attributed to prinomastat were observed. Adverse experiences associated with prinomastat were primarily musculoskeletal complaints observed in a dose- and time-dependent manner. These effects were considered to be evidence of inhibition of MMP-1 and collagen remodeling as well as reassurance of inhibition of MMP-2 and other cancer-associated enzymes against which prinomastat is more potent. Dose limiting complaints were more commonly observed in patients receiving 25 mg (or greater) prinomastat twice daily than at lower doses. The MTD was not identified because dose-limiting joint complaints were rarely observed over the first 4 wk of treatment. The shoulders and the hands were the most frequently affected sites although arthralgia in other sites was also reported. In more advanced cases, joint swelling and range of motion limitations were observed. An effective strategy for dealing with musculoskeletal complaints included treatment rest for 3 to 5 wk followed by dose reduction. The pharmacokinetics of prinomastat administered in the fasted state were linear with increasing dose from 2 to 100 mg twice daily and comparable to healthy volunteers enrolled in earlier studies. Exposure following the 1 mg dose was probably underestimated due to plasma concentrations falling below the limit of quantitation after 4 h. No drug accumulation was noted over time. Pharmacokinetic results of this study are presented in Table 6 and Figure 14. As previously discussed, experiments conducted using preclinical tumor

Table 5
**Demographics of Patients Enrolled in Phase I Prinomastat Dose
Escalation Study (Preliminary Results)**

Patients Enrolled and Treated	75
Patients Summarized	75
Male (%)	44 (59%)
Female (%)	31 (41%)
Race	
Caucasian	72
Black	2
Asian	1
Median Age in Years (range)	54 (25–87)
Diagnosis	
Colorectal	17
Lung	16
Renal	13
Sarcoma	8
Prostate	4
Melanoma	2
Other	15
Prior Therapy	
None or surgery alone	5
Radiotherapy	40
Chemotherapy	63
Other therapies	27

model systems indicated that efficacy was associated with maintenance of a minimum prinomastat plasma concentration rather than peak concentrations or total exposure (29). The mean trough concentration in patients receiving 2 mg or more twice daily exceeded the target trough concentration established in the preclinical model. Although no partial responses were observed (which might have been predicted based on the mechanism of action of prinomastat), 18 of 75 patients experienced stable disease for at least 16 wk. The prinomastat dose assignment at study entry (1 to 100 mg twice daily) did not appear to influence which patients experienced stable disease. Results of this phase I study indicated that prinomastat dose levels between 2 and 25 mg twice daily were candidates for further development.

3.1.3. Pilot Combination Safety Studies

Pilot phase I safety and pharmacokinetic studies of prinomastat (25 mg twice daily) in combination with paclitaxel/carboplatin or mitoxantrone/prednisone (full dose therapy as used in the treatment of lung or prostate cancer, respectively) have been conducted (34–37). In each study, the pharmacokinetics of the

Table 6
Prinomastat Pharmacokinetic Parameters For Ascending Dose
Trial in Patients Having Cancer (Mean ± SD)

Dose (mg BID)	n	AUC_{0-12} (ng*h/mL)	C_{max} (ng/mL)	T_{max} (h)	$t_{1/2}$ (h)
1	5	14 ± 5	10 ± 4	0.70 ± 0.27	0.94 ± 0.26
2	6	86 ± 37	58 ± 24	0.58 ± 0.20	4.76 ± 2.00
5	6	314 ± 173	199 ± 100	0.75 ± 0.42	5.01 ± 1.97
10	6	413 ± 50	291 ± 157	0.88 ± 1.53	2.70 ± 0.55
25	6	1108 ± 518	777 ± 239	0.42 ± 0.30	2.22 ± 0.37
50	5	3107 ± 1603	1861 ± 1296	0.45 ± 0.33	2.08 ± 0.34
100	6	5156 ± 3298	2083 ± 1433	0.79 ± 1.09	2.46 ± 0.68

chemotherapy regimen were evaluated on d 1 of the first course of treatment; prinomastat dosing was initiated on d 15 of the first course with pharmacokinetic evaluation on d 19; the full combination regimen was evaluated on day 1 of the second course. The combination regimens were well-tolerated with all reported adverse events consistent with previous experience with the chemotherapy regimen or prinomastat. The pharmacokinetics of paclitaxel and prednisone were unchanged by coadministration of prinomastat.

The phase I program demonstrated that prinomastat was associated with linear pharmacokinetics within the dose range to be studied in the future and was well tolerated as a single agent and in combination with selected chemotherapy regimens. All adverse effects of prinomastat observed were believed to be mechanism based, associated with inhibition of MMP-1. Moderate severity (potentially dose-limiting) joint complaints were uncommon at doses below 25 mg twice daily.

3.2. Approach to Efficacy Studies Using Prinomastat

The approach to clinical development of prinomastat, like many agents of the MMP and angiogenesis inhibitor classes, required that the traditional paradigms for clinical trial designs be reexamined. Many factors were considered, from what would be the expected outcome of effective MMP inhibition, to hints for optimal use provided by the preclinical experiments. The study designs adopted include what we consider to be applicable elements of traditional designs as well as innovative elements appropriate to the class of agent or prinomastat specifically.

Preclinical work indicated that prinomastat administered as a single agent might reduce the implantation and establishment of new metastases and slow the growth of existing tumors. Patients might benefit from slowed disease progression but tumor shrinkage resulting in partial and complete responses might not be common. Traditional phase II studies estimating response rate in ad-

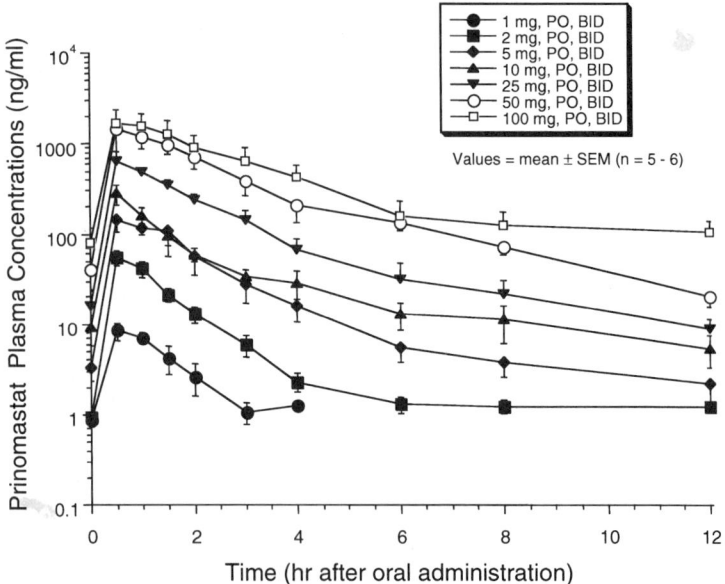

Fig. 14. Prinomastat plasma concentrations (mean ± SD) in cancer patients over a dosing interval of 1–100 mg after 28 d of PO, BID treatment. A single oral dose of prinomastat was given to patients on the morning of the 29th d of study.

vanced diseases were expected to be of limited usefulness. Therefore, endpoints such as time-to-progression and survival were adopted for prinomastat studies. The potential for patient selection bias and the inadequacy of historical controls in many therapeutic settings resulted in the need for randomized, placebo-controlled studies. Because the first efficacy trials were to be relatively large, including a control population and using phase III endpoints, the decision was taken to spend the early years in an actual phase III effort, avoiding the difficulties in interpretation of results that can arise in underpowered studies.

Prinomastat was designed to specifically target MMPs associated with invasive tumors and avoid inhibition of MMP-1, hypothesized to be the cause of musculoskeletal side effects. The K_i value for prinomastat against MMP-2 (a chosen target enzyme) is 166-fold more potent than the K_i for MMP-1. This therapeutic window may provide the opportunity to treat patients without inducing side effects. It is, however, apparent from the phase I experience that dose escalation of prinomastat sufficient to observe joint complaints is possible. Evidence of MMP-1 inhibition would theoretically provide evidence that MMP-2 is well-inhibited. Whereas it might be appealing to use only innocuous doses of prinomastat, traditionally "more is better" in cancer therapy (if for no better reason than to ensure distribution of the agent to the tumor), we chose to err on the side of demonstrating exposure of prinomastat in patients at anticipated therapeutic doses. Whether a treatment regimen associated with uninterrupted therapy would be superior to one requiring occasional treatment rests was unknown. Therefore, the initial efficacy studies with prinomastat attempted to balance these factors; the studies included a dose of prinomastat intended to elicit few, if any, joint complaints, and a higher dose intended to elicit an acceptable degree of this side effect.

In preclinical experiments, prinomastat enhanced the efficacy of nearly all chemotherapy agents without increasing toxicity. Whether the observation was related to increased susceptibility of tumor cells to apoptosis during concurrent exposure to prinomastat or other biological effects is not known. Survey of the pharmacological and toxicological properties of prinomastat did not forewarn for safety interactions with chemotherapy agents. Prinomastat is not highly protein bound, is eliminated by multiple routes, and has a low potential for interactions with chemotherapy agents based on hepatic metabolism. In addition, the side effects of prinomastat do not overlap with those of chemotherapy. Therefore, prinomastat was combined with chemotherapy in the first efficacy studies.

Therapy-induced tumor resistance must be considered in a new light when dealing with MMP inhibitors. Cytotoxic agents are known to induce resistance in tumor cell populations over time, resulting in reduced efficacy. The accepted paradigm is discontinuation of treatment when tumors reach a specified size relative to baseline, and subsequent adoption of treatment with agents having alternative mechanisms of action. Unlike the situation with cytotoxic agents, many of the MMP enzymes contributing to tumor growth and angiogenesis are secreted by stromal cells adjacent to the tumor. The potential for genetic adaptation of these cells is very low. Patients may benefit from a decreased tumor growth rate even if tumor growth is not altogether suppressed. Continued treatment with the MMP inhibitor may result in enhanced survival. Preclinical experiments using prinomastat have not provided evidence of treatment-induced tumor resistance. For these reasons, initial clinical studies with prinomastat allow continued treatment on study beyond disease progression. Initial chemotherapy regimens may be discontinued and alternative regimens instituted in combination with prinomastat or placebo control.

Surveys of MMPs associated with invasive tumors have identified a core group of enzymes implicated in the majority of cancer diseases. Inhibitors targeted at this core group of enzymes may have broad application. Because stromal cells surrounding tumors secrete many of the MMPs involved in tumor growth, investigation of different metastatic patterns will be necessary in establishing broad usefulness. Rational diversification of tumor types in early clinical trial studies is also wise to ensure that investigational therapies are given a chance to demonstrate efficacy. For these reasons, the first diseases chosen for study using prinomastat were nonsmall cell lung and prostate cancer. Together, these two disease targets will provide an array of population subsets for investigation of tumor and disease-specific factors influencing efficacy.

3.3. Phase III Studies Underway using Prinomastat

Three randomized, double-blind phase III trials are underway in patients having advanced cancer. In two studies with patients having metastatic non-small cell lung cancer, patients receive prinomastat or placebo in combination with paclitaxel and carboplatin or gemcitabine and cisplatin as first-line therapy. The primary endpoint of the studies is survival with secondary endpoints including progression-free survival, symptomatic progression-free survival, disease response rate, and quality of life. The third phase III study includes patients having metastatic, hormone-refractory prostate cancer who receive prinomastat or placebo in combination with mitoxantrone and prednisone as first-line chemotherapy. Two of the studies include three treatment arms. Patients are randomized to receive placebo plus chemotherapy or one of two prinomastat doses (one intended to be asociated with few, if any, joint effects and the other intended to be associated with a moderate incidence) plus chemotherapy. Among over 800 patients enrolled in these studies to date, the combination regimens have been well-tolerated. No evidence of increased toxicity during prinomastat dosing has been observed. An unusual element of the studies is the allowance of adoption of second- and subsequent lines of chemotherapy at the time of disease progression. A substantial number of patients have elected to continue study treatment during administration of alternative chemotherapy (i.e., second-line) selected by the investigator or radiotherapy. The variety of regimens being adopted are those commonly utilized in the treatment of lung or prostate cancer. As with the front-line chemotherapy, all alternative combination regimens have been well-tolerated. No efficacy results from these studies are yet available.

3.4. Future Directions

A number of approaches to the therapy of cancer using prinomastat are under consideration. An effort is underway to investigate potential biomarkers of MMP inhibition that can be evaluated in blood, urine, or tissue samples. Disease settings with differing tumor-stromal relationships to those currently under study will be targeted. Assessments of the efficacy of prinomastat in minimal disease settings are also a high priority. The potential utility of an agent such as prinomastat in the treatment of advanced and minimal disease settings appears to be without limits at this time.

ACKNOWLEDGMENTS

We gratefully acknowledge the contributions of the many dedicated members of the preclinical, clinical, regulatory, marketing, graphic arts, and business development teams that have supported the MMP inhibitor projects at Agouron Pharmaceuticals, Inc. We thank John Brekken, Helen Zou, Charles McDermott,

David Gonzalez, and Stanley Robinson for preclinical support of these studies. We also thank Mary Rose Keller, Jill Stuart-Smith, Mary Dixon, and Lei-Ana Caproso for clinical support of these studies. Great appreciation is also expressed to Dr. Steve Margosiak for conducting enzyme binding affinity studies, Dr. Scott Zook for prinomastat synthesis, Dr. Mark Zorbas for conducting prinomastat binding studies, Dr. Ellen Wu for support of development-related pharmacology, Dr. Nissi Varki (U.C., San Diego) for histological and immuno-histochemistry support, and Dr. Alex Wood (Hoffmann-La Roche, Inc.) for helpful discussions.

REFERENCES

1. Birkedal-Hansen H, Moore WGI, Bodden MK, et al. Matrix metalloproteinases: a review. *Crit Rev Oral Biol Med.* 1993;4:197–250.
2. Cottam DW, Rees RC. Regulation of matrix metalloproteases: their role in tumor invasion and metastasis. *Int J Oncol.* 1993;2:861–872.
3. Wojtowicz-Praga, S.M., Dickson, R.B. and Hawkins, M. Matrix metalloproteinase inhibitors. *Investigational New Drugs* 1997;15:61–75.
4. Levy, D.E. and Ezrin, A.M. Matrix metalloproteinase inhibitor drugs. In: *Emerging Drugs: The Prospective for Improved Medicines.* Ashley Publications Ltd., 1997.
5. Sato H, Takino T, Okada Y, Shagawa A, Yamamoto E, Seiki M. A matrix metalloprotease expressed on the surface of invasive tumor cells. *Nature.* 1994;370:61–65.
6. Strongin, A.Y., Collier, I., Bannikov, G., Marmer, B.L., Grant. G.A., and Goldberg, G.I. Mechanism of cell surface activation of 72-kDA type IV collagenase. *J. Biol. Chem.* 1995; 270:5331–5338.
7. Brooks PC, Stromblad S, Sanders LC, et al. Localization of matrix metalloproteinase MMP-2 to the surface of invasive cells by interaction with integrin alpha v beta 3. *Cell.* 1996;85: 683–693.
8. Deryugina EI, Reisfeld RA, Bourdon MA, Strongin A. Cell surface MT1-MMP and alpha v beta 3 jointly govern the activation of MMP-2 proenzyme by human tumor cells. *Proc Am Assoc Cancer Res.* 1998;39:A559.
9. Stetler-Stevenson WG, Aznavoorian S, Liotta LA. Tumor cell interactions with the extracellular matrix during invasion and metastasis. *Ann Rev Cell Biol.* 1993;9:541–573.
9a. Vu TH, Shipley JM, Bergers G, Berger JE, Helms JA, Hanahan D, Shapiro SD, Senior RM, Werb Z. MMP-9/gelatinase B is a key regulator of growth plate angiogenesis and apoptosis of hypertrophic chondrocytes. *Cell* 1998;93:411–422.
9b. Coussens LM, Raymond WW, Bergers G, Laig-Webster M, Behrendtsen O, Werb Z, Caughey GH, Hanahan D. Inflammatory mast cells up-regulate angiogenesis during squamous epithelial carcinogenesis. *Genes Dev* 1999;13:1382–1397.
10. Fini, M.E., Cook, J.R., Mohan, R. and Brinckerhoff, C.E. Regulation of matrix metalloproteases gene expression, *Matrix Metalloproteinases,* Academic Press eds.: Parks, W. C. and Mecham, R.P., 1998;300–339.
11. Nagase, H., Stromelysins 1 and 2. *Matrix Metalloproteinases,* Academic Press, eds: Parks, W.C. and Mecham, R.P., 1998;43–68.
12. Crawford, H.C. and Matrisian, L.M. Mechanisms controlling the transcription of matrix metalloproteinase genes in normal and neoplastic cells. *Enzyme Protein* 1996; 49:20–37.
13. Wilson, C.L., Heppner, K.J., Labosky, P.A., Hogan, B.L. and Matrisian L.M. Intestinal tumorigenesis is suppressed in mice lacking the metalloproteinase matrilysin. *Proc. Natl. Acad. Sci.* 1997; 94:1402–1407.

14. Yocum, S., Lopresti-Morrow, L., Reeves, L., and Mitchell, P. MMP-13 and MMP-1 expression in tissues of normal articular joints. In: *Inhibition of Matrix Metalloproteinases: Therapeutic Applications*. Ed. by Greenwald, Zucker and Golub, *Ann. N. Y. Acad. Sci.,* 1999; 878:583–586.

15. Krane, S.M. Is collagenase (matrix metalloproteinase-1) necessary for bone and other connective tissue remodeling? *Clin Orthop* 1995; 313:47–53.

16. Shalinsky, D.R., Brekken, J., Zou, H., McDermott, C.D., Forsyth, P., Edwards, D., Margosiak, S., Bender, S., Truitt, G., Wood, A., Varki, N.M., and Appelt, K. Broad antitumor and antiangiogenic activities of AG3340, a potent MMP inhibitor undergoing advanced oncology clinical trials. In: *Inhibition of Matrix Metalloproteinases: Therapeutic Applications*. Ed. by Greenwald, Zucker and Golub, *Ann. N. Y. Acad. Sci.,* 1999; 878:236–270.

17. Freije JMP, Diez-Itza I, Balbin M, et al. Molecular cloning and expression of collagenase-3, a novel human matrix metalloprotease produced by breast carcinomas. *J Biol Chem.* 1994;269:16766–16773.

18. Sang QA, and Douglas DA. Computational sequence analysis of matrix metalloproteanases. *J Protein Chem.* 1996;15:137–160.

19. Neri, A., Goggin, B., Kolis, S., Brekken, J., Khelemskaya, N., Gabriel, L., Robinson, S.R., Webber, S., Wood, A.W., Appelt, K. and Shalinsky, D.R. Pharmacokinetics and efficacy of a novel matrix metalloproteinase inhibitor, AG3340, in single agent and combination therapy against B16-F10 melanoma tumors developing in lung after IV-tail implantation in C57BL/6 mice. *Proc. Am. Assoc. Cancer Res.* 1998;39:A2060

20. Himelstein, B.P., Canete-Soler, R., Bernhard, E.J., Dilks, D.W. and Muschel, R. Metalloproteinases in tumor progression: the contribution of MMP-9. *Invasion Metastasis:* 1994;14:246–258.

21. Koop, S., Khoka, R., Schmidt, E.E., MacDonald, I.C., Morris, V.L., Chambers, A.F and Groom, A.C. Overexpression of metalloproteinase inhibitor in B16F10 cells does not affect extravasation but reduces tumor growth. *Cancer Res.* 1994;54:4791–4797.

22. Shalinsky, D.R., Brekken, J., Zou, H., Bloom, L., McDermott, C., Varki, N.M and Appelt, K. Marked antiangiogenic and antitumor efficacy of AG3340 in chemoresistant human NSCLC tumors: Single agent and combination chemotherapy studies. *Clin Cancer Res.* 1999; 5:1905–1917.

23. Price, A., Shi, Q., Morris, D., Brasher, P.M.A., Wilcox, M.E., Rewcastle, N.B., Shalinsky, D., Zou, H., Appelt, K., Johnston, R.N., Yong, V.W., Edwards, D., and Forsyth, P. Marked inhibition of tumor growth in a malignant glioma tumor model by the novel, synthetic matrix metalloproteinase (MMP) inhibitor, AG3340. *Clin. Cancer Res.* 1999;5:845–854.

24. Johnston, M., Mullen, J.M., Pagura, M., Brekken, J., Zou, H. and Shalinsky, D.R. AG3340 and carboplatin increase survival in an orthotopic nude rat model of primary and metastastic human lung cancer. *Proc. Am. Assoc. Cancer Res.* 1999;40:A1946.

25. Kelner, M.J., McMorris, T.C., Estes, L., Starr, R., Sampson, K., Varki, N. and Taetle, R. Nonresponsiveness of the metastatic human lung carcinoma MV522 xenograft to conventional anticancer agents. *Anticancer Res.* 1995;15:867–871.

26. Favaloro, E.J., Moraitis, N., Bradstock, K. and Koutts, J. Co-expression of haemopoietic antigens on vascular endothelial cells: a detailed phenotypic analysis. *Br. J. Haematol.* 1990; 74:385–394.

27. Weidner, N. Folkman, J. Tumoral vascularity as a prognostic factor in cancer. In: *Important Advances in Oncology,* eds. DeVita, V., Hellman, S. and Rosenberg, S.A. Lipincott-Raven Press, Philadelphia, 1997.

28. O'Leary, J., Young, D., Shalinsky, D., Carroll, P. and Shuman, M. Identification of membrane type matrix metallorproteinase-1 (MT-MMP-1) in human prostate cancer and in vivo inhibition of PC3 cell invasion and angiogenesis by AG3340 [Abstract]. *Proc. Am . Soc. Clin. Oncol.,* 1999;A1198.

29. Shalinsky, D.R., Brekken, J., Zou, H., Kolis, S., Wood, A., Webber, S. and Appelt, K. Antitumor efficacy of AG3340 associated with maintenance of minimum effective plasma concentrations and not total daily dose, exposure or peak plasma concentrations. *Investigational New Drugs,* 1999; 16:4, 303–313.

30. Zou, H., Brekken, J. and Shalinsky, D.R. Human tumors retain sensitivity to AG3340, a selective metalloprotease inhibitor, after extended treatment and serial passage in vivo. *Proc. Am. Assoc. Cancer Res.* 1999; 40:A4886.

31. Collier, M.A., Yuen, G.J., Bansal, S.K., Kolis, S., Chew, T.G., Appelt, K. and Clendeninn, N.J. A Phase I study of the matrix metalloproteinase inhibitor (MMP) inhibitor, AG3340 given in single doses to healthy volunteers. *Proc. Am. Assoc. Cancer Res.* 1997; 38:A1491.

32. Collier, M.A., Yuen, G.J., Bansal, S., Kolis, S., Petersen, A.K., Chew, T.G., and Clendeninn, N.J. Phase I studies of the matrix metalloproteinase (MMP) inhibitor AG3340 administered as an oral tablet in single and multiple doses [Abstract]. *Intl. J. Oncol., Proc 2nd World Congress Advances in Oncology.* 1997;11:A308.

33. Hande, K., Wilding, G., Ripple, G., Fry, J., Arzoomanian, R., Dixon, M., Yuen, G., Collier, M.A. Phase I study of AG3340, a matrix metalloproteinase (MMP) inhibitor, in patients having advanced cancer [Abstract]. *Proc NCI/EORTC.* 1998; Amsterdam, The Netherlands.

34. Wilding, G., Small, E., Ripple, G., Keller, M.R., Yuen, G., and Collier, M. Phase I study of AG3340, a matrix metalloproteinase inhibitor, in combination with mitoxantrone/prednisone in patients having advanced prostate cancer. *Proc NCI/EORTC.,* 1998; Amsterdam, The Netherlands.

35. Wilding, G., Small, E., Collier, M., Dixon, M., and Pithavala, Y. A phase I pharmacokinetic evaluation of the matrix metalloprotease (MMP) inhibitor AG3340 in combination with mitoxantrone and prednisone in patients with advanced prostate cancer. *Proc. Amer. Soc. Clin. Oncol.* 1999;18:A1244.

36. D'Olimpio, J., Hande, K., Collier, M., Michelson, G., Paradiso, L., and Clendeninn, N. Phase I study of the matrix metalloprotease inhibitor AG3340 in combination with paclitaxel and carboplatin for the treatment of patients with advanced solid tumors. *Proc. Amer. Soc. Clin. Oncol.* 1999;18:A615.

37. Collier, M., Shepherd, F., Ahmann, F.R., Keller, M.R., Michelson, G., Paradiso, L., Clendeninn. N., and the Lung and Prostate Cancer Study Groups. A novel approach to studying the efficacy of AG3340, a selective inhibitor of matrix metalloproteinases. *Proc. Amer. Soc. Clin. Oncol.* 1999;18:A1861.

38. Shi, Z.O., Raithatha, S., Spencer, D.P., Rewcastle, N.B., Brasher, P.M., Morris, D., Feeley, R., Brekken, J., Shalinsky, D.R., Johnston, R., Edwards, D.R., Forsyth, P. Enhanced effectiveness of a novel MMP inhibitor, prinomastat (AG3340) with radiotherapy (RT) in a glioma model. *Proc. Am. Assoc. Cancer Res.* 2000;41:A2071.

7

A Potent Nonpeptidic Matrix Metalloproteinase Inhibitor
Discovery of BAY 12-9566

G. Clemens, *PhD*, B. Hibner, *PhD*,
R. Humphrey, *MD*, H. Kluender, *PhD*,
and S. Wilhelm, *PhD*

CONTENTS

1. INTRODUCTION

Inhibitors of matrix metalloproteinases (MMPs) are comprised of a zinc-binding functional group which targets the inhibitor to the catalytic zinc within the active site of the enzyme, and a peptidomimetic portion which increases the affinity of the inhibitor to the enzyme active site, thereby mimicking the natural peptide substrate. The majority of first generation inhibitors of MMPs were first described in the literature in the late 1980s. These matrix metalloproteinase inhibitors (MMPIs) were designed as inhibitors of fibroblast interstitial collagenase (MMP-1) and consisted of a hydroxamic acid as the zinc-binding functional group and a LeuLeuPhe or LeuPhe as a mimetic of the preferred substrate of MMP-1 (Fig. 1) *(1)*. These early compounds were often broad-spectrum MMPIs, with potent inhibitory activity against fibroblast collagenase, stromelysin-1 (MMP-3), and the gelatinases (MMP-2 and MMP-9). As pep-

From: *Cancer Drug Discovery and Development:*
Matrix Metalloproteinase Inhibitors in Cancer Therapy
Edited by: Neil J. Clendeninn and Krzysztof Appelt © Humana Press Inc., Totowa, NJ

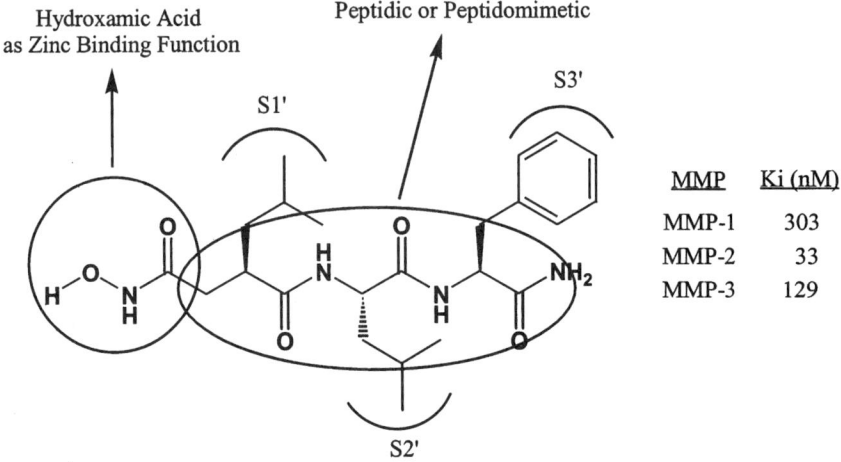

Fig. 1. An early MMP inhibitor from an ICI (Stuart) team.

tides, they suffered from low bioavailability and rapid metabolism, and as hydroxamic acids they were potentially mutagenic.

In spite of these weaknesses, several research teams discovered peptidomimetic hydroxamic acids as clinical candidates with reasonable bioavailability, longer $T_{1/2}$, and relatively minimal toxicity (in preclinical studies). Most of these second generation compounds share the same broad-spectrum activity of the original leads. Beckett and Whittaker (2) have recently reviewed broad-spectrum as well as selective MMPIs that are known to be in the clinic for the treatment of cancer, arthritis, and several other indications.

2. RANDOM SCREENING AT BAYER

In an effort to move beyond the peptidomimetic hydroxamic acid strategy, a team of scientists at Bayer Corporation (Pharmaceutical Division, West Haven, CT) conducted a random high throughput screen of repository compounds for novel inhibitors of MMPs. The strategy used by Bayer was to identify novel inhibitors that were selective for the MMPs believed to be implicated in the etiologies of osteoarthritis (MMP-3) and various cancers (MMP-2, MMP-9). Inhibitory activity against MMP-1 was negatively selected against because of its widespread expression and potential for adverse effects.

The search was initially conducted using heat-activated truncated recombinant human stromelysin-1 (3) (MMP-3) together with a thiopeptolide spectrophotometric substrate (structure below), following the assay methods of Weingarten (4). Human gelatinase B (MMP-9) was isolated from polymorphonuclear leukocytes following a modification of the methods of Hibbs et al. (5) and Wilhelm et al. (6), and subsequently used in a similar thiopeptolide assay to identify the hits from the first search that were also inhibitors of MMP-

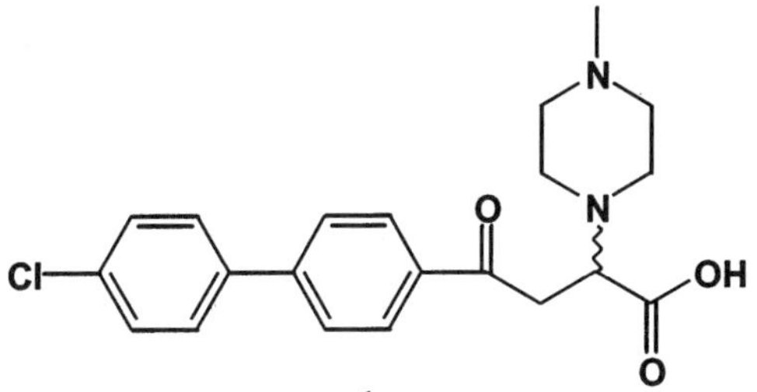

IC$_{50}$ (as hydrochloride)
2 μM (MMP-3)
ca. 5 μM (MMP-9)
inactive (MMP-1)

Fig. 2. An MMP inhibitor from a random screen.

9. Human gingival fibroblast MMP-1 was obtained from Dr. Jack Windsor *(7)* (University of Alabama at Birmingham), human recombinant MMP-2 was obtained from Dr. William Stetler-Stevenson *(8)* (National Cancer Institute, Bethesda, MD), human recombinant MMP-13 was obtained from Dr. Gillian Murphy *(9)* (Strangeways Research Laboratory, Cambridge, UK), human recombinant MMP-8 and MMP-14 were obtained from Dr. Harold Tschesche *(10,11)* (Universitat of Bielefeld, Bielefeld, GR).

A superior assay was later developed as a modification of procedures first described by Knight et al *(12)*. This assay used a more sensitive and stable fluorogenic substrate (our identifying code P218, structure below) at enzyme and substrate concentrations that were low enough to determine the K$_m$'s for a larger bank of MMPs, calculate the K$_i$'s, and thereby measure selectivity of our lead substances. Each assay was automated in 96-well plates using a Hamilton Microlab AT Plus robotic system together with a Biotek Ceres UV Spectrophotometer (thiopeptolide substrate) or Perceptive Systems Cytoflour 2300 plate reader (fluorogenic substrate).

Thiopeptolide substrate: Ac-Pro-Leu-**Gly-S-Leu**-Leu-Gly-OC$_2$H$_5$

Fluorogenic substrate (P218): MCA-Pro-Lys-Pro-**Leu-Ala**-Leu-DPA-Ala-Arg-NH$_2$

A particularly attractive hit that emerged from the MMP-3 based random screen was the substituted 3-biphenoyl propionic acid (1) shown in Figure 2. This compound, a substituted derivative of the antiinflammatory compound fenbufen *(13)*, is neither a hydroxamic acid nor a peptide and is thus novel as an MMP inhibitor. Subsequent studies indicated that compound 1 was a competitive and selective inhibitor of MMPs with activity vs MMP-3 and MMP-9, but insignificant activity vs MMP-1 at 5 μM.

Although compound 1 had many positive features as a lead, it suffered from questionable reactivity, as it was prone to a β-elimination that yielded inactive decomposition products, especially when it was stored as the water soluble (and thus easier to assay) hydrochloride.

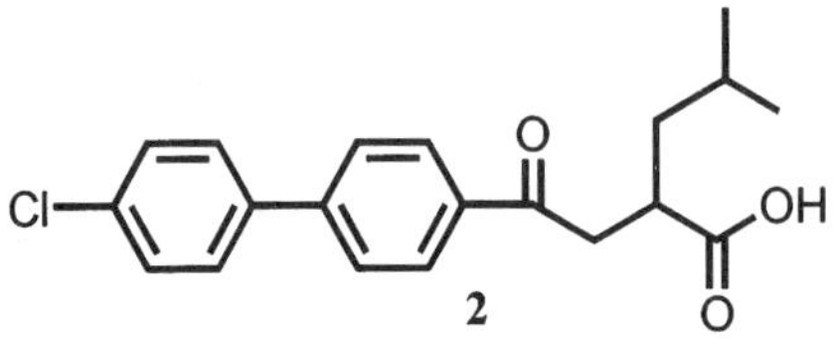

RS - IC_{50} 0.59 μM (MMP-3)
1.0 μM (MMP-9)
very weak (MMP-1)
S - IC_{50} 0.28 μM (MMP-3)
R - IC_{50} weak (MMP-3)

Fig. 3. A nonreactive 3-biphenoyl propionic acid MMP inhibitor is discovered.

3. OPTIMIZATION OF THE SCREENING HIT

A major breakthrough occurred when it was discovered that the reactive N-methylpiperazine side chain could be replaced with an isobutyl group *(14)*. The resultant compound 2, shown in Figure 3, had both increased MMPI activity and increased stability compared with compound 1. Chiral syntheses of the two isomers of compound 2 indicated that most MMPI activity resided in the 2S enantiomer *(15)*. As with compound 1, this compound was active as an inhibitor of MMP-3 and MMP-9, but only weakly active vs MMP-1.

Classical medicinal chemistry methodologies, together with an appreciation of drug/protein interactions on an atomic level obtained through structures determined by nuclear magnetic resonance (NMR) and X-ray, led to the discovery of BAY 12-9566, which was to become a clinical candidate for the treatment of osteoarthritis and cancer. The synthesis and in vitro MMP inhibition exhibited by BAY 12-9566 are shown in Figure 4 and Table 1 *(14)*.

Attempts to determine the structures of complexes of various 3-biphenoyl propionic acids and MMP-3 by either high field NMR or X-ray studies of crystals were ongoing in parallel with the classical medicinal chemistry approaches. Whereas the complex of BAY 12-9566 with MMP-3 eluded our best attempts at crystallization, the structures of several related MMP inhibitor complexes were determined by either or both of the techniques. Figure 4 is a cartoon which depicts the structure of an analog of BAY 12-9566 as determined by high field NMR experiments *(16)*. As with all of our 3-biphenoyl propionic acids, the biphenyl group was bound deep into the P1′ pocket and the 1-carboxyl group was bound to the zinc which resides in the active site. As is the case for many of the biphenyl MMPIs, the carboxyl group appeared to form bidentate bonds with the zinc atom, and sometimes the binding was increased by the additional interaction of the carboxy OH with Glu 202 of the enzyme. The 4-carbonyl group consistently formed bifurcated hydrogen bonds to the backbone NH of Ala 165 and Leu 164, and the side chain phenyl group was found in the P2 pocket. These novel compounds thus bridge the catalytic site of MMP-3. In every case, the biologically active bound isomer was found to have the 2S absolute configuration, even when racemates were used in the NMR or X-ray studies. An X-ray study of pure BAY 12-9566 crystals confirmed the 2S configuration of this single enantiomer, as shown in Figure 5 *(17)*. Figure 6 shows the X-ray structure of crystals of BAY 12-9566.

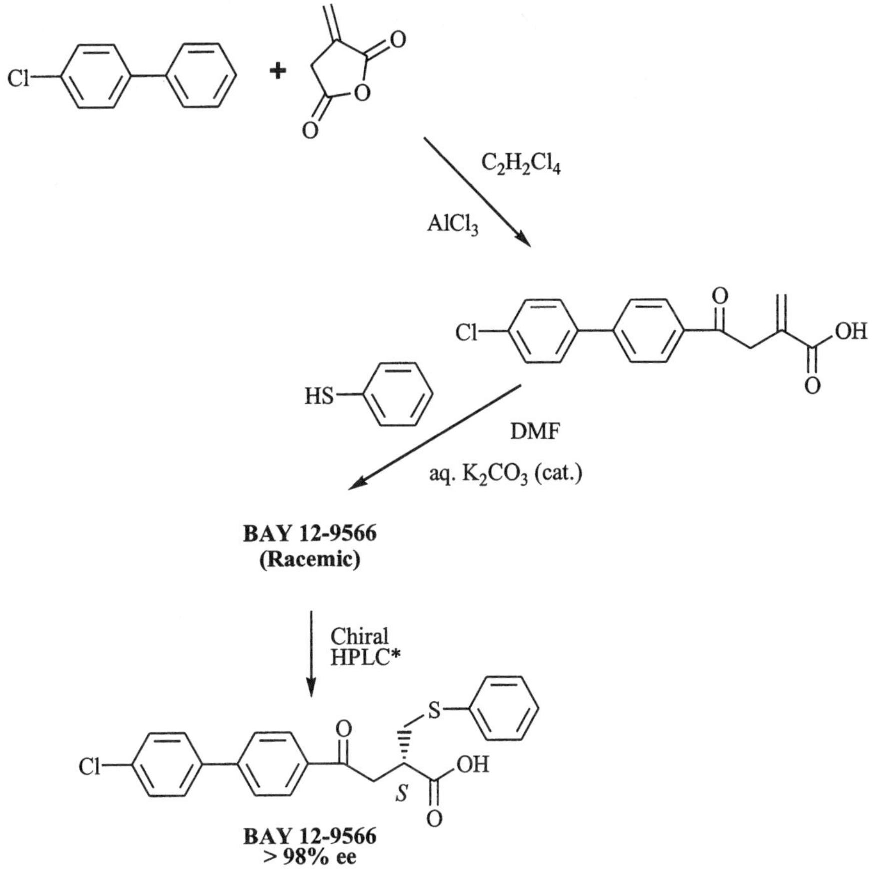

Fig. 4. Preparation of BAY 12-9566. *A proprietary chiral stationary phase was used for good resolution. Large quantities can be obtained by classical resolution using (+)-cinchonine

Table 1
In Vitro Inhibitory Activity of BAY 12-9566[a]

MMP	MMP-1 K_i (nM)	MMP-2 K_i (nM)	MMP-3 K_i (nM)	MMP-8 IC_{50} (nM)	MMP-9 K_i (nM)	MMP-13 IC_{50} (nM)	MMP-14 IC_{50} (nM)
value	> 5,000	11	134	51	301	1470	400

[a]Assays were performed at 6 μM substrate and 0.1–0.5 nM active MMPs at pH 6.5 for 30 min at room temperature. MMP-1 was isolated from human gingival fibroblasts; MMP-2, MMP-3, MMP-8, MMP-9, MMP-13, and MMP-14 are recombinant human enzymes.

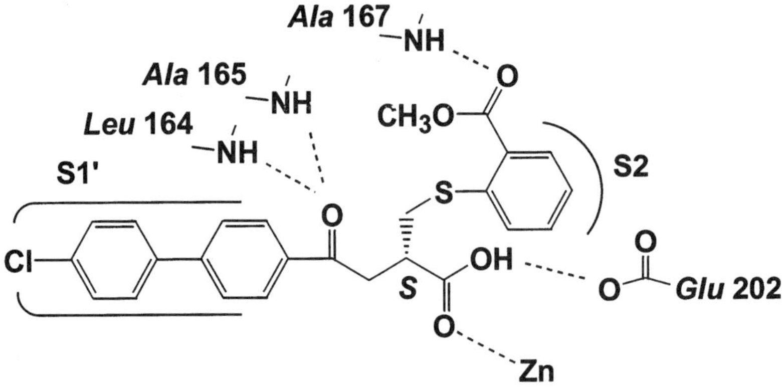

Fig. 5. Interactions of a representative 4-biphenoyl propionic acid MMPI with MMP-3 *(16)*.

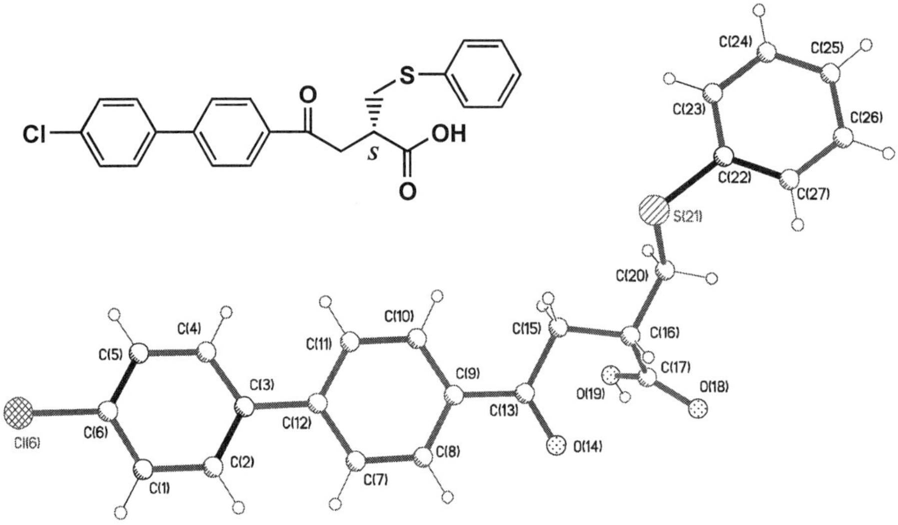

Fig. 6. X-ray structure of crystals of pure BAY 12-9566 *(17)*.

The remainder of this chapter presents the results of preclinical experiments designed to assess the antitumor activity and toxicolgy of this novel MMPI, as well as the results of the initial phase I studies in patients with cancer.

4. PRECLINICAL ACTIVITY

4.1. Activity Against Invasion and Angiogenesis

BAY 12-9566 has been tested in both in vitro and in vivo experimental models to determine whether it can inhibit cell invasion and angiogenesis. In one experiment, human umbilical vein endothelial cells (HUVEC) were treated with BAY 12-9566 to examine antiangiogenic activity in vitro *(18)*. There was a dose-dependent decrease in the ability of HUVEC to invade through matrigel, a solution of matrix proteins, in a modified Boyden chamber assay, with an IC_{50} of 9.1×10^{-7} M. In contrast, the motility of the endothelial cells, which was not dependent on matrix degradation, was not inhibited at these concentrations, indicating that the decreased invasion was not a toxic effect on the cells. In addition, treatment of HUVEC with BAY 12-9566 for 6 h did not inhibit proliferation in a 3 d assay.

The effect of BAY 12-9566 on the angiogenic response was also assessed in vivo in the matrigel model. Matrigel was mixed with bFGF at 150 ng/pellet as the angiogenic stimulus, and 0.5 mL of the solution was injected subcutaneously into C57BL/6 mice. Over the course of 4–7 d, new blood vessels invaded the gel, and this response was quantified by determining blood content (hemoglobin) and/or by counting vessels. Treatment with 200 mg/kg BAY 12-9566 orally for 4 d resulted in a significant reduction in hemoglobin content *(19)*. A second experiment using 25, 50, and 200 mg/kg BAY 12-9566 orally for 7 d demonstrated significant decreases in hemoglobin content at both 50 and 200 mg/kg, with no effect at 25 mg/kg *(18)*. Histological analysis of the matrigel pellets confirmed that in the animals treated with BAY 12-9566, endothelial cells were poorly organized, and there was a reduced number of mature vessels.

BAY 12-9566 was also tested for antiinvasive activity in a cell based assay. Similar to human endothelial cells, tumor cells require matrix degradation to invade and metastasize. When tested in an in vitro invasion assay similar to that described previously, BAY 12-9566 inhibited HT1080 tumor cell invasion by 38% and 66% at 2.5 and 55 μM, respectively *(19)*. At these concentrations, BAY 12-9566 did not inhibit tumor cell motility or the proliferation of HT1080 cells in a 3 d assay.

4.2. Activity Against Metastasis in Murine Models

BAY 12-9566 was tested in two murine models used to assess tumor growth and metastatic capabilities, the B16 murine melanoma and the murine Lewis Lung Carcinoma (LLC) models. In an experiment performed at Southern Research Institute, B16 tumors maintained in serial passage were implanted subcutaneously into C57BL/6 female mice. Oral administration of BAY 12-9566 at 100 mg/kg twice daily for 14 d inhibited the subcutaneous growth of B16 melanoma tumors by 50%, presumably by decreasing blood vessel support, as the compound did not demonstrate antiproliferative or cytotoxic properties in vitro *(20)*. To mimic part of the metastatic cascade, B16.F10 cells were injected into the tail vein of female BDF1 mice, and animals were monitored for lung colony growth. BAY 12-9566 was administered at doses up to 100 mg/kg orally. At four timepoints (day −1 to day +2) obtained around the time

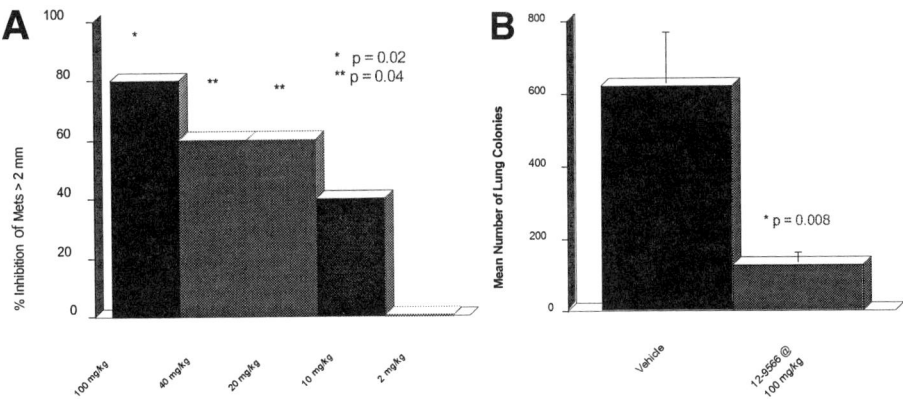

Fig. 7. (A) A forced metastasis model showing the inhibitory effect of BAY 12-9566 on the development of large metastases. **(B)** A forced metastasis model showing the inhibitory effect of 100 mg/kg BAY 12-9566 on the overall development of metastases.

of tumor cell inoculation, BAY 12-9566 inhibited the growth of lung nodules by a maximum of 58% at 100 mg/kg. When analyzed by size, the growth of lung colonies larger than 2 mm^3 was inhibited by 80% at 100 mg/kg (Fig. 7a) *(21)*. Increasing the length of treatment with 100 mg/kg once daily to 14 d led to an 80% inhibition in the overall number of lung colonies (Fig. 7b), with an 87% inhibition of colonies larger than 2 mm^3.

In the LLC model, untreated, subcutaneous LLC tumors spontaneously metastasize to the lungs and grow in this secondary site, providing a model that reproduces the entire metastatic pathway of local tumor growth, tumor cell invasion, and spread through the vasculature to a secondary metastatic site. Treatment with BAY 12-9566 administered orally at 100 mg/kg once daily from d 3 through d 20 after tumor implantation significantly inhibited subcutaneous LLC tumor growth by 50% *(20)*. In this experiment, treatment with BAY 12-9566 resulted in a maximum reduction in the number of lung metastases of 86% and in the number of lung metastases > 3 mm^3 of 90%. A higher dose of BAY 12-9566 (200 mg/kg) did not inhibit either subcutaneous tumor growth or lung metastasis.

4.3. Activity Against Metastasis in Xenograft Models

The activity of BAY 12-9566 was also examined in a human subcutaneous xenograft model. Fragments of the human colon cell line HCT 116, maintained by serial passage in nude mice, were implanted into CD-1 nu/nu female mice. Animals were dosed orally with BAY 12-9566 beginning on d 2 through day 44. Maximal inhibition of subcutaneous growth was 40% at a dose of 30 mg/kg daily *(22)*. Histological analysis of these tumors revealed that the tumors were

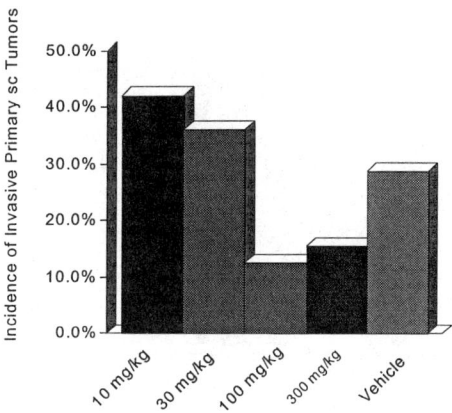

Fig. 8. Treatment with BAY 12-9566 reduced the incidence of tumor invasion by a maximum of 60%.

poorly differentiated, and the majority were moderately vascularized around the periphery. No significant differences in vascularization or degree of necrosis was observed in this experiment; however, the mitotic index was qualitatively reduced in all treatment groups compared with vehicle controls. In addition, although no tumors were noted to have invaded through the peritoneal wall or to have metastasized, as is consistent with this model, there was a significant dose-dependent inhibition in the incidence of tumor cell invasion into the surrounding subcutaneous connective tissue (Fig. 8).

BAY 12-9566 has also been tested in human tumor metastatic xenograft models. In one model, fragments of serially passaged HCT 116 tumors were implanted onto the cecums of CD-1 nude mice *(23)*. Treatment with BAY 12-9566 at 100 mg/kg from day 5 through the end of the study resulted in a 35% inhibition in the growth of the primary tumor, similar to that observed with subcutaneously growing HCT 116 tumors. Within all groups, hematogenous, lymphatic, and intraperitoneal metastases were identified. Metastases tended to be more poorly differentiated than the primary tumors. The most common metastatic sites were the liver, pancreas, lungs, intestinal mesentery, and mesenteric lymph nodes. Liver, pancreas, and lungs were evaluated histologically for the presence of metastases, using 2–3 sections/organ. A dose-dependent inhibition in the overall incidence of metastases was observed for both liver (55% decrease in incidence at 50 and 100 mg/kg) and pancreas (46% decrease in incidence at 100 mg/kg) (Fig. 9). A decrease in the incidence of metastases compared with control animals was not observed in the lungs; however, the incidence of metastases in the lungs of control animals was below that expected. A dose-dependent decrease in metastasis did occur in the drug-treated groups,

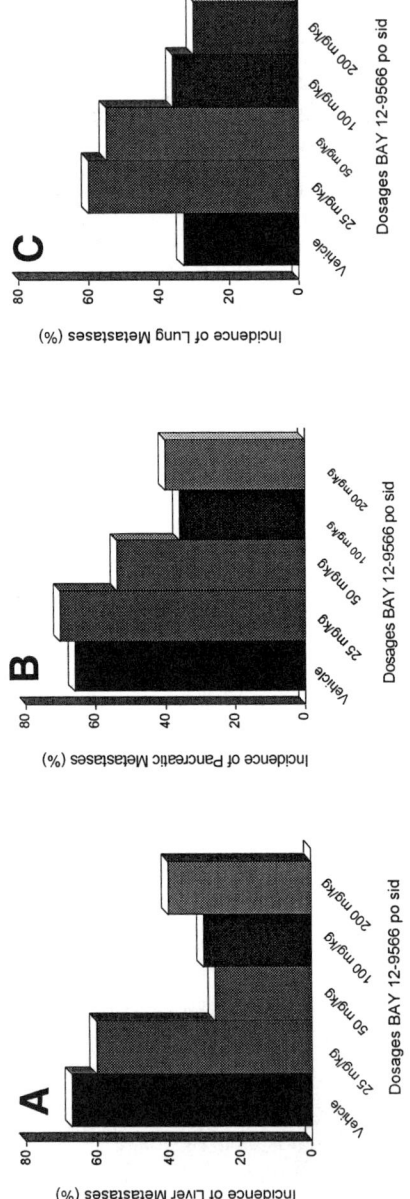

Fig. 9. (**A**) The incidence of liver metastases was reduced with BAY 12-9566 treatment. (**B**) The incidence of pancreatic metastases was reduced with BAY 12-9566 treatment. (**C**) The incidence of lung metastases was not reduced by BAY 12-9566 compared with vehicle.

with a maximal inhibition of 67% at a dose of 200 mg/kg. In addition, lung metastases that were present in the drug-treated groups were typically fewer in number and smaller in size.

Experiments using a second human orthotopic metastatic model were performed in the laboratory of Dr. G. Sledge at Indiana Cancer Research Institute. In this model, the human breast carcinoma MDA MB-435 was implanted into the mammary fat pad of nude mice *(24)*. After 8 wk, the tumor, which by this time had metastasized to the lung, was resected and the animals were treated orally daily with BAY 12-9566 or vehicle alone for 7 wk. Animals receiving 100 mg/kg BAY 12-9566 demonstrated a 51% decrease in the regrowth of the primary tumor, and a 57% inhibition in the number of lung metastases. In addition, the overall size of the lung metastases was reduced by 88%.

As mentioned above, a clear dose-proportional response to treatment with BAY 12-9566 was not observed in several experiments. In the HCT 116 colon orthotopic experiment described above, blood samples were obtained from the mice in the study on day 14. Pharmacokinetic analysis indicated that although the dose was increased eightfold, exposure (AUD_{0-24}) increased less than twofold. The less than dose-proportional increase in drug exposure may be due to a saturation of oral absorption in mice as the dose is escalated, and/or an increase in drug metabolism through the induction of liver enzymes.

In conclusion, BAY 12-9566 is a potent inhibitor of MMPs and has demonstrated antiangiogenic, antiinvasive, and antimetastatic activity in a variety of cell based assays and murine tumor models, including models of murine and human tumor metastasis.

5. PRECLINICAL DRUG SAFETY ASSESSMENT

In addition to the experiments described above, acute, multidose (subacute, subchronic, and chronic), and reproductive toxicology studies have also been performed with BAY 12-9566 in rodents and nonrodents *(25)*. Other studies have been undertaken in vitro and in vivo to assess mutagenicity and/or clastogenicity and safety pharmacology.

BAY 12-9566 has little potential for acute oral toxicity, with dose-limiting toxicity values above 2000 mg/kg in both rats and mice and 1000 mg/kg in the dog. The Ames test (with 5 tester strains), an in vitro mammalian chromosome aberration test, the HGPRT forward mutation assay (all with and without metabolic activation), and the mouse micronucleus test have revealed no evidence for mutagenic and/or clastogenic potential. Numerous safety pharmacology studies, including those assessing the central nervous system, pulmonary function, intestinal motility, ileal contractions, hemodynamics and cardiac contractility, and renal function, as well as studies for photoreactive and antigenic potential, did not reveal safety concerns for BAY 12-9566.

Multidose oral subacute (2- and 4-wk), subchronic (13-wk) and chronic (6-mo rat and 12-mo dog) toxicity studies have been performed with BAY 12-9566. In the multidose program, the highest dose levels tested were 400 mg/kg in rats, 300 mg/kg in dogs, and greater than 800 mg/kg in mice. These studies have identified the erythron, kidney (rodent only), and liver as primary targets for toxicity. The effects on the liver ranged from an adaptive, hepatocellular hypertrophy in the rat liver to distinct elevations of serum transaminase levels (particularly alanine aminotransferase) in the dog. Elevations in serum transaminase activity in the dog rapidly returned to normal values posttreatment. Single cell necrosis of hepatocytes was observed only at doses nearing the maximum tolerated dose. In vitro studies of P450 subfamilies suggested that BAY 12-9566 would be only a weak inducer in humans, if at all.

Decreases in red blood cells, hemoglobin, and hematocrit were observed in all 3 species, but only at the higher dose levels tested. In the Wistar rat, a degenerative renal tubulopathy was observed in both males and females, whereas in the NCI BR strain, tubulopathy was observed only in female rats. In the male rats, the nephropathy was attributed to the presence of $\alpha 2\mu$-globulin. The nephropathy did not occur in the male NCI BR strain of rat, which is a strain deficient in $\alpha 2$ μ-globulin. Since the $\alpha 2$ μ-globulin nephropathy is specific to the rat, it is not considered relevant in human risk assessment. The renal findings and changes in hematologic values were reversible upon discontinuation of the drug. There was no evidence for tendonitis following chronic administration of BAY 12-9566, although tendonitis is known to occur with some matrix metalloproteinase inhibitors. On the basis of chronic studies, the dose levels at which no adverse events were observed have been established at 15 mg/kg for the rat and 75 mg/kg for the dog.

Fertility and reproductive performance were unaffected, even at maternal and paternal toxic dose levels. In developmental toxicity studies in the rat and rabbit, there was no evidence for selective targeting of the developing conceptus at doses below those causing overt maternal toxicity.

6. PHASE I CLINICAL RESULTS

6.1. Pharmacokinetics

The clinical trials completed thus far with BAY 12-9566 consist of five phase I studies initiated in the United States and Canada. These studies were designed to examine the safety and pharmacokinetics of BAY 12-9566 in humans. The first study, U.S. D95-024, was a randomized, double-blind, placebo-controlled, parallel group study exploring the safety and pharmacokinetics of ascending multiple dose levels of BAY 12-9566 (26). Participants in the study were healthy subjects of both sexes, 45–70 years of age. At each dose level, subjects received BAY 12-9566 or placebo. Plasma samples were collected at each dose level on d 1 and at steady state on d 16.

A comparison of the plasma levels of BAY 12-9566 at the various doses revealed that increases in plasma concentrations were less than dose-proportional above the 100 mg/d dose of BAY 12-9566. For example, the AUC_{0-24h} value at steady-state for the 400 mg dose (2150 mg mg*h/L) was only approximately twice the corresponding d 16 value at the 100 mg/d dose (1080 mg*h/L), and not fourfold as would be predicted if plasma levels were proportional to dose. The same trend was observed in values of C_{max} and C_{min}. Values of AUC_{0-24h} and C_{max} (AUC_{0-24h} norm. and C_{max} norm.) normalized for dose and weight were similar for doses up to 100 mg/d, but decreased for 200 mg/d and 400 mg/d dose levels, again demonstrating the less than dose-proportional increase beyond the 100 mg dose level. The nonlinearity in pharmacokinetics above the 100 mg dose level was also observed on d 1.

The d 16/d 1 AUC_{0-24h} accumulation ratios for all dose levels (10–400 mg/d) were approx 4 to 5. These observations suggested that enzyme induction was not the explanation for the nonlinear pharmacokinetics at the higher dose levels. Saturation of absorption, possibly related to the low aqueous solubility of BAY 12-9566, seemed to be the most likely explanation for the nonlinear pharmacokinetics above the 100 mg dose level.

Four phase I studies in patients with cancer have been conducted in the United States and Canada *(27–30)*. In total, 89 individuals with cancer received BAY 12-9566 in doses ranging from 100 mg daily to 800 mg twice daily. Eligible patients must have had evidence that their tumor was progressing in spite of all known standard-of-care therapy. Patients remained on BAY 12-9566 unless they experienced significant side effects or their tumor progressed.

As with the healthy volunteers in the D95-024 study, cancer patients in the phase I studies had less than dose-proportional increases in plasma concentrations above the 100 mg/d dose level. In the cancer patients, doubling the dose from 100 mg once daily to 200 mg once daily resulted in an increase in the steady-state trough concentration of approx 50%. Doubling the daily dose from 200 mg to 400 mg resulted in an increase in the steady-state trough concentration of only 34%. By extrapolation, it was estimated that increasing the dose from 400 mg once daily to 800 mg once daily would produce an increase in the steady-state trough concentration of only about 20%. Thus, it could be predicted that the steady-state trough concentration at a dose of 800 mg once daily was unlikely to be notably higher than 100 mg/L.

Based on the overall data which suggested that the less than dose-proportional increase in plasma levels of BAY 12-9566 was due to a limitation in absorption, doses higher than 400 mg were administered as split doses in an attempt to increase absorption and achieve higher trough concentrations and AUC_{0-24h} at steady-state. Administration of 400 mg two times daily (bid) resulted in a mean steady state trough concentration of 115 mg/L and mean steady-state AUC_{0-24h} of 2300 mg*h/L. These values were significantly higher than corresponding values at 400 mg once daily, and values predicted for 800 mg administered as a single dose.

Since the administration of 400 mg bid produced notably higher steady-state trough and AUC_{0-24h} values compared with 400 mg given once daily, it was decided to evaluate dose levels of 400 mg three times daily (tid) and 400 mg four times daily (qid). A dose of 400 mg tid produced notable increases in the steady-state trough concentration and AUC_{0-24h} compared with 400 mg bid, but 400 mg qid was not different from 400 mg tid. It therefore appeared that increasing the daily dose of BAY 12-9566 beyond 1200–1600 mg/d was unlikely to produce meaningful increases in the plasma concentration of BAY 12-9566.

The administration of BAY 12-9566 at a dose of 800 mg bid produced steady-state trough concentrations and AUC_{0-24h} similar to 400 mg tid, while offering the convenience of a twice daily regimen. Overall systemic exposure was similar at the 800 mg bid and 400 mg tid doses. Therefore, BAY 12-9566 800 mg bid was determined to be the best dose based on overall exposure and dosing schedule considerations.

6.2. Safety

BAY 12-9566 was well-tolerated in the phase I studies. Few patients discontinued therapy due to adverse events that could not be attributed to tumor progression. The musculoskeletal syndrome described with first generation MMPIs (hydroxamates) was not observed in any patient.

Grade 1 and 2 decreases in platelet counts were noted in 13 (29%) of the patients receiving the highest doses of BAY 12-9566 (400 mg tid, 400 mg qid, 800 mg bid), whereas only 3 (7%) of the patients at the highest doses experienced grade 3 and 4 decreases in platelet counts. Of these three patients, two were noted to have platelet counts of approx 50,000 cells/mm^3 and one was noted to have a platelet count that steadily decreased to a nadir of 29,000 cells/mm^3. This latter patient had cancer-related disseminated intravascular coagulation that had been noted in the months prior to the start of treatment with BAY 12-9566. Moreover, the rate of decline of her platelet count was not affected by the initiation of treatment with BAY 12-9566. None of the patients with thrombocytopenia experienced bleeding related to the drop in platelets and all had rapid increases in the platelet count when treatment with BAY 12-9566 was completed or the dose reduced. The relationship of the thrombocytopenia to prior anticancer therapy remains unclear.

A close examination of the patients in the phase I studies revealed that nearly all patients experienced some dose-dependent decrease in platelet count that remained within the normal range. In general, the platelet nadir occurred approx 2 wk after the initiation of therapy with BAY 12-9566, which corresponded to the onset of steady-state plasma levels of BAY 12-9566. Typically, the platelet count remained stable or, in some cases, began to increase even in the continued presence of BAY 12-9566. It is currently unclear whether this dose-dependent depression in the platelet count represents a biological effect of BAY 12-9566. Studies to define the role of MMPs in the transfer of platelets from the bone marrow to the circulation are planned.

Studies designed to test the safety of BAY 12-9566 in combination with standard chemotherapy agents are ongoing and are expected to be completed soon. Available data suggest that there are no safety concerns or pharmacokinetic interactions with BAY 12-9566 and paclitaxel or carboplatin.

6.3. Anticancer Activity

In phase I studies that test conventional chemotherapy agents, shrinkage of tumors provides an early indication of anticancer activity. Unlike standard chemotherapy agents, however, MMPIs such as BAY 12-9566 are not expected to cause a tumor to shrink but rather to slow the growth and spread of the tumor. The pace with which cancer progresses varies substantially from patient to patient, and it may be unclear whether stabilization of the growth of a tumor represents a true effect of the drug or the slow-growing nature of the tumor itself. As such, it is difficult to determine whether patients receiving BAY 12-9566 during the phase I studies derived benefit. Well-controlled phase III clinical trials are the only means to truly determine the efficacy of an MMPI such as BAY 12-9566.

Of the 89 eligible patients that were enrolled into the four phase I studies in patients with cancer, 32 (36%) patients with a variety of cancers remained on BAY 12-9566 for 100 days or more, 11 (12%) remained on BAY 12-9566 for 200 days or more, and 5 (6%) remained on BAY 12-9566 for greater than one year. As of December 28, 1998, one patient has been on study without toxicity or cancer progression for 13 mo and another for 18.6 mo. Thus, although tumor shrinkage was not expected or observed, many patients remained stable on BAY 12-9566 for longer than would normally be expected.

One patient who remains on BAY 12-9566 to date was diagnosed with mesothelioma 3 mo prior to entry into a BAY 12-9566 phase I study. The patient's cancer progressed quickly through his first regimen of cisplatin and he has remained on BAY 12-9566 (400 mg daily) for 18.6 mo without evidence of tumor progression. This is highly unusual for mesothelioma, which tends to be very aggressive and rapidly fatal. The other patient who remains on therapy (800 mg bid) has colorectal cancer and has remained stable after more than 13 mo of treatment with BAY 12-9566. This patient underwent an abdominal aortic aneurysm repair while on study without perioperative complications.

Other patients also remained stable on prolonged treatment with BAY 12-9566. Such patients include a woman with omental cancer who started therapy with paclitaxel in February, 1997; she progressed after only 2 mo. She was then entered into a BAY 12-9566 phase I study at a dose of 400 mg tid. She remained on BAY 12-9566 without toxicity for more than 15 mo before small bowel obstruction (possibly related to tumor progression) prompted discontinuation of therapy. A patient with renal cell cancer and multiple lung lesions was enrolled into a phase I study at a dose of 400 mg bid. He remained on treatment with BAY 12-9566 with no apparent change in his tumor burden or toxicity before formally progressing on study after 1 year of therapy.

Phase III clinical studies have been designed to determine whether BAY 12-9566 can prolong the time of remission and improve survival in patients who have responded to chemotherapy and/or radiation for lung cancer and ovarian cancer. Other studies are evaluating whether patients with pancreatic cancer can survive longer and have an improved quality of life on oral BAY 12-9566 compared with patients receiving the intravenous chemotherapy agent gemcitabine. Additional studies in patients with a variety of other cancer types will open in 1999.

REFERENCES

1. Caputo, C.B., Wolanin, D.J., Roberts, R.A., Sygowski, L.A., Patton, S.P., Caccese, G.G., Shaw, A., and DiPasquale, G. Proteoglycan Degradation by a Chondrocyte Metalloprotease—Effects of Synthetic Protease Inhibitors. *Biochem. Pharm.* 1987: 36:995–1002.
2. Beckett R.P. and Whittaker, M. Matrix metalloproteinase inhibitors 1998. *Expert Opinion on Therapeutic Patents* 1998; 8(3):259–282.
3. Housley, T.J., Baumann, A.P., Braun, I.D., Davis, G., Seperack, P.K., and Wilhelm, S.M. Recombinant Chinese Hamster Ovary Cell Matrix Metalloprotease-3 (MMP-3, Stromelysin-1). *J. Biol. Chem.* 1993; 268:4481–4487.
4. Weingarten, H. and Feder, J. Spectrophotometric Assay for Vertebrate Collagenase. *Anal. Biochem.* 1985; 147:437–440.
5. Hibbs, M.S., Hasty, K.A., Seyer, J.M., Kang, A.H., and Mainardi, C.L. Biochemical and Immunological Characterization of the Secreted Forms of Human Neutrophil Gelatinase. *J. Biol. Chem.* 1984; 260:2493–2500.
6. Wilhelm, S.M., Collier, I.E., Marmer, B.L., Eisen, A.Z., Grant, G.A., and Goldberg, G.I. SV40-transformed Human Lung Fibroblasts Secrete a 92-kDa Type IV Collagenase Which is Identical to That Secreted by Normal Human Macrophages. *J. Biol. Chem.* 1989; 264:17213–17221.
7. Birkedal-Hansen, B., Moore, W.G., Taylor, R.E., Bhown, A.S., and Birkedal-Hansen, H. Monoclonal Antibodies to Human Fibroblast Procollagenase. Inhibition of Enzymatic Activity, Affinity Purification of the Enzyme, and Evidence for Clustering of Epitopes in the NH2-Terminal End of the Activated Enzyme. *Biochemistry* 1988; 27:6751–6758.
8. Fridman, R., Bird, R.E., Hoyhta, M., Oelkuct, M., Komarek, D., Liang, C.M., Berman, M.L., Liotta, L.A., Stetler-Stevenson, W.G., and Fuerst, T.R. Expression of Human Recombinant 72 kDa Gelatinase and Tissue Inhibitor of Metalloproteinase-2 (TIMP-2): Characterization of Complex and Free Enzyme. *Biochem. J.* 1993; 289:411–416.
9. Knauper, V., Lopez-Otin, C., Smith, B., Knight, G., and Murphy, G. Biochemical Characterization of Human Collagenase-3. *J. Biol. Chem.* 1996; 271:1544–1550.
10. Schnierer, S., Kleine, T., Gote, T., Hillemann, A., Knauper, V., and Tschesche, H. The Recombinant Catalytic Domain of Human Neutrophil Collagenase Lacks Type I Collagen Substrate Specificity. *Biochem. Biophys. Res. Comm.* 1993; 191:319–326.
11. Lichte, A., Kolkenbrock, H., and Tschesche, H. The Recombinant Catalytic Domain of Membrane-type Matrix Metalloproteinase-1 (MT1-MMP) Induces Activation of

Progelatinase A and Progelatinase A Complexed with TIMP-2. *FEBS Lett.* 1996; 397:277–282.

12. Knight, G.C., Willenbrock, G., and Murphy, G. A Novel Coumarin-labelled Peptide for Sensitive Continuous Assays of the Matrix Metalloproteinases. *FEBS Lett.* 1992; 296:263–266.

13. Child, R.G., Osterberg, A.C., Sloboda, A.E., and Tomcufcik, A.S. Fenbufen, a New Anti-Inflammatory Analgesic: Synthesis and Structure-Activity Relationships of Analogs. *J. Pharm. Sci.* 1977; 66:466–476.

14. Kluender, H.C.E., Benz, G.H.H.H., Brittelli, D.R., Bullock, W.H., Combs, K.J., Dixon, B.R., Schneider, S., Wood, J.E., Van Zandt, M.C., Wolanin, D.J., and Wilhelm, S.M. Substituted 4-Biarylbutyric or 5-Biarylpentanoic Acids and Derivatives as Matrix Metalloprotease Inhibitors WO 9615096, Nov 15, 1994.

15. An Evans chiral auxiliary route starting with N-acylation of (*R*)-(+)-4-Isopropyl-2-oxazolidinone with 4-methylpentanoyl chloride followed by α-alkylation with *tert*-Butyl bromoacetate and ending with hydrolysis by $H_2O_2/LiOH/H_2O/THF$ followed by TFA/CH_2Cl_2 yielded (S)-2-isobutyl succinic acid. This enantiomerically pure acid was cyclized to the anhydride by treatment with acetyl chloride and then used in a Friedel-Crafts reaction with 4-chlorobiphenyl as described in patent reference 11 to yield the *S* isomer of compound 2. Similarly, (S)-(-)-4-Isopropyl-2-oxazolidinone led to the *R* isomer of compound 2. A manuscript to describe the details of these syntheses is in preparation.

16. The authors wish to thank all the members of the X-ray and high field NMR labs of Bayer, West Haven for their efforts in solving the structures of the complexes of several Biphenyl MMP inhibitors related to BAY 12-9566 together with MMP-3. The structure of the complex represented by the cartoon shown in Figure 4 was determined using NMR techniques by Drs. Sarah Heald and Paul Blake.

17. The authors wish to thank the efforts of Dr. Wolfgang Kreiss and colleagues of Bayer, A.G., Leverkusen, Germany for their efforts to crystallize and determine the X-ray structure of BAY 12-9566 as shown in Figure 5.

18. Gatto, C., Rieppi, M., Borsotti, P., Drudis, T., and Hibner, B. Anti-Angiogenic Activity of BAY 12-9566, an Inhibitor of Matrix Metalloproteinases. *Annals of Oncology* 1998; 9(suppl 2):74.

19. Hibner, B., Card, A., Flynn, C., Casazza, A.M., Taraboletti, G., Rieppi, M., and Giavazzi, R. BAY 12-9566, a Novel, Biphenyl Matrix Metalloproteinase Inhibitor, Demonstrates Anti-Invasive and Anti-Angiogenic Properties. *Proceedings of the American Association for Cancer Research* 1998; 39:302.

20. Bull, C., Flynn, C., Eberwein, D., Casazza, A.M., Carter, C.A., and Hibner, B. Activity of the Biphenyl Matrix Metalloproteinase Inhibitor BAY 12-9566 in Murine In Vivo Models. *Proceedings of the American Association for Cancer Research* 1998; 39:302.

21. Hibner, B., Bull, C., Flynn, C., Eberwein, T., Garrison, A., Casazza, A.M., Carter, C., and Gibson, N. Activity of the Matrix Metalloproteinase Inhibitor BAY 12-9566 Against Murine Subcutaneous and Metastatic in vivo Models. *Annals of Oncology* 1998; 9(suppl 2):75.

22. Flynn, C., Bull, C., Matherne, C., Eberwein, D., Gibson, N., and Hibner, B. Anti-Invasive and Anti-Metastatic Activity of the Novel MMP Inhibitor BAY 12-9566 In Subcutaneous and Orthotopic Models Using the Human Colon Carcinoma, HCT 116. *Annals of Oncology* 1998; 9(suppl 2):75.

23. Flynn, C., Bull, C., Eberwein, D., Matherne, C., and Hibner, B. Anti-metastatic Activity of BAY 12-9566 in a Human Colon Carcinoma HCT116 Orthotopic Model. *Proceedings of the American Association for Cancer Research* 1998; 39:301.

24. Nozaki, S., Sissons, S., Casazza, A.M., and Sledge, G.W. Jr. Inhibition of human breast cancer regrowth and pulmonary metastases by BAY 12-9566 in athymic mice. *Proceedings of the American Association for Cancer Research* 1998; 39:301.

25. Clemens, G., Detzer, K., and Bomhard, von Keutz E. Pre-clinical Drug Safety Profile for the Antimetastatic Matrix Metalloprotease Inhibitory Agent BAY 12-9566. *Annals of Oncology* 1998; 9(suppl 2):74.

26. Shah, A., Sundaresan, P., Humphrey, R., and Heller, A.H. Comparative pharmacokinetics (PK) of BAY 12-9566, a metalloproteinase (MMP) inhibitor, in healthy volunteers and cancer patients. *Proceedings of the American Association for Cancer Research* 1998; 39:521.

27. Grochow, L., O'Reilly, S., Humphrey, R., Sundaresan, P., Donehower, R., Sartorius, S., Kennedy, M.J., Armstrong, D., Carducci, M., Sorensen, J.M., and Kumor, K. Phase I and Pharmacokinetic Study of the Matrix Metalloproteinase Inhibitor (MMPI), BAY 12-9566. *Proceedings of American Society of Clinical Oncology* 1998; 17:213a.

28. Rowinsky, E., Hammond, L., Aylesworth, C., Humphrey, R., Siu, L., Smith, L., Thurman, A., Rodriguez, G., Sorensen, M., Von Hoff, D., and Eckhardt, G. Prolonged administration of BAY 12-9566, an oral nonpeptidic biphenyl matrix metalloproteinase inhibitor: A Phase I and PK Study. *Proceedings of American Society of Clinical Oncology* 1998; 17:216a.

29. Erlichman, C., Adjei, A., Alberts, S., Sloan, J., Goldberg, R., Pitot, H., and Rubin, J. Phase I Study of BAY 12-9566- A Matrix Metalloproteinase Inhibitor (MMPI). *Proceedings of American Society of Clinical Oncology* 1998; 17:217a.

30. Goel, R., Hirte, H., Shah, A., Major, P., Waterfield, B., Holohan, S., Bennett, K., Elias, I., and Seymour, L. Phase I Study Of The Metalloproteinase Inhibitor BAYER 12-9566. *Proceedings of American Society of Clinical Oncology* 1998; 17:217a.

8 D1927 and D2163
Novel Mercaptoamide Inhibitors of Matrix Metalloproteinases

A.D. Baxter, PhD, *J.B. Bird,* PhD,
R. Bannister, PhD, *R. Bhogal,* PhD,
D.T. Manallack, PhD, *R.W. Watson,* PhD,
D.A. Owen, PhD, *J. Montana,* PhD,
J. Henshilwood, PhD, *R.C. Jackson,* PhD

CONTENTS

1. INTRODUCTION AND OBJECTIVES

This chapter aims to provide a historical perspective of the Chiroscience matrix metalloproteinase inhibitor (MMPI) program, including the medicinal chemistry strategy which culminated in the clinical candidates D1927 and D2163. We shall focus on the design of substrate-based inhibitors utilizing a novel zinc-binding group, and the discovery of novel MMPIs that display selectivity for the matrix metalloproteinases (MMPs) over the related metalloproteinase enzymes that mediate cellular shedding events will be reviewed.

The MMP program at Chiroscience was initiated in November 1993. At that time most competitor activity was focused on peptoid inhibitors based on the potency enhancing hydroxamic acid zinc-binding group *(1,2,3)*. None of the compounds in the public domain had demonstrated oral activity and this was believed to be a key element to the successful identification of an MMPI drug.

From: *Cancer Drug Discovery and Development:*
Matrix Metalloproteinase Inhibitors in Cancer Therapy
Edited by: Neil J. Clendeninn and Krzysztof Appelt © Humana Press Inc., Totowa, NJ

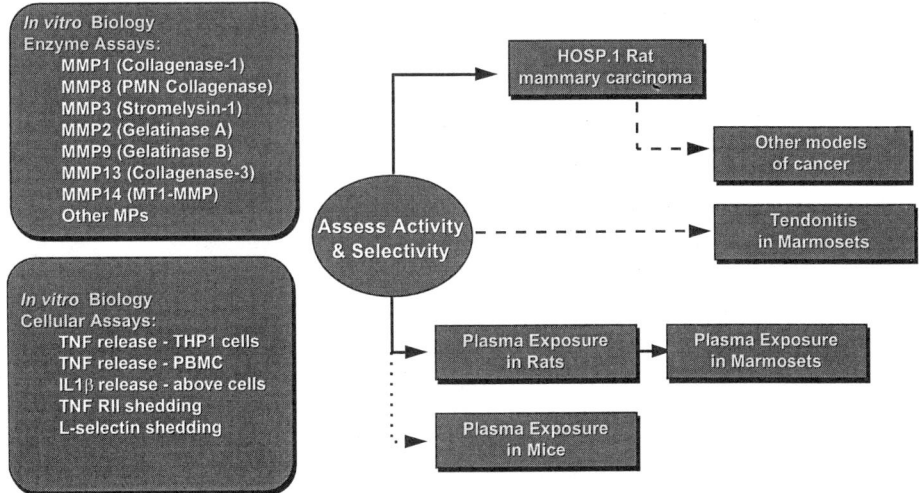

Fig. 1. Oncology Screening Protocol for MMPIs.

Chiroscience's program has therefore focused on providing novel, potent, orally active inhibitors of the MMP enzymes. By making extensive use of computer-aided drug design (CADD) and high speed chemistry it was shown that a large library of compounds could be prepared furnishing MMPIs that would display a range of different selectivity profiles within the MMP gene family.

The initial strategy of the program was aimed at providing broad spectrum inhibitors of MMPs that were also capable of inhibiting the release of TNFα in a whole cell assay. A combined inhibition of MMPs and TNF convertase (TACE), an enzyme which is known to be closely related to MMPs, was believed to provide a particularly attractive profile for the inflammatory end-points in which MMPs are implicated *(4)*. This selectivity profile was not thought, however to be optimal for oncology endpoints where the TNFα inhibitory activity may not be desirable. A screening protocol was put in place with these objectives in mind, providing access to a range of MMPI enzyme assays and also cellular assays to assess the activity of compounds against membrane-shedding events such as TNFα processing and L-selectin shedding (Fig. 1). Compounds with an interesting selectivity profile were then evaluated in pharmacokinetic studies alongside investigation in animal models of inflammation (lipopolysaccharide-stimulated rat or mouse and the adjuvant arthritic rat model) and cancer (HOSP.1 rat mammary carcinoma and B16 melanoma).

Evidence has recently emerged from the more clinically advanced MMPIs that treatment in clinical trials has led to a succession of dose-limiting musculo-skeletal side effects *(5)*. It is believed that this tendonitis effect is closely related to a phenomenon observed in marmoset toxicology. Pharmacokinetics and toxicology were therefore carried out in marmosets to determine the side effect potential of exploratory development compounds.

2. INHIBITOR DESIGN

Substrate-based inhibitors of the MMP enzymes are designed around the cleavage site of the natural substrate. The most potent inhibitors have traditionally been designed around a hydroxamic acid zinc-binding group with peptide recognition being provided by occupation of the S1′ and S2′ pockets (1,6). Further interactions are then provided by hydrogen bonding interactions between the amide characteristics present in the inhibitor and residues present in the backbone of the enzyme active site (Fig. 2). Hydroxamic acids have become associated with very broad spectrum activity and poor oral activity (7). In addition competitor activity in the area is very intense and obtaining an intellectual property position for substrate-based compounds containing hydroxamic acids would have been very difficult to secure at the time of initiating our program. The challenge was to provide compounds with an alternative zinc-binding group that display these same potency enhancing characteristics.

It was postulated that if a novel zinc-binding group could be identified, we could make use of the X-ray crystal structure data, published for hydroxamic acids, in the CADD of novel, potent inhibitors of MMP-8 (Fig. 3) (8). Note that the interaction of the hydroxamic acid with the zinc is achieved in a bidentate manner. The coordination state of the zinc atom is fulfilled by the three active site histidine residues. The P1′ leucine isostere occupies the lipophilic S1′ pocket but interestingly the P2′ phenylalanine residue is orientated away from the enzyme backbone toward the surrounding solvent. As a result of this the P3′ methylamide of the inhibitor is able to realize two key hydrogen bonding interactions whereas three other hydrogen bonding interactions are achieved between the amide bonds in the inhibitor and the surrogate amide bonds along the backbone of the enzyme. This is a classical substrate-based inhibitor.

It appeared from the literature that the mercaptoamide zinc-binding group could provide a potential opportunity. This zinc-binding function had been utilized by several groups in order to provide combined inhibitors of angiotensin-converting enzyme (ACE) and neutral endopeptidase (NEP) (Fig. 4) (9). Such compounds could be demonstrated to be potent inhibitors of this class of metalloproteinases and showed oral activity comparable to captopril in models of hypertension. We therefore had good confidence that this zinc-binding group could provide the vehicle for achieving the initial objective of oral activity.

Interestingly the mercaptoamide zinc-binding group had never been used as a template for MMP inhibitors. A strong patent position in this area would provide the springboard for the success of our MMPI program. Synthesis of the sim-

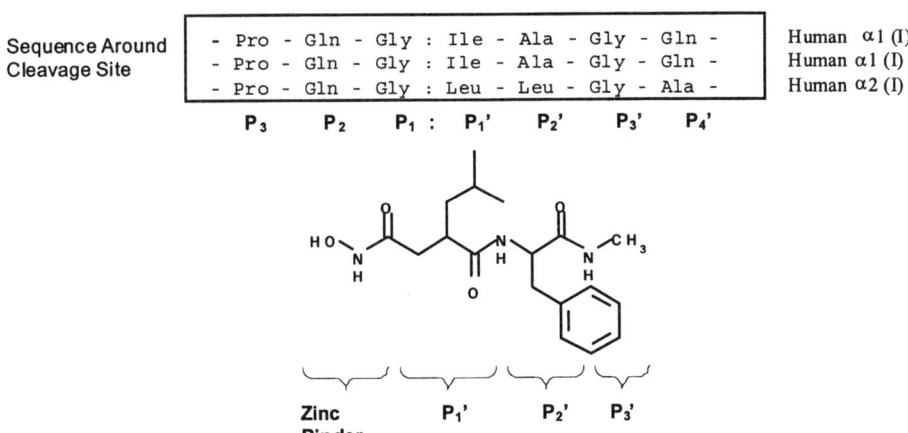

Fig. 2. The Design of Substrate Based MMPIs Around the Substrate Cleavage Site.

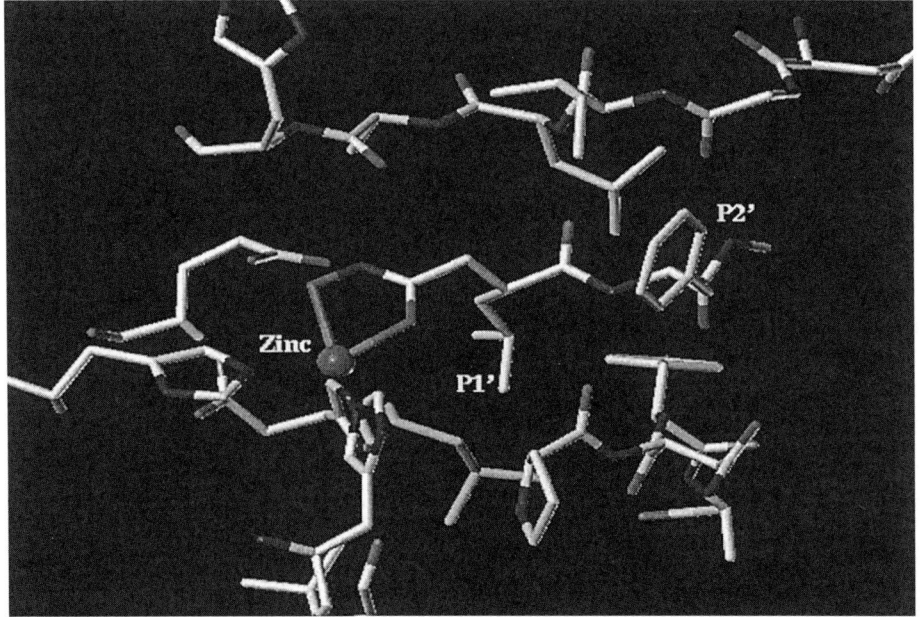

Fig. 3. The X-ray Crystal Structure of a Classical Substrate Based MMPI Showing a Prototypical hydroxamic Acid in the Active Site of Neutrophil Collagenase.

plest mercaptoamide-based compound (CH104) provided a modestly potent, but nevertheless, broad spectrum inhibitor of the MMP enzymes (Table 1). Interestingly the compound was also capable of inhibiting the release of TNFα in a whole cell system. We were gratified to observe that CH104 demonstrated oral

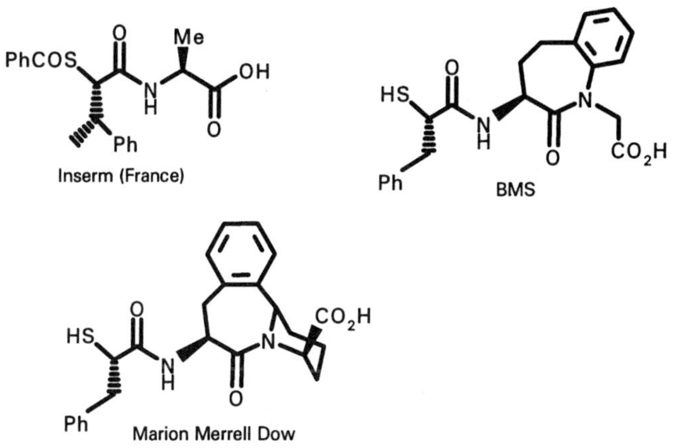

Fig. 4. Orally Active, Mercaptoamide Based Inhibitors of ACE/NEP.

Table 1
The In vitro Profile of CH104, a Prototypical Mercaptoamide Based MMPI

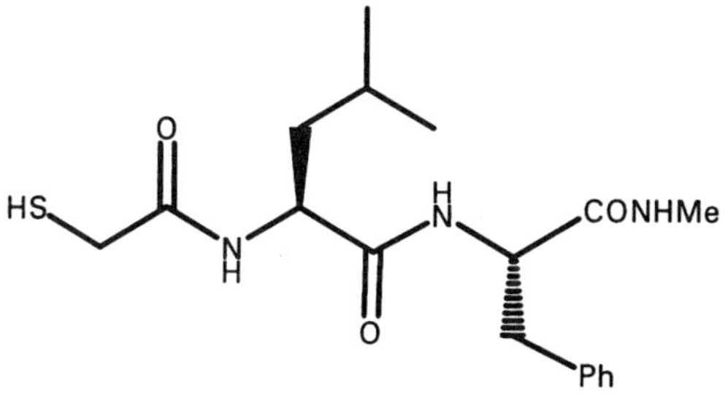

Activity (IC$_{50}$, µM)

CH No.	MMP-1	MMP-8	MMP-3	MMP-2	MMP-9	TNF
104	0.410	0.060	2.63	1.01	0.09	20

activity in the adjuvant arthritic rat model and in the lipopolysaccharide(LPS)-induced mouse model of TNFα release.

CH104 represented an ideal template for the development of more potent compounds and since at this time the focus of the program was on both arthritis and cancer endpoints these results, from only a modestly potent compound, were particularly encouraging. The peptoid structure ideally lends itself to a positional scanning approach to high speed analog synthesis and as such both solution and solid phase combinatorial chemistry techniques assisted by CADD technology were used to optimize this lead compound *(10)*.

A molecular model of CH104 docked in the active site of MMP-8 was obtained by overlaying the molecule with the X-ray crystal structure of the corresponding basic hydroxamic acid (Fig. 5). Assuming a bidentate interaction of the mercaptoamide with the zinc this prototypical inhibitor can realize a similar binding orientation to the hydroxamic acid molecule. However, the mercaptoamide-based inhibitor is unable to achieve a hydrogen bond corresponding to the -NH of a hydroxamic acid residue. The lack of this hydrogen bond, which may help to augment the interaction of a hydroxamic acid with the active site zinc, may be partially responsible for the reduced activity observed with the base mercaptoamide when compared to the analogous hydroxamic acid. However, it is also noteworthy that the mercaptoamide is likely to be a less potent zinc chelator than a hydroxamic acid. It would therefore be necessary to identify additional enzyme-inhibitor interactions in order to improve the potency of this early compound.

Initial work was aimed at identifying the binding characteristics of the mercaptoamide moiety and it was quickly established that further separation of the thiol and amide carbonyl group was detrimental to activity *(11)*. As expected the free thiol group was required for activity, but the S-acetate functionality was capable of providing a pro-drug for CH104 both in vitro and in vivo. Our attention was now focused on how the potency of CH104 could be improved.

It is well known, from structure based drug design of hydroxamic acid-based MMPIs, that the S1′ pocket provides a significant opportunity for potency optimization, whereas the P2′ substituent provides no significant interactions with the enzyme and a wide range of substituents are tolerated. Some examples of P1′ variation are provided (Table 2) and represent a summary of examples from the positional scanning compound library. Most of the structure-activity relationships (SAR) in this series appear consistent with literature examples based on hydroxamic acid inhibitors *(1–3)*.

Replacing the P1′ leucine residue with S-methyl cysteine provides a significant improvement in potency against the MMP enzymes, an effect which is consistently observed in several series of mercaptoamide-based compounds from our database. Interestingly though, whereas the methanesulphonylmethyl substituent gives a significant increase in potency against gelatinase A, a reduction in TNFα inhibitory activity is observed. The corresponding sulphoxide derivative displayed poor activity in keeping with other polar or hydrogen-bonding substituents that are not tolerated by the S1′ pocket of the MMP enzymes. The straight chain alkyl residue (norvaline) in P1′ conferred an improvement in potency against the collagenases but had little effect on stromelysin or gelatinase inhibitory activity, whereas O-methyl serine provided good selectivity for gelatinase B over gelatinase A. The poor potency of the P1′ threonine compound was a surprise for two reasons: first MMP-1 is known to terminate its self-digestion process when a threonine residue occupies the S1′

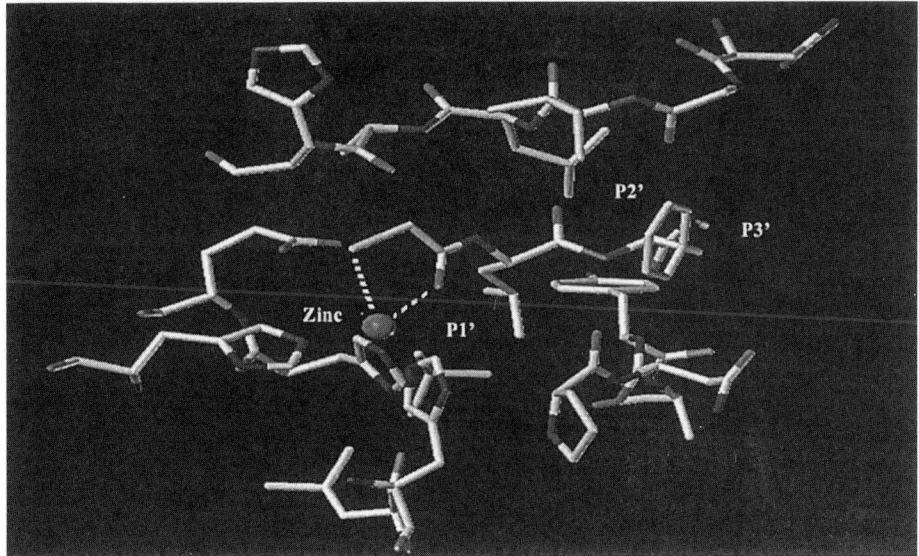

Fig. 5. A Molecular Model of CH104 Docked into the Active Site of MMP-8.

Table 2
Variation of the P1′ Substituent[a]

Activity (IC$_{50}$, µM)

R	MMP-1	MMP-8	MMP-3	MMP-2	MMP-9	TNF
i-Bu	0.410	0.057	2.63	1.01	0.093	20
CH$_2$SMe	0.073	0.021	0.587	0.400	0.013	37
CH$_2$SO$_2$Me	0.170	0.060	3.20	0.046	0.187	ia
CH$_2$SOMe	1.40	0.480	8.50	3.80	0.350	ia
(CH$_2$)$_2$Me	0.076	0.038	1.04	0.064	0.202	47
CH$_2$OMe	0.621	0.274	ia	3.03	0.095	ia
CH$_2$OH	11.9	ia	5.52	ia	27.8	ia
CH(Me)OH	2.60	4.10	ia	ia	1.70	ia
(CH$_2$)$_2$CONH$_2$	3.30	3.40	ia	5.60	6.80	ia

[a]ia = inactive at 50 µM.

pocket *(12)* and secondly a recent X-ray crystal structure of TIMP-1 in complex with the active site domain of MMP-3 shows a threonine—S1' interaction *(13)*. Both of these observations indicate that threonine should be well tolerated in P1' perhaps indicating that the template may not be binding in a totally traditional manner. In summary, a modest increase in potency can be achieved by manipulating the P1' residue and interesting selectivity data can be gained from this positional scanning approach. In order to realize a further improvement in potency additional sites of substitution should be sought.

Significant effort has been invested in evaluating the key structural requirements of the mercaptoamide group (Fig. 6). Investigation of the area accessible to an α-substituent (R^1) is not possible using a hydroxamic acid zinc-binding group. However, since the chemistry of the mercaptoamide series of compounds allows facile elaboration of this position, the preparation of a large library of compounds has provided the essential structural requirements required for potency optimization and improvements in selectivity. The position of substitution is important, because although α-substitution (R^1) generally provides potent MMP inhibitors, N-substitution (R^2) is detrimental to MMP potency. Interestingly some of these N-substituted compounds retain activity against TNFα in the whole cell assay system.

Again, CADD played a key role in designing compounds with improved MMP potency. By searching the active site region for potential hydrogen-bonding interactions it was felt that by introducing a hydrogen bond acceptor residue into the α-position (R^1), a hydrogen bond could be realized to serine-172 in the collagenases. This residue is only mutated to tyrosine in the gelatinases, so we had good confidence that if the chain length were optimized, a potent, broad spectrum inhibitor could be achieved. An ester group was used for the purpose of designing the optimum chain length that might be required to realize this key hydrogen-bonding interaction. The molecular model based on the published X-ray crystal structure of hydroxamic acids bound in the active site of MMP-8 provided the proposed mode of binding of the basic mercaptoamide template. It was suggested that the potential hydrogen bond to serine-172 could be achieved by means of the ester linked to the backbone by a three carbon chain (Fig. 7). The ester and also a phthalimide group were therefore chosen as hydrogen bond acceptor residues in order to probe the structure–activity relationships (SAR) around this region of the active site. Phthalimide had been used by other groups to realize a hydrogen bonding interaction to asparagine-80 in another part of the active site *(14)* (Table 3). It is clear that in the case of phthalimide a three carbon spacer is indeed optimum, both for MMPI activity and potency against TNFα in the whole cell assay. In the case of the ester group a three or four carbon spacer provided good inhibitory potency and as expected an increase in potency over the unsubstituted chain (i-propyl).

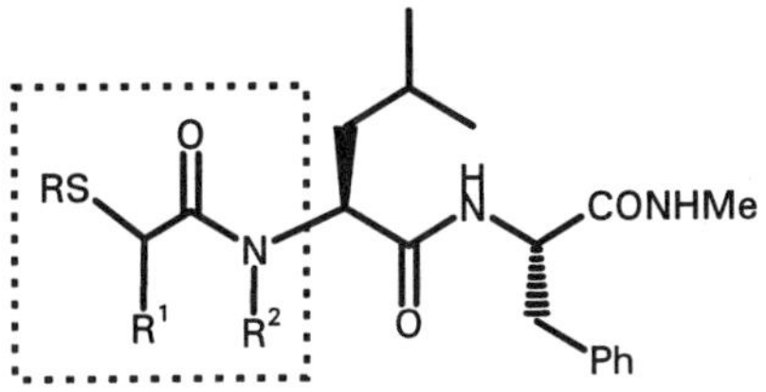

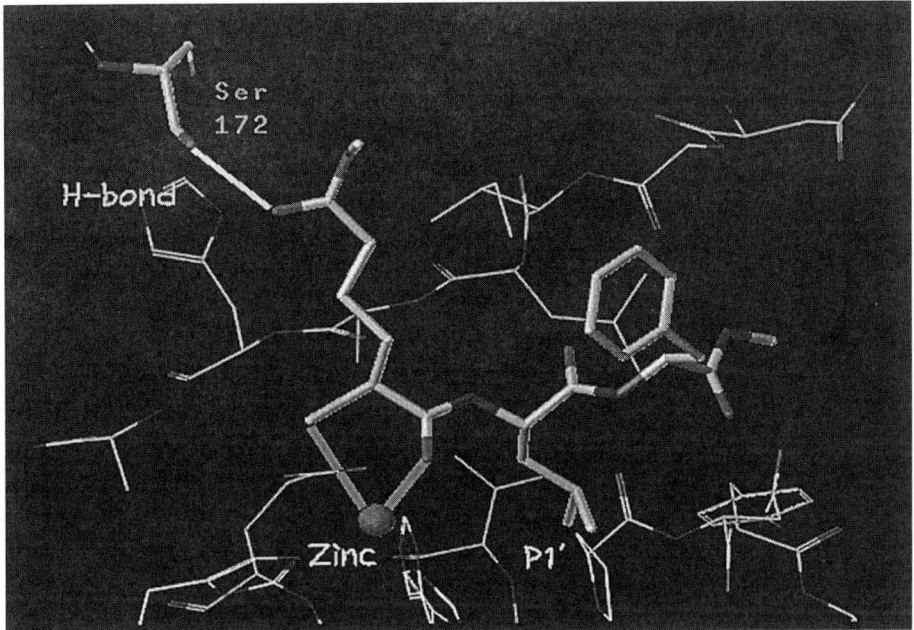

Fig. 6. Exploring the Requirements around the Mercaptoamide Moiety.

Fig. 7. A Molecular Model Showing the Potential of a Hydrogen Bond Interaction Between Serine-172 in MMP-8 and a Hydrogen Bond Acceptor Attached to the α Position of the Mercaptoamide Template.

One of the problems often associated with a phthalimide group is the lack of aqueous solubility it generally confers on the compound and as such one of the key goals of the medicinal chemistry strategy at this time was to evaluate compounds with improved physicochemical properties. Converting the phthalimide to a succinimide group improved the aqueous solubility of the compound 100-fold. In this case MMPI potency was retained but the transformation was detrimental to TNFα activity (Table 3). This observation would prove to be very important to the future of the program as it provided a consistent handle for achieving MMP selectivity over other metalloproteinases such as membrane sheddases (e.g., TACE) a profile

Table 3
Variation of the α-Substituent[a]

Activity (IC$_{50}$, μM)

R	MMP-1	MMP-8	MMP-3	MMP-2	MMP-9	TNF
H	0.410	0.057	2.63	1.01	0.093	20
i-Pr	0.220	0.077	1.41	0.730	0.067	ia
(CH$_2$)$_2$NPhth	0.160	0.015	0.870	0.150	0.031	23
(CH$_2$)$_3$NPhth	0.043	0.036	0.160	0.042	0.012	9.0
(CH$_2$)$_4$NPhth	0.480	0.130	0.500	0.170	0.034	ia
(CH$_2$)$_3$NSucc	0.098	0.018	0.320	0.058	0.002	69
(CH$_2$)$_3$CO$_2$Me	0.080	0.014	0.500	0.077	0.002	16
(CH$_2$)$_3$CO$_2$H	0.068	0.011	1.00	0.280	0.036	ia
(S)-(CH$_2$)$_3$NPhth	0.079	0.008	0.078	0.017	0.005	6.1

[a]ia = inactive at 50 μM.

that was felt to be particularly appropriate for oncology endpoints in order to provide compounds with a low side effect potential. A similar improvement in solubility was achieved by replacing the ester group with a carboxylic acid residue; in this case activity against the gelatinases and stromelysin was reduced but potency against the collagenases retained. This may reflect the fact that introducing a carboxylic acid now provides a hydrogen bond donating group in the area of serine-172 (collagenases) or tyrosine-172 (gelatinases). Since serine is a better hydrogen bond acceptor than tyrosine, a reduction in gelatinase activity would be expected.

Consistent with other series of substrate-based MMPIs it was demonstrated that the majority of the enzyme inhibitory activity was contributed by a single diastereoisomer. In several structurally different series of molecules the MMPI and TNFα inhibitory activity resided in the (S)-α-isomer.

3. LEAD OPTIMIZATION OF PROTOTYPE MMP INHIBITORS

At this time the MMP program was directed toward developing compounds for oncology endpoints and it was decided that the desired selectivity profile should be a potent, broad spectrum MMPI displaying no effect on the release of proinflammatory cytokines mediated by the cell membrane shedding metalloproteinases (i.e., TACE). This selectivity had proved difficult to achieve by other companies working on hydroxamic acid-based inhibitors, and would delineate Chiroscience compounds from those of other companies in the field.

To determine whether the early lead MMPIs would be active in models of cancer we tested CH264 (I), an early MMP/TNF inhibitor against the HOSP.1 rat mammary carcinoma model, and observed activity in this system.

The HOSP.1 is a cell line produced at the Institute of Cancer Research (London) which produces mainly activated MMP-2 and some MMP-9 *(15)*. These cells are used in a model of metastasis where tumor cells are injected by the iv route and lung colonies examined 35 d later. In this model of tumor cell invasion compound was administered at 30mg/kg both orally (po) and intraperitoneally (ip), initially 4 h prior to administration and then 1, 6, 24, 48, and 72 hours post administration of the tumor cells. Using this standard protocol CH264 had good activity when administered by the ip route (70% inhibition), inhibiting both tumor colony weight and number (Fig. 8). However, when administered orally at 30mg/kg CH264 had substantially weaker activity (28% inhibition) possibly indicating that this compound was poorly absorbed. Nevertheless CH264 was a promising lead compound that could be optimized to provide good oral activity in this model.

An area where the overall properties of the compound could be improved was in the P2′ group. CADD had previously demonstrated that the P2′ residue made no important interactions with the enzyme backbone. Indeed it was believed that this residue behaved more as a conformational lock, allowing the P3′ amide group to realize essential hydrogen bonding interactions. Extensive use of combinatorial chemistry has allowed the probing of this residue utilizing a range of unnatural α-amino acids. It was a key element of the medicinal chemistry strategy to use this residue to improve the metabolic stability, by protecting the potentially vulnerable P3′ amide group, and physicochemical properties of the molecule, to enhance oral absorption, rather than improve potency or selectivity. It was clear that the P1′ group and α-substituent could be used to fine-tune selectivity and potency once oral activity had been optimized.

Introducing a range of sterically demanding α-amino acids (i.e., tert-leucine and S-methylpenicillamine) provided compounds which retained MMPI potency. Solubility-enhancing phenylalanine replacements also retained some MMPI activity but interestingly these compounds were less active against stromelysin and gelatinase-A and against TNFα in the whole cell assay (Table 4). It seemed that in order to maintain good broad spectrum activity the tert-leucine residue would offer an opportunity to improve the metabolic stability of the molecule. It would however not provide any improvement in the physicochemical properties of the molecule. Nevertheless, CH1766 (R = t-Bu, Table 4), a lead compound from this series has consistently demonstrated good oral

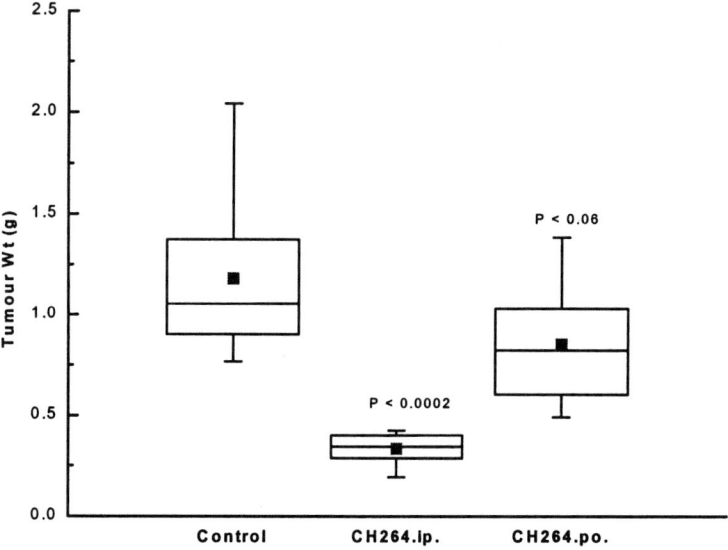

Fig. 8. Activity of CH264 in the HOSP.1 Rat Mammary Carcinoma Model of Tumour Invasion.

Table 4
Modification of the P2′ Substituent[a]

Activity (IC$_{50}$, μM)

R	MMP-1	MMP-8	MMP-3	MMP-2	MMP-9	TNF
CH$_2$Ph	0.079	0.008	0.078	0.017	0.005	6.1
CH$_2$ 2-Pyr	0.100	0.009	0.528	0.110	0.012	ia
CH$_2$ 4-Thiaz	0.120	0.011	0.435	0.170	0.007	53
tert-Bu	0.028	0.009	0.079	0.021	0.005	10
C(Me)$_2$SMe	0.047	0.011	0.325	0.047	0.006	18
C(Me)$_2$SO$_2$Me	0.009	0.004	0.222	0.019	0.005	15

[a]ia = inactive at 50 μM.

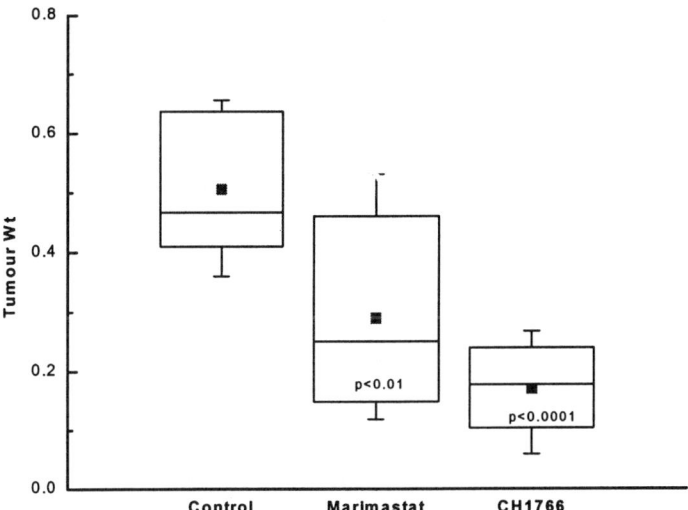

Fig. 9. A Comparison Between CH1766 and Marimastat in the HOSP.1 Rat Mammary Carcinoma Model.

activity in animal models. In the adjuvant arthritic rat model, CH1766 inhibited paw swelling by 56% at 1mg/kg po bid. In the HOSP.1 rat mammary carcinoma model of tumor cell invasion described earlier, CH1766 demonstrated excellent oral activity, inhibiting both tumor colony weight and number (55% inhibition). This activity compares to that reported in the literature for the British Biotech compound, Marimastat (II), which inhibited by ~70% when dosed at 30 mg/kg po in this model using the same dose regimen as indicated for CH1766 and CH264 previously *(16)*.

When the two compounds were compared directly in this model, CH1766 proved to be slightly better than Marimastat when dosed equivalently (30 mg/kg po) (Fig. 9). Therefore, CH1766 represented a key lead compound in the search for a MMPI directed toward oncology endpoints. Furthermore, around this time it was becoming clear that Marimastat was demonstrating dose-limiting side effects, of joint pain and tendonitis in phase II clinical trials. These side effects were severe enough to cause patients to require dosing holidays and then physiotherapy before treatment could be resumed *(17,18)*. There is clearly an opportunity for second generation MMPIs, which lack these debilitating side effects, to provide a compound superior to Marimastat. Marimastat is a broad spectrum inhibitor of MMPs with a similar profile to CH1766. However, Marimastat, and indeed other clinically advanced hydroxamate-based MMPIs, such as the Novartis compound CGS27023 (III) and the Agouron compound, AG3340 (IV) are also known to inhibit the shedding of cell membrane macromolecules from the cell surface *(19)*.

Table 5
Activity of MMPIs Against Membrane Shedding
Events in a Whole Cell Assay System[a]

Compound	TNFα	IL-1β	TNF RII	IL-1 RII	IL-6 R	L-Selectin
			Activity (IC$_{50}$, μM)			
CH1766	10	ia	ia	ia	ia	ia
Marimastat	4.0	Stim	6.0	3.4	3.6	1.0
CGS27023	8.0	ia	7.0	5.0	6.5	11
AG3340	1.6	ia	14	1.8	12	0.8

[a]ia = inactive at 50 μM.

These shedding events include, not only the processing of TNFα, but also the shedding of cytokine receptors, such as the type-II TNF and IL-1 receptors and the IL-6 receptor and the shedding of adhesion molecules, such as L-selectin (Table 5). These events are mediated by membrane-bound sheddase enzymes that are known to be metalloproteinases. It is possible that the joint pain problems demonstrated by Marimastat may well be as a result of the inhibition of these sheddase enzymes. It has also been demonstrated that Marimastat, in keeping with some other first generation hydroxamic acids (20,21), is capable of elevating levels of the proinflammatory cytokine, IL-1β, in whole cell systems (R. Wills, J. Bird, personal communication). Although the therapeutic relevance of this is not known, the observation augments the fact that Marimastat has a less than ideal enzyme inhibition profile. In contrast to this, although CH1766 is capable of inhibiting the production of TNFα in whole cell systems this compound does not elevate IL-1β, and does not inhibit the other metalloproteinase-driven shedding events. In this respect CH1766 would seem to have a unique profile.

In order to put this theory to the test, a medicinal chemistry strategy was put in place to provide MMPIs lacking activity against TNFα and the sheddase enzymes. Again making extensive use of combinatorial chemistry, regions of the molecule were systematically varied in order to achieve selectivity over membrane sheddases. Returning to the P1′ group, an area of the molecule previously demonstrated to be potency-enhancing for the MMPs, it was found that TNFα activity could not be abolished without also significantly reducing MMPI activity. It was therefore decided to conduct any future SAR studies utilizing the potency enhancing S-methyl cysteine residue in P1′. It was identified that TNFα inhibitory activity could be abolished by the introduction of bulky amide substituents in P3′. Thus, replacing the methyl amide with either tert-butyl or phenyl amides resulted in compounds which retained good MMPI potency but were devoid of activity against TNFα (Table 6).

Table 6
Reduction in TNFα Inhibitory Potency by Providing
Sterically Demanding Residues in P3′[a]

Activity (IC$_{50}$, μM)

R	MMP-1	MMP-8	MMP-3	MMP-2	MMP-9	TNF
Me	0.006	0.002	0.011	0.005	0.002	9
t-Bu	0.130	0.008	0.035	0.028	0.006	ia
Ph	0.038	0.023	0.032	0.080	0.037	ia
(CH$_2$)$_3$NMe$_2$	0.056	0.008	0.059	0.056	0.002	8
CH$_2$ 2-Pyr	0.040	0.005	0.042	0.070	0.001	4

[a]ia = inactive at 50 μM.

Note that in general these modifications to the P3′ amide substituent resulted in a substantial decrease in activity against collagenase-1 and gelatinase A, but activity was retained against gelatinase B and collagenase-2. Interestingly TNFα inhibitory activity was enhanced by the introduction of a pyridylmethyl substituent in this position.

While investigating the variation of the α-substituent it was identified that replacing the phthalimido group by succinimido, not only improved the aqueous solubility of the molecule by over 100-fold, but also significantly reduced activity against TNFα. Furthermore, reducing the spacer length from three to two carbon atoms in this series, totally abolished activity against TNFα although retaining a potent, broad spectrum profile against the MMP enzymes. Replacing the succinimide with a 1,2,2-trimethyl-4-hydantoin moiety provided a similar profile. This is significant because this hydantoin ring is likely to be more metabolically stable than the relatively labile succinimide (Table 7).

These factors provided the foundations for the discovery of D1927 (V) and D2163 (VI), the two compounds which were ultimately chosen for clinical evaluation.

Table 7
Reduction in TNFα Inhibitory Potency by Modification of the α-Substituent[a]

Activity (IC$_{50}$, μM)

R	MMP-1	MMP-8	MMP-3	MMP-2	MMP-9	TNF
(CH$_2$)$_3$NPhth	0.003	0.002	0.100	0.009	0.001	5
(CH$_2$)$_3$NSucc	0.013	0.008	0.110	0.008	0.004	31
(CH$_2$)$_2$NSucc	0.002	0.008	0.071	0.008	0.002	ia
(CH$_2$)$_2$NHyd	0.007	0.008	0.180	0.010	0.016	ia

[a]ia = inactive at 50 μM.

4. PROCESS OPTIMIZATION

4.1. Introduction

The matrix metalloproteinase inhibitor D2163 (VI) appears at first sight to be a reasonably complex molecule, containing three stereogenic centres with a maximum of eight possible isomeric forms. Our screening protocols identified the all-natural S,S,S configuration as the active isomer. To facilitate rapid and cost-effective preclinical and clinical development we chose to pursue this compound in its single isomer form. Upon closer inspection the molecule is revealed as a synthetically simple tripeptoid, the stereogenic centers of which can be considered separately. The two amino acid components, tertiary leucine and leucine can clearly be derived from commercial sources. Indeed tertiary leucine is a reasonably common component of modern drugs conferring metabolic stability upon molecules in which it is contained. We had already developed our own proprietary supply position for this unusual amino acid *(22)*. The thiol-containing portion of the molecule could clearly be related to an amino acid precursor by some double displacement functional group chemistry. Alternatively, syntheses involving generation of the stereogenic center from achiral precursors may be preferred. It is with these general considerations that we embarked upon the evaluation and planning of our synthesis and supply of these materials to our clinical program.

4.2. D2163 And D1927: General Considerations

As is often the case with chiral pharmaceutical products one is wrong to consider chirality the key overriding factor in the synthesis. There are additional challenges that were presented by D2163. The thiol group must be introduced in an environmentally sensitive and low cost manner, and any additional processing and analysis must minimize the formation of the homodisulphide. Both molecules contain no acidic or basic subunits which may assist in crystallinity and allow purification through salt formation. This was a very significant obstacle given that these molecules were initially isolated as impure low melting "glasses" which defied crystallization. Control of the byproduct profile could be envisaged as a major obstacle. Both inhibitors (V) and (VI) have a lack of chromophoric groups and their involatile nature excludes the easy use of both reverse phase high-performance liquid chromatography (HPLC) and gas chromatography (GC) techniques, both workhorse tools for materials supply scientists. Any processing of the isomeric products must preserve the stereogenic centers so carefully installed and our analytical methods must be able to verify that this is indeed the case. Finally, MMP inhibitors are envisaged as being used chronically by cancer sufferers for many years. We therefore sought a supply position that would allow these materials to be made in a cost-effective manner to help minimize daily treatment costs.

4.3. Synthetic Strategy

We could choose to investigate the synthesis of D2163 in a "left to right," or "right to left" manner. However, from a perspective of economics and speed we chose to employ a convergent strategy. We were able to satisfy ourselves through synthesis that the key dipeptide (VII) could be considered as a bulk available chirality pool starting material (Fig. 10). The dipeptide could then be coupled with the thiol-containing side chain. There were then three approaches we could pursue:

1. We could carry out this coupling with racemic sidechain (VIII) to give rise to D2163 in the S,S,S configuration as a mixture (we may get some selective coupling induced by the dipeptide) with its diastereomer (R,S,S). We could then carry out a crystallization-based separation of the diasteromers. This approach would almost certainly be successful, but would clearly be wasteful in product and uneconomic in the long run.
2. We could prepare the sidechain (VIII) in single isomer form, either by asymmetric synthesis, from the chirality pool or by resolution. We could envisage a number of opportunities for introducing chirality to the molecule at an intermediate stage. Armed with this material we could then perform one of the many mild coupling reactions to form the final product.
3. A more elegant approach is to realize that D2163 is an all-natural configuration tripeptoid structure and as such should be amenable to formation of the amide bonds through an enzyme-mediated coupling. Such couplings in well tailored

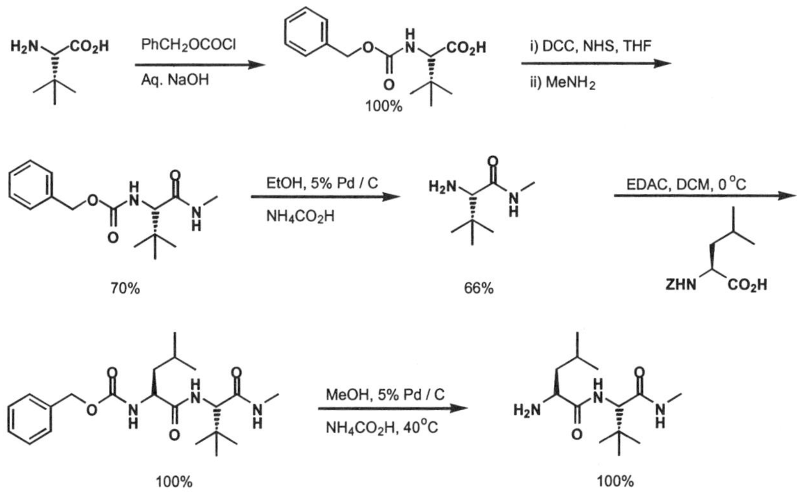

Fig. 10. An early supply route of dipeptide (VII).

and optimized processes are high yielding volume-efficient substrate-specific reactions. We would clearly have the option to carry this out with enantiomerically pure sidechain or with the racemic intermediate.

We chose to pursue the third approach with a clear fallback position that we could divert into single isomer (VIII) and mild coupling with dipeptide (VII) if a stereospecific enzyme-mediated coupling approach was not achievable. We decided at an early stage that we would mask the thiol group as a carbonyl-protected thioloester. This would then greatly simplify all processes and minimize unwanted side reactions in any coupling or resolution steps. In addition we could then envisage the sulphur atom being derived from a nonvolatile source. The final step of all of our approaches was to reveal the sensitive thiol functionality in a mild deprotection step. We had evidence from other programs in this area *(10,11)* that such chemistry is highly flexible, being amenable to a number of mild acid and base deprotection methods. Our synthesis is outlined in Fig. 11. The key to our synthetic strategy was therefore to prepare the side chain (VIII) in either racemic or single isomer form with the sulphur atom suitably protected.

4.4. Synthesis of Side Chain (VIII)

The synthesis of racemic side chain is shown in Fig. 11. Butyrolactone as solvent is heated with trimethyl hydantoin (IX) (commercially available) to effect ring opening and provide the amino butyric acid (X). Excess butyrolactone

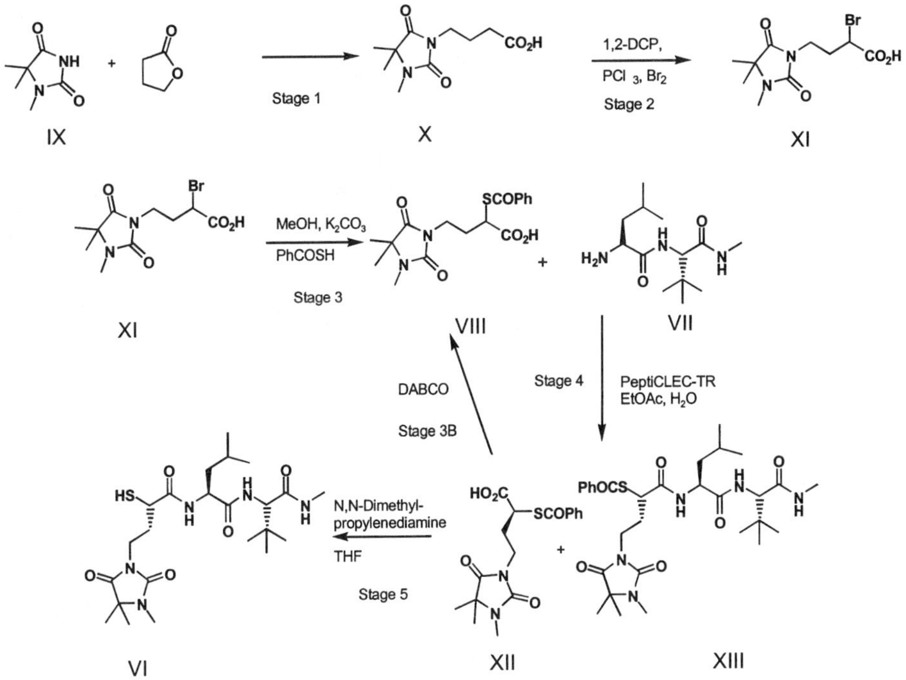

Fig. 11. Synthetic route to D2163 (VI).

is distilled off to isolate the product. However second generation ring opening byproducts are formed by addition of further molecules of butyrolactone. The product held in these "oligomeric byproducts" is recovered by hydrolysis with sodium hydroxide in the work up to obtain (X) in over 70% yield as a highly crystalline colorless solid.

Bromine is introduced adjacent to the carboxylic acid group to furnish (XI) using the well known Hell-Volhard-Zelinsky reaction. The reaction, using sequential addition of phosphorus trichloride and bromine in dichloropropane proceeds well at 95°C. Typically yields above 80% are achieved of this highly crystalline colorless product. The benzoyl-protected side chain (VIII) is prepared by bromine displacement using dropwise addition of thiobenzoic acid to a methanolic solution of (XI) containing potassium carbonate. The fine white crystalline product is obtained in over 80% yield.

The racemic side chain could thus be obtained in good overall yield in three synthetic steps. Moreover the two racemic acids, (XI) and (VIII) could well be amenable to separation either by bioresolution (of their esters or amides), or chemoresolution through a diastereomeric salt should access to the optical isomers be necessary. Secondarily, chirality induced by substitution adjacent to an acid can often either be lost through racemisation or inverted through nucle-ophilic displacement, and so we felt that a potential recycle route could also be achieved. However, our first approach was to use an enzymatic coupling of the racemic sidechain (VIII) with dipeptide (VII).

4.5. Enantiospecific Enzyme-Mediated Coupling Reactions

The criticism is sometimes made that organic reactions using enzymatic reagents are dilute, aqueous, slow, and difficult to work up. This need not be the case in processes thoughtfully designed and optimized. An elegant solution to many of the perceived problems has been provided by Altus and their proprietary Cross-Linked Enzyme Crystals (CLEC). For our purposes PeptiCLEC-TR (a cross-linked thermolysin reagent) had a number of very desirable features. The reagent performs the key coupling of side chain (VIII) to dipeptide (VII) in very high selectivity giving rise to a low level of the RSS diastereomer. This one reac-tion had therefore simultaneously generated the key molecular structure, and the remaining element of asymmetry. Hence our need to make single isomer sidechain (VIII) was no longer necessary. From the processing perspective these reagents are ideal: being heterogeneous, they are easily recovered by filtration and recycled many times; they are stable to, and work best in, organic solvent under concen-trated conditions and reactions proceed rapidly in a few hours. The byproduct R enriched sidechain (XII) as discussed above can easily be recycled and returned to the synthetic sequence. Initially we chose the acetyl protecting group for the sul-phur atom, however under the CLEC coupling conditions a small amount of hy-drolytic deprotection occurred. The released thiol group led to poisoning of the enzymatic catalyst. Since we felt that recycle of the catalyst was likely to be key to the longer term process economics we sought an alternative, more stable, pro-tecting group. It is a constant dilemma in protection strategy that groups that are easier to append and more stable are often more difficult to remove, and a delicate balance has to be struck. The benzoyl protecting group offered a number of ad-vantages including low cost and a low odor method of introduction of sulphur through potassium thiobenzoate. However, hydrolysis using acidic reagents was found to proceed slowly with significant racemization, and ammonia also led to secondary reactions compromising both yield and quality. Rather than carry out an extensive search for alternative protecting groups, we sought to refine the hydrol-ysis reagent and conditions. We found that N,N-dimethylpropyl-1,3-diamine to have exactly the right characteristics for the hydrolysis of the final precursor (XIII) to furnish D2163 (VI) in 85% yield. In addition the tertiary amine function of this reagent ensured that byproducts could easily be removed through an aqueous wash protocol and hence aid product quality. After final crystallization we were able to supply D2163 in high quality in good overall yield by a five stage synthetic route that could form the basis of longer term supply.

5. PRECLINICAL EVALUATION OF D1927 AND D2163

In this section the clinical candidates, D1927 (V) and D2163 (VI) are described in more detail. As described in Heading 3, CH1766, a prototypical mercaptoamide-based inhibitor, has consistently demonstrated good activity in the HOSP.1 rat mammary carcinoma model. This compound has also shown consistent activity in the adjuvant arthritic rat model even though its physico-chemical properties are not ideal. The transition from CH1766 to the clinical candidates D1927 (V) and D2163 (VI) was also described in Heading 3 and it is the purpose here to focus more on the preclinical information which has been accumulated on these compounds during this transition phase of the discovery process. Important considerations in this process were:

1. Inhibitor selectivity.
2. The physicochemical parameters of the molecules, including aqueous solubility and LogP.
3. The plasma exposure of the compounds in both rats and marmosets.
4. The efficacy of the compounds in animal models of cancer.
5. The tolerability and long term safety of the compounds, particularly with reference to the joint pain side effect seen with first generation MMPIs.

D1927 (V) and D2163 (VI) are broad spectrum inhibitors of the MMP enzymes (Table 8). Note that D1927 in particular is much less active against the gelatinases than the first generation hydroxamic acid-based inhibitors exemplified here by Marimastat (II), CGS27023 (III) and AG3340 (IV). In general the mercaptoamide-derived compounds deselect on stromelysin, an effect which is less pronounced for the hydroxamic acids.

These compounds are unique amongst the more clinically advanced MMPIs in that they do not inhibit the release of TNFα in whole cell systems and they do not inhibit the shedding of cytokine receptors or the shedding of L-selectin (Table 9). CH1766 demonstrated an interesting profile since it is capable of inhibiting TNFα but lacks effects on the other shedding events. This observation provided the basis for developing inhibitors more selective for the MMPs and the SAR which allowed TNFα and unwanted sheddase activity to be designed out of the compounds was presented in the previous section. As can be seen D1927 and D2163 are delineated from the first generation compounds in that they exhibit a much cleaner inhibition profile. Marimastat, for instance, is known to inhibit a whole range of events in which metalloproteinases are thought to play a crucial role. It is possible that this nonideal profile associated with Marimastat is responsible for the side effects observed with this compound in clinical trials. The observation that Marimastat can apparently stimulate the release of IL-1β may not be crucial since this is observed at a reasonably high concentration. This effect of hydroxamic acids has, however,

Table 8
A Comparison of the Enzyme Activities of D1927 and D2163 with those of First Generation Inhibitors

Compound	MMP1	MMP8	MMP13	MMP3	MMP7	MMP2	MMP9	MMP14
				Activity (IC_{50}, μM)				
Marimastat	0.003	0.004	0.002	0.036	0.007	0.009	0.007	0.014
CGS27023	0.024	0.007	0.025	0.018	0.250	0.017	0.007	0.025
AG3340	0.017	0.002	0.0002	0.030	0.060	0.002	0.004	0.008
CH1766	0.028	0.009	0.002	0.179	0.024	0.021	0.005	0.035
D1927	0.012	0.010	0.010	0.381	0.036	0.130	0.053	0.058
D2163	0.026	0.010	0.004	0.157	0.023	0.041	0.025	0.040

Table 9
Activity of MMP Inhibitors Against Sheddases in a Whole Cell System[a]

	Activity in PBMC cell line (IC$_{50}$, μM)					
Compound	TNFα	IL-1β	TNF RII	IL-1 RII	IL-6 R	L-Selectin
Marimastat	4	Stim	6	3.4	3.6	1.0
CGS27023	8	ia	7	5	6.5	11
AG3340	1.6	ia	14	1.8	12	0.8
CH1766	10	ia	ia	ia	ia	ia
D1927	ia	ia	ia	33	ia	ia
D2163	ia	ia	ia	ia	ia	ia

[a]PBMC = peripheral blood mononuclear cells; ia = inactive at 50 μM.

been observed by other workers using monocyte and synovial cell cultures although in these cases other structurally related MMPIs, not Marimastat, were being studied (20,21).

Another area for improvement in respect of CH1766 was that of its physico-chemical properties. The physico-chemical properties of any molecule play an important role in oral absorption. One of these parameters is aqueous solubility and as can be seen improvements have been made in D1927 and D2163 over that exhibited by CH1766 (Table 10). We have also made use of a parameter called ΔLogP, which is a measure of the hydrogen bonding capacity of the molecule and derives from a study by an Abbott group while evaluating endothelin A antagonists (23). These workers demonstrated a correlation between ΔLogP and oral absorption where a value of this parameter in the range of 3.5 to 4.5 was considered to be particularly favorable. Working to these principles CH1766 was shown to be outside this range whereas both D1927 and D2163 fall at either end of the favorable range. However, the test of the applicability of ΔLogP values to this series of compounds is the plasma exposure exhibited by animals following oral dosing.

Using a bioassay method based on the analysis of samples in a standard gelatinase-B assay, the plasma exposure of Marimastat was evaluated (Fig. 12) in the rat following an oral dose of 30 mg/kg. In our hands the C$_{max}$ of Marimastat in the rat was observed at 116 ng/mL with an AUC of 51. This compares reasonably well with data presented for this compound at conferences (C$_{max}$ = 280 ng/mL) (16).

It is often stated that the metabolism of MMPIs is unique in the rat and that marmosets are a more predictive species for the human situation. When considering the Roche MMPI for arthritis (Ro 32,3555) it has been claimed that the metabolism of that compound is the same in man and marmoset and markedly different in the rat (1996 Inflammation Research Association Conference, Hershey, PA). For this reason and due to the fact that the tendonitis side effect can be evaluated in marmosets we have also performed analogous experiments in this primate species,

Table 10
Physicochemical Parameters of D1927 and D2163 in
Comparison with CH1766[a]

Compound	Aqueous solubility (mg/mL)	LogP	ΔLogP
CH1766	0.090	2.9	5.7
D1927	3.6	0.7	3.6
D2163	0.46	1.7	4.3

[a]ΔLogP = Partition Coeff (octanol/H_2O) — Partition Coeff (cyclohexane/H_2O)

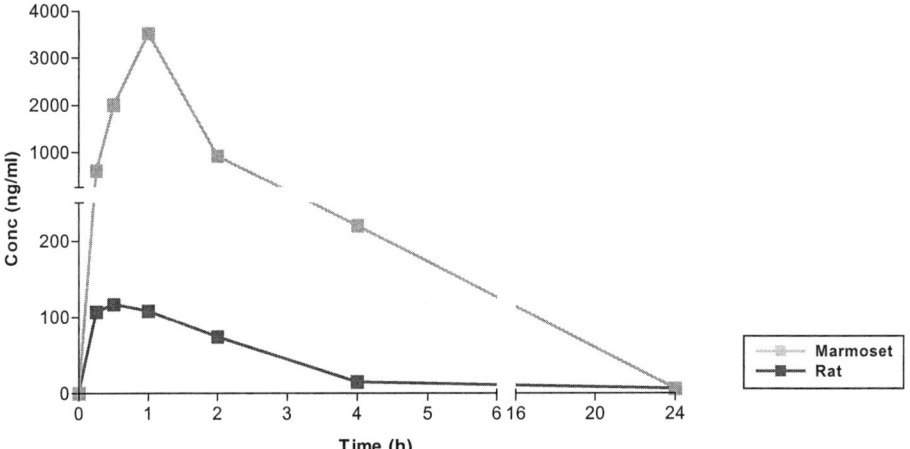

Fig. 12. The Plasma Exposure Profile of Marimastat in Rats and Marmosets Determined by Bioassay Following Oral Dosing at 30 mg/kg.

where an improvement in overall plasma exposure is indeed observed (C_{max} = 3520 ng/mL, AUC = 350). Again these results compare favorably with data presented by British Biotech for this compound (C_{max} = 4000 ng/mL) (24).

An evaluation of D1927 and D2163 under an identical protocol revealed greatly improved plasma exposure for both compounds over Marimastat (Fig. 13). When evaluated side by side D1927 had a C_{max} of 846 ng/mL and an AUC of 197, compared to the much higher C_{max} of 11,000 ng/mL and AUC of 635 for D2163. By comparison, Marimastat in this experiment displayed a C_{max} of 142 ng/mL and a relatively poor AUC of 49.

A similar evaluation in marmosets provided a similar picture (Fig. 14) with D2163 reaching a peak plasma concentration of 54,400 ng/mL, greater than that observed for D1927 (C_{max} = 22,300 ng/mL) which is in turn much greater than that determined for Marimastat (C_{max} = 3520 ng/mL). We were pleased to ob-

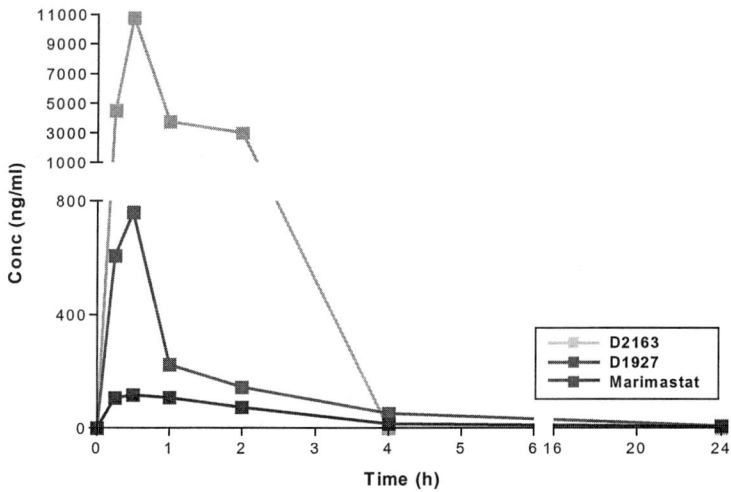

Fig. 13. A comparison of the Plasma Exposure Profiles of D1927 and D2163 with Marimastat in Rats Determined by Bioassay Following Oral Dosing at 30 mg/kg.

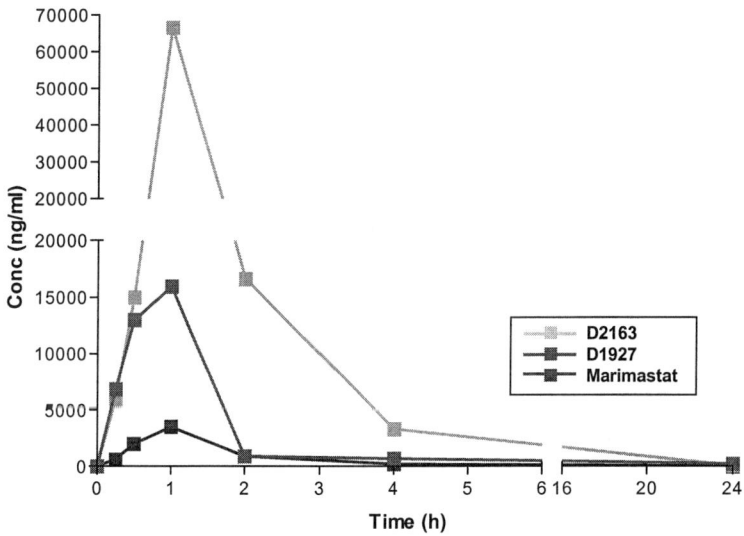

Fig. 14. A comparison of the Plasma Exposure Profiles of D1927 and D2163 with Marimastat in Marmosets Determined by Bioassay Following Oral Dosing at 30 mg/kg.

serve that the same plasma exposure profile for D1927 and D2163 was observed when these compounds were subjected to a bioanalytical assay. Using this LC-MS-MS assay the bioavailability of D1927 and D2163 was calculated as 53% and 57% respectively, much higher than that observed for Marimastat (21%).

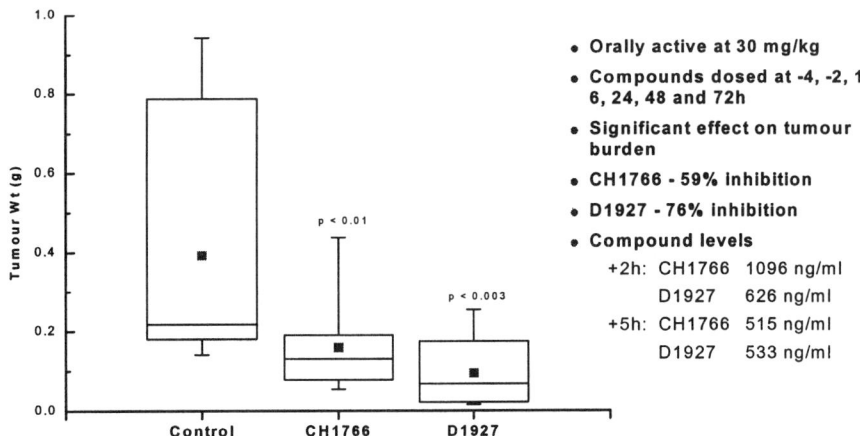

Fig. 15. A Comparison of D1927 with CH1766 in the HOSP.1 Model.

A consideration in any therapeutic regimen will be the maintenance of plasma levels to ensure biological effect. This may be particularly true for MMPIs since it is assumed that relatively high plasma levels are required to be maintained to prevent metastasis. It has been observed following a single oral dose of 30 mg/kg both in the rat, but especially in the marmoset, plasma levels of D1927 and D2163 are maintained well above the concentration required to inhibit the enzymes. The next phase of this work would be to demonstrate that these encouraging results are translated into good oral activity in animal models.

From the preceding experiments it should be apparent that both D1927 and D2163 display a good in vitro profile and are bioavailable. Initially the HOSP.1 rat mammary carcinoma model described previously was employed as a primary model of in vivo efficacy. In one such experiment D1927 had comparable activity to CH1766 which was employed as an internal standard and had been previously shown to be at least as good as Marimastat in this model (Fig. 15).

Using the standard dosing regimen the plasma compound levels were well maintained as indicated by bioassay of plasma samples taken at 2 and 5 h post injection of the tumor cells. In a similar experiment D2163 also had comparable activity to CH1766 (Fig. 16).

Both of these compounds have also demonstrated good activity in the B16 melanoma model in mice. In a side by side comparison using a similar dosing protocol to that used for the HOSP.1 model D1927 and D2163 were more effective than Marimastat and equivalent in activity to AG3340.

A primary focus of the program around D1927 and D2163 has been to demonstrate that these compounds do not display joint pain or tendonitis in marmosets. In order to evaluate this the compounds were dosed orally at 30 and 100 mg/kg uid for 90 days. Animals were observed throughout the study and

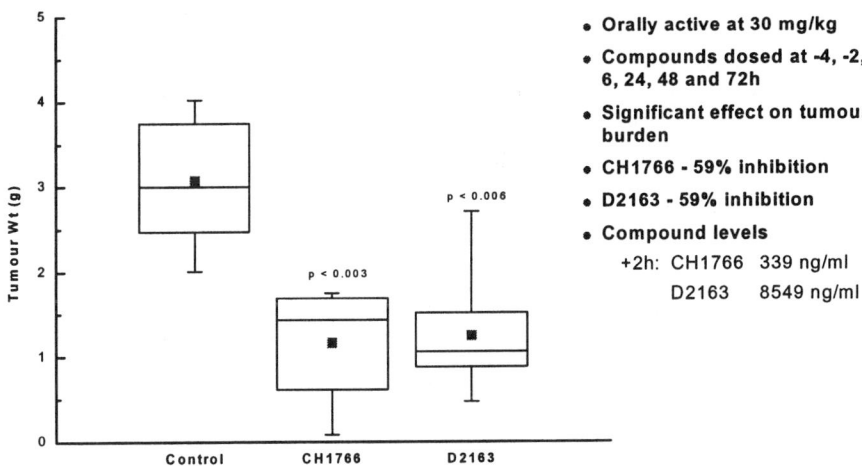

Fig. 16. A Comparison of D2163 with CH1766 in the HOSP.1 Model.

clinical signs rated as slight, moderate, or marked. Finally, histopathology was performed on sections of selected tissues and scored. The results on D1927 and D2163 were as follows:

Sustained plasma levels were achieved throughout the study, well in excess of enzyme IC_{50} up to 9 h post dosing. No adverse effects due to the treatment were observed and this was transferred to a clean histopathology of joints and tendons. Also the parent compound, CH1766, was without effect in this model indicating that this novel class of compounds was free of the side effects in animal models which have been observed with the first generation inhibitors. In order to prove this principle in humans, D1927 and D2163 were selected for clinical development.

ACKNOWLEDGMENTS

We thank all our colleagues at Chiroscience who have contributed to the matrix metalloproteinase inhibitor project. We also acknowledge with thanks the contribution of Dr. David Gregory and Professor Stephen Neidle (Institute of Cancer Research, Sutton, UK) to the molecular modeling work.

REFERENCES

1. Beeley NRA, Ansell PRJ, Docherty AJP. Inhibitors of matrix metalloproteinases (MMPs). *Curr Opin Ther Patents* 1994; 4:7–16.
2. Brown PD, Giavazzi R. Matrix metalloproteinase inhibition: a review of antitumour activity. *Annals of Oncology* 1995; 6:967–974.
3. Stetler-Stevenson WG. 1997. Matrix metalloprotease inhibitors, in *Cancer Therapeutics: Experimental and Clinical Agents* (Teicher, B., ed), Humana, Totowa, NJ, pp. 241–261.

4. Gearing AJH, Beckett P, Christodoulou M, Churchill M, Clements J, Davidson AH, Drummond AH, Galloway WA, Gilbert R, Gordon JL, Leber TM, Mangan M, Miller K, Nayee P, Owen K, Patel S, Thomas W, Wells G, Wood LM, Woolley K. Processing of tumour necrosis factor-α precursor by metalloproteinases. *Nature* 1994; 370:555–557.

5. Mousa SA. Mechanisms of angiogenesis in vascular disorders: potential therapeutic targets. *Drugs of the Future* 1998; 23:51–60.

6. Bird J, De Mello RC, Harper GP, Hunter DJ, Karran EH, Markwell, RE, Miles-Williams AJ, Rahman SS, Ward RW. Synthesis of novel N-phosphonoalkyl dipeptide inhibitors of human collagenase. *J Med Chem* 1994; 37:158–169.

7. Porter JR, Millican TA, Morphy JR. Recent developments in matrix metalloproteinase inhibitors. *Exp Opin Ther Patents* 1995; 5:1287–1296.

8. Stams T, Spurlino JC, Smith DL, Wahl RC, Ho TF, Qoronfleh MW, Banks TM, Rubin B. Structure of human neutrophil collagenase reveals large S1′ specificity pocket. *Nature Struct Biol* 1994; 1:119–123.

9. Wyvratt MJ, Patchett AA. Recent developments in the design of angiotensin-converting enzyme inhibitors. *Med Res Rev* 1985; 5:483–531.

10. Baxter AD, Bird J, Bhogal R, Massil T, Minton KJ, Montana J, Owen DA. A novel series of matrix metalloproteinase inhibitors for the treatment of inflammatory disorders. *BioMed Chem Lett* 1997; 7:897–902.

11. Baxter AD, Bhogal R, Bird JB, Buckley GM, Gregory DS, Hedger PC, Manallack DT, Massil T, Minton KJ, Montana JG, Neidle S, Owen DA, Watson RJ. Mercaptoacyl matrix metalloproteinase inhibitors: the effect of substitution at the mercaptoacyl moiety. *BioMed Chem Lett* 1997; 7:2765–2770.

12. Lovejoy B, Hassell AM, Luther MA, Weigl D, Jordan SR. Crystal structures of recombinant 19-kDa human fibroblast collagenase complexed to itself. *Biochemistry* 1994; 33 (27): 8207–8217.

13. Gomis-Ruth FX, Maskos K, Betz M, Bergner A, Huber R, Suzuki K, Yoshida N, Nagase H, Brew K, Bourenkov GP, Bartunik H, Bode W. Mechanism of inhibition of the human matrix metalloproteinase stromelysin-1 by TIMP-1. *Nature* 1997; 389 (6646), 77–81.

14. Brown P (1994). Inhibitors of matrix metalloproteinases, at SCI Fine Chemicals Group Symposium, New Horizons in Anti-inflammatory Therapy. 11th May 1994, Scientific Societies Lecture Theatre, New Burlington Place, London, W1.

15. Eccles SA, Box GM, Court WJ, Bone EA, Thomas W, Brown PD. Control of lymphatic and hematogenous metastasis of a rat mammary carcinoma by the matrix metalloproteinase inhibitor batimastat. *Cancer Research* 1996; 56 (12), 2815–2822.

16. Drummond AH, Beckett P, Bone EA. BB-2516: an orally bioavailable matrix metalloproteinase inhibitor with efficacy in animal cancer models. *Proc Am Assoc Cancer Res* 1995; 36:100 (abstract).

17. Millar A, Parsons S, Primrose J, Poole C, Evans J 1996. Phase II clinical trials of marimastat. Proceedings of the 21st Congress of the European Society for Medical Oncology, Vienna, Austria.

18. Wojtowicz-Praga S, Torri J, Johnson M, Steen V, Marshall J, Ness E, Dickson R, Sale M, Rasmussen HS, Chiodo TA, Hawkins MJ. Phase I trial of Marimastat, a novel matrix metalloproteinase inhibitor, administered orally to patients with advanced lung cancer. *J. Clin. Oncology* 1998; 16:2150–2156.

19. Lombard MA, Wallace TL, Kubicek MF, Petzold GL, Mitchell MA, Hendges SK, Wilks JW. Synthetic matrix metalloproteinase inhibitors and tissue inhibitor of metalloproteinase (TIMP)-2, but not TIMP-1, inhibit shedding of tumor necrosis factor-α receptors in a human colon adenocarcinoma (Colo 205) cell line. *Cancer Res* 1998; 58:4001–4007.

20. McGeehan GM, Becherer JD, Bast RC, Boyer CM, Champion B, Connolly KM, Conway JG, Furdon P, Karp S, Kidao S, McElroy AB, Nichols J, Pryzwansky KM, Schoenen F, Sekut L, Truesdale A, Verghese M, Warner J, Ways JP. Regulation of tumour necrosis factor-α processing by a metalloproteinase inhibitor. *Nature* 1994; 370:558–561.

21. Williams LM, Gibbons DL, Gearing A, Maini RN, Feldmann M, Brennan FM. Paradoxical effects of a synthetic metalloproteinase inhibitor that blocks both p55 and p75 TNF receptor shedding and TNF alpha processing in RA synovial membrane cell cultures. *J Clin Invest* 1996; 97:2833–2841.
22. Tiffen P and Adger B, *Tetrahedron Letters* 1997; 38:2153.
23. von Geldern TW, Hoffman DJ, Kester JA, Nellans HN, Dayton BD, Calzadilla SV, Marsh KC, Hernendez L, Chiou W, Dixon DB, Wu-Wong JR, Opgenorth TJ. Azole endothelin antagonists 3: Using D log P as a tool to improve absorption *J. Med. Chem.* 1996; 39,982–991.
24. Drummond AH. Paper given at the CHI conference on 'Protease inhibitors: new therapeutics and approaches'. Baltimore, USA, November 1996.

9 Research on MMP Inhibitors with Unusual Scaffolds

*Frank Grams, PhD, Hans Brandstetter, PhD,
Richard A. Engh, PhD, Dagmar Glitz, PhD,
Hans-Willi Krell, PhD, Valeria Livi, PhD,
Ernesto Menta, PhD, Luis Moroder, PhD,
J. Constanze D. Müller, PhD,
Erich Graf v. Roedern, PhD,
Gerd Zimmermann, PhD*

1. INTRODUCTION

Synthetic inhibitors of matrix metalloproteases have been developed using hydroxamate, N-carboxyalkyl, phosphonamidate, phosphinate, thiol, and other groups, each as a ligand for the active-site zinc atom of metalloproteases. Several of these inhibitors have been crystallized in complexes with the catalytic domains of various matrix metalloproteinases (MMPs).

The MMP inhibitor design program at Boehringer Mannheim (which is now Roche Diagnostics) was started when other companies had already well established and advanced research programs in this field. Due to this fact, we avoided hydroxamic acid inhibitors, and instead we concentrated on new compounds with new binding behavior, either of the whole inhibitor or of the

From: *Cancer Drug Discovery and Development:
Matrix Metalloproteinase Inhibitors in Cancer Therapy*
Edited by: Neil J. Clendeninn and Krzysztof Appelt © Humana Press Inc., Totowa, NJ

Malonic acid derivatives

Discovery of new binding mode by X-ray	$\Rightarrow$ Design and synthesis of new inhibitors according to the X-ray structure

Cysteine derivatives

Knowledge about cysteine and thiol compounds as MMP inhibitors	$\Rightarrow$ Synthesis of 1st inhibitors	$\Rightarrow$ Drug design based on results of the 1st compounds. Synthesis of further inhibitors

Barbiturates

		$\Rightarrow$ Optimization of one residue by drug design and classical chemistry	
Lead identified in regular screening	$\Rightarrow$ Model of binding and finally X-ray structure		$\Rightarrow$ Merger of both residues and further optimization
		$\Rightarrow$ Optimization of the other residue by structure-based combinatorial chemistry	

Fig. 1. Simplified comparison between the different strategies for drug optimization of the malonic acid derivatives, cysteine derivatives and barbiturates.

zinc chelating group. This approach promised completely different pharmacological profiles. Our strategy was further to overcome the low specificity of most of the known compounds in order to reduce the associated side effects.

In the following we highlight three very different strategies for MMP inhibitor optimization used at Boehringer Mannheim, two of them in collaboration with MPI of Biochemistry (Martinsried, Germany) (Fig. 1). In the malonic acid series the lead compound came from X-ray crystallography information, whereas the cysteine series was derived from the knowledge of metalloprotease inhibition by thiols. Here, lacking X-ray structure information a pragmatic approach using knowledge-based drug design was chosen. Finally the barbiturate lead came from regular high-throughput screening. Here, a two track optimization strategy was chosen: one key binding residue was optimized by classical chemistry in combination with drug design, whereas the other was optimized by drug design guided combinatorial chemistry.

2. INHIBITOR DESIGN STRATEGIES

2.1. Malonic Acid Derivatives

2.1.1. MONOSUBSTITUTED MALONIC ACID DERIVATIVES

For most of the known synthetic inhibitors of MMPs, a substrate-like binding mode was postulated on the basis of X-ray crystallographic structures of MMP/inhibitor complexes. Conversely, the malonic acid-based inhibitor HONH-CO-CH(i-Bu)-CO-Ala-Gly-NH$_2$ was found to bind in a surprisingly different manner *(1)*.

This type of inhibitor containing a malonic acid hydroxamate moiety had originally been designed for the metalloproteinase thermolysin *(2)* and was reported in early stages of the MMP inhibitor research *(3)*.

The binding mode of HONH-Mal(i-Bu)-Ala-Gly-NH$_2$ to MMP-8 is schematically outlined in Fig. 2. The hydroxamate acts as bidentate chelator to the active-site Zn^{2+} ion. The hydrophobic substituent at the malonic acid moiety in the S configuration points toward the edge strand of the enzyme active-site cleft. In contrast to the binding mode of well known succinate inhibitors like batimastat or marimastat (Fig. 2), there is no spacer between the chelating and the hydrophobic group in the malonic acid-based inhibitors. Correspondingly, the position of the side chain of the subsequent amino acid residue becomes similar but not identical to that of P2' residues of substrate like binding inhibitors, whereas the residual peptidic tail is inserted into the S1' pocket, thus leading to an overall ß turn-like conformation of the inhibitor in the enzyme-bound state.

The discovery of this unique binding mode led us to explore the new lead structure in terms of stabilization of the bent conformation and modifications at the various interaction sites to improve the inhibitory potency of such malonic acid hydroxamate-based compounds *(4)*.

The observation of nonsubstrate-like binding also explains some older data that are inconsistent with substrate-like binding *(5)*.

2.1.1.1. Chemistry. The malonic acid-based inhibitors are composed of two parts, i.e., the malonic acid hydroxamate moiety and a CO-linked tail. The Cα-substituted diethyl malonates were prepared by standard procedures and then hydrolyzed to produce the malonate monoethyl esters which were condensed with (benzyloxy)amine and saponified. The resulting benzyl-protected malonic acid hydroxamates were amidated with the R2-NH$_2$ moieties consisting of amino acid derivatives or aryl- and alkylamines. Finally, acidolytic removal of side chain protecting groups, when required, followed by hydrogenolytic cleavage of the benzyl group from the hydroxamate over Pd/C catalyst gave the target hydroxamic acids. Among all compounds only HONH-Mal(i-Bu)-AspNHBn (**6**, Table 1) was obtained as a single diastereomer by crystallization of the protected precursor from diethyl ether. There is strong support for the

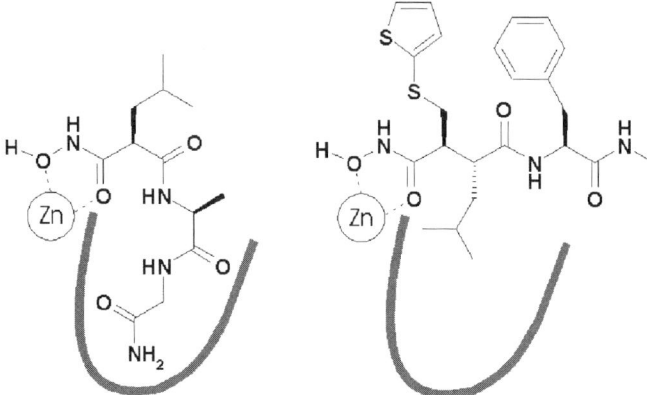

Fig. 2. Comparison of binding modes of malonic acid based and succinic acid based inhibitors.

S configuration of the 2-isobutylmalonic acid residue of this diastereomer, since it is a more potent inhibitor than the diastereomeric mixture **5**, and in crystals of the related compounds **1** and **8** with MMP-8 *(1,5)* the enzyme-bound malonic acid moiety is unequivocally in the S-configuration, whereas in crystals of the **5**/MMP-8 complex *(5)* an unambiguous assignment of the configuration was not possible. For the remaining compounds, the composition of the diastereomeric ratios was determined by ^{1}H NMR spectroscopy *(4)*.

2.1.1.2. Peptidic Malonic Acid-Based Inhibitors. Using the binding mode of HONH-Mal(i-Bu)-Ala-GlyNH$_2$ (**1**) as lead structure, positions A–D outlined in Fig. 3 were the targets of our attempts to optimize such malonic acid-based hydroxamic acids for MMP inhibition.

Replacement of the Gly-NH$_2$ tail of **1** with the more hydrophobic benzylamide led to improvement of the inhibitory potency by a factor of about 3–4 (Table 1). Therefore, in a first series, benzylamide derivatives were synthesized for exploration of position B in Fig. 3. The side chain of Ala in **1**, (Table 1) in the **1**/MMP-8 complex is pointing toward the S2′ subsite of the enzyme without apparent interactions. A change of the chirality of the Ala residue (**2** and **3**) was found to completely reverse the beneficial effects of the hydrophobic tail leading to a K$_i$ value similar to that of just the malonic acid moiety, i.e., of HONH-Mal-(i-Bu)-OEt (**16**) (Table 1). Correspondingly, in all subsequent modifications the L-configuration was retained for this residue, and Ala was replaced by the amino acids Ser (**4**), Asp (**5**), and Asn (**7**), which according to modeling experiments were expected to form hydrogen-bonding networks with Tyr219N and Glu158O of the active-site cleft of MMP-8. Since the additional hydrogen bonds do contribute to binding, the failure to improve the binding en-

Table 1

Compound	Formula	Residues		Diastereo-meric Ratio	K_i [μM]
1		-		36:64	121
2		X: Ala		40:60	50
3		D-Ala		25:75	194
4		Ser		28:72	35
5		Asp		43:57	136
6		Asp		100:0	88
7		Asn		34:66	55
8		-		44:56	26
		R1:	R3:		
9		i-Butyl	CH_3	23:77	1.4
10		i-Butyl	OH	24:76	12
11		i-Butyl	$COOCH_3$	22:78	9.6
12		i-Butyl	COOH	50:50	20
13		CH_2-Ph	CH_3	43:57	1.7
14		$(CH_2)_2$-Ph	CH_3	25:75	4.0
15		OH	CH_3	45:55	1.6
		R1:	R2:		
16		i-Butyl	O-ethyl		190
17		Ph	O-ethyl		98
18		CH_2Ph	O-ethyl		53
19		$(CH_2)_2$-Ph	O-ethyl		189
20		CH_2Ph	N-morpholide		50
21		CH_2Ph	$NHCH_2Ph$		3.1
22		$(CH_2)_2$-Ph	$NHCH_2Ph$		2.3
23		i-Butyl	$NH(CH_2)_3Ph$		0.54
24		CH_2Ph	$NH(CH_2)_3Ph$		0.56
25		$(CH_2)_2$-Ph	$NH(CH_2)_3Ph$		0.49
26		OH	$NH(CH_2)_3Ph$		2.3
27		i-Butyl	NH-n-octyl		0.24

ergy may be due to a correspondingly increased solvation of the unbound inhibitor. Introduction of a further potential hydrogen bond from the meta position of the P1′ benzyl to either Tyr216O and Leu214O in a bidentate manner or

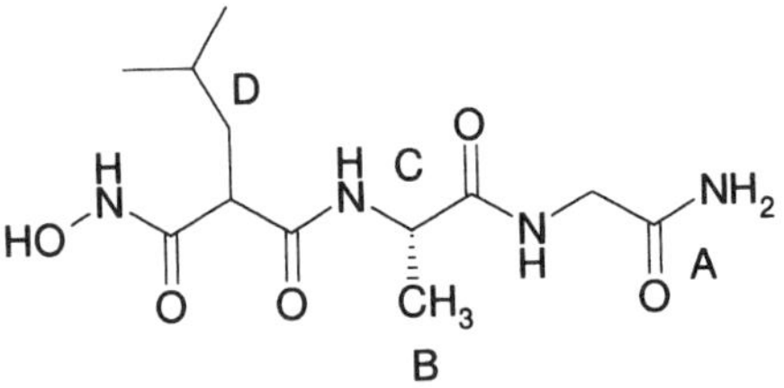

Fig. 3. General formula of malonic acid based inhibitors.

to Leu193O yielded a twofold improvement in binding (**8**). Because the addition of hydrogen bonds improved binding only modestly, new strategies to increase the extent of hydrophobic bonding were used. One idea was to fill the entire volume of the S1′ pocket by the C-terminal fragment NH-CH$_2$-CH$_2$-(C$_6$H$_4$)-p-CH$_3$, another was to occupy the hydrophobic binding area in the S2′ site with the benzene moiety of a homo-Phe. The result was an inhibitor (**9**) with highly improved affinity (ca. 100-fold over HONH-Mal(i-Bu)-Ala-Gly-NH$_2$ *(4,5)*. Similar P1′ residues have been used in succinylic type inhibitors, which also display high affinity. However, due to the different binding mode these residues are in "the front part" of the inhibitor, whereas in case of the malonic acid type inhibitors this moiety forms the "inhibitor tail."

The strategy of increased hydrophobicity (compound **9**) seemed in general more successful than, for example, specific hydrogen bonds, despite the likely unfavorable entropy effect due to the additional loss of flexibility upon binding.

Further attempts to improve the binding affinities of the homophenylalanine (hPhe) analogue **9** by introduction of hydrophilic moieties in the para position of the 2-phenylethyl group, like the hydroxyl (**10**), carboxyl (**12**), or methyl ester function (**11**), to possibly favor hydrogen bond or salt bridge interactions with the Arg222 residue on the bottom of the S1′ pocket, failed. In fact the potencies were 10- to 20-fold reduced *(4)*.

2.1.1.3. Modifications in Position D. Omission of the pseudo-P1 isobutyl group in the Asp derivative **5** led to a 10-fold increase of the K$_i$ to about 1 m*M*. Therefore, we replaced the isobutyl moiety in compound **9** with the benzyl or 2-phenylethyl group (compounds **13** and **14**); both compounds showed (slightly) reduced inhibition of MMP-8 (Table 1). Substitution of the hydrophobic isobutyl group in **9** with an hydroxyl function (**15**) had practically no effect on inhibitory potency *(4)*.

2.1.1.4. Nonpeptidic Malonic Acid-Based Inhibitors. In the first series of MMP-8 inhibitors **1–15** the pseudo P1 residue is linked to the pseudo P1′ residue via a three- and four-atom (compound **16**) spacer formed by an α- or β-amino acid residue. The results obtained with the variously C2-substituted ma-

Ionic acid derivatives **16–19** (Table 1) were compelling to attempt direct linkage of the P1 and P1′ groups. Correspondingly, the malonic acid derivatives **18** and **19** were converted to the morpholide and benzylamides. While with the morpholide **20** no improvement was observed, the benzylamides **21** and **22** were found to exhibit inhibitory potencies comparable to those of the best peptidic inhibitors with K_i values of 3.1 and 2.3 μM, respectively (Table 1) *(4)*.

To allow for deeper insertion of the C-terminal aromatic group into the S1′ subsite, the benzyl group was replaced by 3-phenylpropyl as a longer pseudo P1′ residue (compounds **23–26**) with a sixfold decrease in the K_i values. Finally, as a result of modeling studies we found an aliphatic C8 amide substituent (**27**), which further decreases the K_i to 0.24 μM, also suggesting a certain degree of flexibility for the substituents as an important feature for optimal occupancy of the deep hydrophobic S1′ subsite of MMP-8.

To conclude, taking advantage of the information gained with the X-ray structures of a few selected malonic acid based hydroxamate inhibitors, about 500-fold improved inhibition of MMP-8 to submicromolar K_i values could be achieved in comparison to the lead structure **1**. This was done by stepwise optimization of the interaction sites and finally by conversion of the peptidic structures into low molecular weight nonpeptidic malonic acid derivatives *(4)*.

2.1.2. *Bis*-Substituted Malonic Acid Derivatives

The previously described mono-substituted malonic acid hydroxamates (*see* Subheading 2.1.1.4.) are racemates and thus enantioselective synthesis are required for the production of the *R* or *S* isomers. We have also investigated unsymmetrical and symmetrical malonic acids, the latter being achiral.

2.1.2.1. Chemistry. Monoalkylation of diethyl malonate at the C2 position was performed by standard methods with alkyl halides. In a subsequent alkylation step the 2,2-*bis*-substituted diethyl malonates were obtained. The cyclic *bis*-substituted malonic acid diethyl esters were prepared in one step employing suitable dibromo derivatives. The resulting 2,2-*bis*-substituted malonic acid diethyl esters were then hydrolyzed to produce the monoethyl esters which then were condensed with (benzyloxy)amine. After saponification, the resulting benzyl-protected malonic acid hydroxamates were amidated with arylamines. Finally, hydrogenolytic cleavage of the benzyl group from the hydroxamate over Pd/C catalyst led to the target hydroxamic acids. (For details *see* ref. *6*.)

2.1.2.2. MMP-8 Inhibition by *Bis*-Substituted Malonic Acid Hydroxamates. In an attempt to further exploit the S1 binding site, we synthesized *bis*-substituted malonic acid derivatives *(6)* (Table 2). To determine whether the *bis*-substituted derivatives retain the binding mode of the mono-substituted malonic acid-based inhibitors, an X-ray crystallographic analysis of the **28**/MMP-8 complex was performed. Apparent disorder in the crystals of **28**/MMP-8 prevented the unambiguous determination of a single structure, possibly because both

Table 2

Compound	R1	R2	R3	Ki [μM]
28	Me	CH$_2$Ph	O-ethyl	11
29	Me	CH$_2$Ph	NH-Ph	44
30	Me	CH$_2$Ph	NH-CH$_2$-Ph	1.1
31	Me	CH$_2$Ph	NH-(CH$_2$)$_2$-Ph	9.6
32	Me	CH$_2$Ph	NH-(CH$_2$)$_3$-Ph	0.24
33	Me	CH$_2$Ph	NH-(CH$_2$)$_4$-Ph	0.38
34	Me	CH$_2$Ph		41
35	NH-COCH$_3$	CH$_2$Ph	NH-CH$_2$-Ph	2.3
36	OH	CH$_2$Ph	NH-CH$_2$-Ph	1.9
37			NH-CH$_2$-Ph	1.5
38			NH-(CH$_2$)$_3$-Ph	0.30

stereoisomers may be bound in the crystals. However, it was clear that the typical binding mode is preserved. In a first series of compounds the methyl/benzyl substitution pattern at the malonic acid was retained and the effect of different C-terminal derivatizations for interaction with the S1′ subsite of MMP-8 was analyzed. Taking into account the beneficial effect of C-terminal aromatic amides

R1	R2	IC50 [µM]
Me	NH-Ph	44
Me	NH-CH$_2$-Ph	1.1
H	NH-CH$_2$-Ph	3.1
Me	NH-(CH$_2$)$_2$-Ph	9.6
Me	NH-(CH$_2$)$_3$-Ph	0.24
H	NH-(CH$_2$)$_3$-Ph	0.56
Me	NH-(CH$_2$)$_4$-Ph	0.38

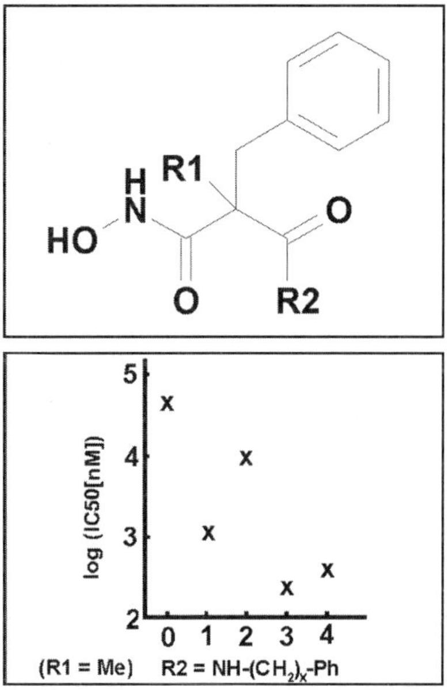

Fig. 4. Chain length dependence of MMP-8 inhibition by malonic acid based inhibitors.

observed for monosubstituted malonic acid hydroxamates, the amides **29–33** were synthesized which differ in the number of methylene groups as spacers of the phenyl group from the amide. Although the anilide **29** showed a fourfold weaker inhibitory potency (K_i = 44 µM) than the ester **28**, with the benzyl amide **30** (K_i = 1.1 µM) a remarkably more potent inhibitor with a 10-fold enhanced binding affinity was obtained. Indeed there is a clear dependence on the length of the residue as shown in Fig. 4. Affinity also depends on the number of CH$_2$ groups being even or odd. The odd numbers have a clear advantage over the even. This might derive from the fact that the S1′ pocket of MMP-8 is not perfectly symmetrical and there might be in general a better fit of the phenyl tail on one side of the pocket than on the other. Extension of the C-terminus with three methylene groups (**32**) finally resulted in a significantly improved inhibitory potency with a K_i value of 0.24 µM. Attempts to similarly improve inhibition of MMP-8 with para-, meta-, or ortho-chloro substitutions in the benzyl amide **30** failed (K_i values in the range of 1.8–1.7 µM). Similarly, with para-, meta, or ortho-methyl derivatives of **30** the K_i values remained in the range of 1.4–9 µM. Introduction of a para-carboxyl group into the benzyl amide **30**, as a potential interaction partner for the Arg222 residue on the bottom of the S1′ pocket of MMP-8, led to a K_i value of 41 µM (**34**). This result would suggest that a buried salt bridge between the para-carboxyl group and the Arg side chain does not occur and that interactions with the S1′ subsite are significantly reduced.

Attempts to improve the solubility of the inhibitors as well as the hydrogen-bonding network with the edge strand of the active-site cleft of MMP-8 led us to replace the 2-methyl group of compound **30** with an acetamido (**35**) or hydroxy (**36**) group. Both hydroxamates showed an approx twofold reduced inhibitory potency compared with the parent compound **30** (Table 2) *(6)*.

2.1.2.3. MMP-8 Inhibition by Achiral Cyclic 2,2-*bis*-Substituted Malonic Acid Hydroxamates. The *bis*-substituted malonic acid derivatives described above were all obtained as racemates. Since enantioselective synthesis is required for the production of the *R* or *S* isomers we have also investigated symmetrical malonic acids, thus achiral inhibitors *(6)*. For this purpose the indan-2,2-dicarboxylic acid was prepared as a mimetic of the 2-benzyl-2-methylmalonic acid and converted to the hydroxamate benzyl amide **37**. As expected from modeling experiments, it showed an inhibitory potency that compared well to that of compound **30** (Table 2).

In crystals of the **37**/MMP-8 complex the structure of the achiral inhibitor could be unambiguously determined (Fig. 5). Minor adjustments of the malonic acid moiety and of the substituent, correlated with the indan pucker, might be a reasonable explanation. A comparison of the position of inhibitor **37** in the active-site cleft of the enzyme with that of the mono-substituted compound **1** (Fig. 3) shows a very similar binding behavior; however, hydrogen bonding of the malonic acid carbonyl to Leu160NH is retained and the indan group interacts with the hydrophobic surface formed mainly by the side chain of Ile159, whereas the C-terminal benzyl group inserts into the S1′ pocket.

In agreement with the results obtained for the 2-benzyl-2-methyl-substituted derivatives, replacement of the C-terminal benzyl residue with the 3-phenylpropyl group (**38**) leads to improved interactions in the hydrophobic S1′ site ($K_i = 0.3 \ \mu M$).

2.2. Cysteine Derivatives

The thiol group has long been known to be a good Zn-chelator for metalloproteases. A prominent example is the inhibitor of the angiotensin converting enzyme (ACE) Captopril, which belongs to the most often sold drugs worldwide. It was known that cysteine is able to inhibit MMPs. Also, cysteine containing inhibitors have been described which were based on the propeptide approach. This approach uses the knowledge that the MMP propeptide in the latent pro-MMP binds to the catalytic zinc atom by the thiol group of a cysteine. In contrast to normal substrates, the propetide binds parallel to the active site edge strand of the enzyme *(7)*. Correspondingly, the design of the thiol-based MMP inhibitors proposed so far, besides relying on the binding mode of the substrate, has more recently also been derived from cysteine-containing propeptide mimetics. In contrast to these propeptide approaches, we have derivatized both L- and D-cysteine with its chelating thiol group in an iterative manner at the amino and carboxyl

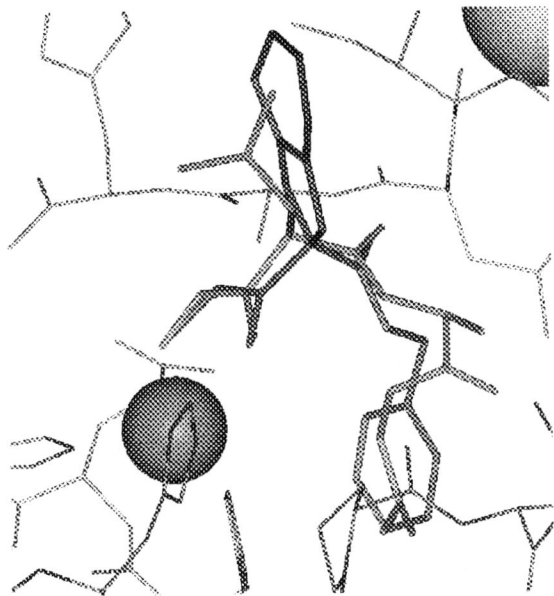

Fig. 5. Comparison of the binding modes of the inhibitors **1** and **38** to the active site of MMP-8.

function to non-peptidic structures *(8)*. Very simple compounds showed promising results for further investigation. By exploiting the thiol function of L-cysteine as a chelating group of the active-site zinc atom of matrix metalloproteases (MMPs), N- and C-terminal derivatization of this amino acid with aliphatic and aromatic groups allowed us to explore the selectivity of the S and/or S′ binding subsites of human neutrophil collagenase (MMP-8) and stromelysin (MMP-3). With N-benzyloxycarbonyl-L-cysteine-(2-phenyl)ethylamide a submicromolar inhibitor of MMP-8 was discovered *(8)*.

2.2.1. CHEMISTRY

All cysteine derivatives used in this study were synthesized by classical procedures of amino acid chemistry. As shown in Scheme 1, cystine was suitably acylated and amidated, and the resulting cystine derivatives were then converted to the cysteine compounds by reduction with tributylphosphine in trifluoroethanol containing water as hydrogen donor. Thereby particular attention was paid to avoid desulfuration, which was observed to occur to a certain extent unless fresh phosphine was used (for details *see* ref. *8*).

2.2.2. EFFECTS OF THE SYNTHETIC COMPOUNDS ON MMP-8 AND -3

Since all structures of MMP/inhibitor complexes show occupancy of the S1′ subsite by more or less bulky hydrophobic residues, we have examined the effect

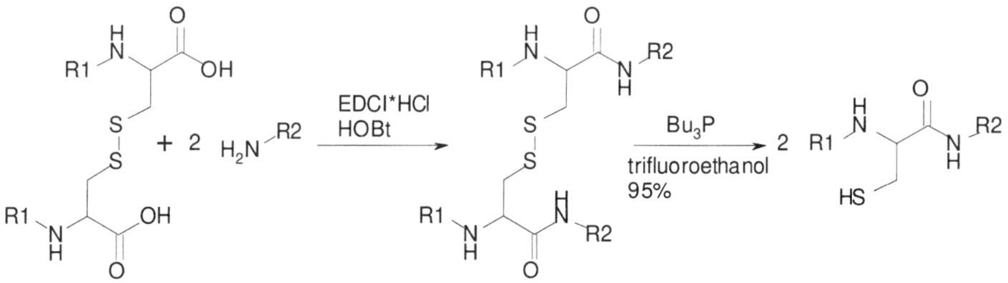

Scheme 1. General route for the synthesis of the N- and C-substituted cysteine derivatives.

of aromatic substituents at the amino and carboxyl function of cysteine, respectively. The introduction of an N-terminal benzyloxycarbonyl group (**40**, Table 3) enhanced the binding affinity to MMP-8 drastically compared with pure cysteine (**39**; IC_{50} 15 μM and 450 μM, respectively). An equivalent C-terminal derivatization to L-cysteine-benzylamide (**41**) was found to improve inhibition although to lower extents. To analyze the effect of the negative and positive charge of compounds **40** and **41**, compound **40** has been converted to the methyl ester, whereas compound **41** has been acetylated or *tert*-butyloxycarbonylated. Although these derivatizations had only marginal effects on the K_i values (data not shown), the related formyl derivative **42** was found to exhibit a 10-fold enhanced inhibition. With the incorporation of a second aromatic group into compound **41**, i.e., with N-benzyloxycarbonyl-L-cysteine-benzylamide (**43**), a significant improvement of the inhibitory potency ($K_i = 0.70$ μM) was achieved. This value, however, was only marginally affected by the type of the aromatic acyl moiety introduced, e.g., benzoyl, tosyl. Similarly, amidation of benzyloxycarbonyl-L-cysteine with 4-, 3-, or 2-aminomethylpyridine to possibly induce hydrogen bond formation in the S1′ pocket, was without marked effects on the inhibitory potency (data not shown).

Replacement of the benzylamide with (2-phenyl)ethylamide (**45**) yielded in a fourfold lower K_i value (0.16 μM). Further attempts to improve the inhibition with substituents in the (2-phenyl)ethylamide moiety, e.g., with the para-hydroxy or para-chloro group, failed (data not shown). Replacement of the (2-phenyl)ethylamide group with the (3-phenyl)propylamide (**46**) led unexpectedly again to an increase of the K_i value to 0.85 μM. But the tryptamine derivative **47** showed an inhibition of MMP-8 almost identical to that of compound **45** although the phenyl moiety of the indole group in **47** is spaced from the amide group as in compound **46**.

In order to analyze the role of the absolute configuration of the cysteine residue in the inhibition potency, compounds **43** and **47** were synthesized as D-cysteine derivatives (**44** and **48**). In both cases the K_i values were found to be not that much affected (2.6 μM for **44** vs 0.7 μM for **43** and 0.5 μM for **48** vs 0.17 μM for **47** in the case of MMP-8).

Table 3
R1-Cys-R2

Compound	R1	R2	Cys configuration	IC50 / Ki; MMP8 [μM]	IC50 / Ki; MMP3 [μM]
39	H (image)	,,,OH	L	450/n.d.	n.d./n.d.
40	(image)	,,,OH	L	15.0/13.0	n.d./n.d.
41	H (image)	(image)	L	150*/130*	n.d./n.d.
42	(image)	(image)	L	2.1/1.7	20.8/14.8
43	(image)	(image)	L	0.80/0.70	18.2/12.9
44	(image)	(image)	D	3.0/2.6	n.d./n.d.
45	(image)	(image)	L	0.18/0.16	17.3/12.3
46	(image)	(image)	L	0.98/0.85	4.2/3.0
47	(image)	(image)	L	0.2/0.17	1.9/1.4
48	(image)	(image)	D	0.6/0.5	n.d./n.d.

Regarding the specificity of the cysteine derivatives reported above, all were found to inhibit MMP-8 more efficiently than MMP-3, whereby compound **45**, besides being the most potent inhibitor of MMP-8 in this series, was also found to be the most selective, with a factor of about 80 (K_i's) referred to the inhibition of MMP-3. Interestingly, among the phenylalkylamine substituted cysteine derivatives compound **46**, with the largest spacer between the phenyl moiety and the amide group, proved to be the most potent inhibitor of MMP-3.

Among the synthesized cysteine derivatives the most potent inhibitors contain two aromatic groups that may interact with the hydrophobic S1′ protein pocket as well as with additional sites of the active-site cleft *(8)*. The X-ray structural analysis of N-biphenylmethyl-Cys-Gly-Val-OMe with MMP-3 revealed a binding mode of the inhibitor consisting of insertion of the aromatic N-terminus into the S1′ pocket of stromelysin and of an interaction of the residual peptide in a substrate-like manner with subsites of the primed region *(9)*. A similar binding mode was recently proposed on the basis of docking calculations for N-acyl-L-cysteinyl-L-phenylalanine-amide derivatives *(10)*. Superposition of compound **45** onto one of these dipeptide derivatives, i.e., to (3-phenyl)propionyl-L-cysteinyl-L-phenylalanine-amide, places the aromatic residues at identical positions. Correspondingly, at least compound **45** of our series of inhibitors could bind in an analogous manner to the MMP-8 with the benzyloxycarbonyl group inserted into the S1′ pocket and the C-terminal aromatic group interacting along the S′ cleft.

To analyze the binding of our inhibitors, we have performed some docking experiments to MMP-8 *(8)*. The calculations were done as all other modeling studies mentioned in this chapter with the program package INSIGHT/DISCOVER (version 2.96, MSI Technologies, San Diego, USA). By keeping the protein structure fixed and a 0.23–0.19 nm distance restraint between the cysteine sulfur and the active-site zinc, alternative orientations and conformations of the inhibitor were generated and energy-minimized to convergence. Binding of N-benzyloxy-carbonyl-L-cysteine-(2-phenyl)ethylamide (**45**) to MMP-8 with the benzyloxy-carbonyl group inserted into the S1′ pocket brings the urethane group into an unfavorable hydrophobic environment, but the C-terminal amide group into hydrogen bonding distance to Leu160 NH and Pro217 CO. Conversely, insertion of the C-terminal (2-phenyl)ethylamide moiety into S1′, as shown in Fig. 6, allows for better accommodation of the amide group at the entrance of the S1′ pocket with the Cys CO in hydrogen bonding distance to Ala161 NH, and the urethanyl moiety with the carbonyl group in hydrogen bonding distance to Leu160 NH. Moreover, the urethanyl amide is located in hydrogen bond distance to the Pro217 CO. Although the calculated surface contact areas in the binding modes are very similar, insertion of the C-terminus of compound 45 into the S1′ appears to be more probable. This inverted binding mode, if compared to those of the biphenyl-tripeptide *(9)* and (3-phenyl)propionyl-dipeptide *(10)* derivatives, may be attrib-

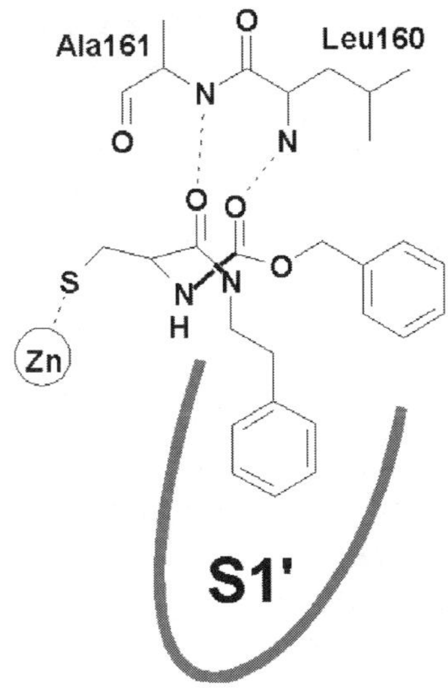

Fig. 6. Putative binding mode of cysteine inhibitors.

uted to the replacement of a methylene moiety with an oxygen atom in the ure-thanyl cysteine derivative and to the lack of additional amide groups in the C-terminus of our derivatives. This type of binding mode would also better cor-relate with the observed relatively strong inhibition of MMP-3 by compound **46**.

2.3. Barbiturates

We have identified 5-[4-(2-hydroxyethyl)]piperidino-5′-phenyl-barbituric acid as MMP-8 inhibitor by using a high-throughput screening assay. Carboxylic acids, hydroxamic acids, thiols, and phosphinates have been de-scribed as MMP inhibitors long ago. Here we describe barbiturates as new zinc chelators for metalloproteases and their optimization to nanomolar inhibitors. Barbiturates have been used for other purposes for decades. They are used as sedatives (e.g., Nervolitan, Resedorm, and Neodorm), narcotics (Methoxyhexital [Brevimytal©], Thiopental [Trapanal©]) and as antiepileptica (Phenobarbital and Methylphenobarbital). However, these typical barbiturate effects are strongly dependent on the barbiturate substituents and are not found with in-hibitors of our series. Furthermore, barbiturates in general show good adsorp-tion features which makes them attractive drug pharmacophores.

Modeling and an X-ray structure of our lead structure with different MMPs identified the binding mode of this class of compounds. We initiated an exten-sive program including modeling and combinatorial chemistry, which finally yielded barbiturate derivatives with in vitro activities toward the gelatinases A and B similar to marimastat, batimastat, and other compounds. Indeed these compounds are much more specific toward the gelatinases than our reference compounds. Docking experiments to the active site of MMP-8 suggested two different modes of binding. The binding to the catalytic zinc ion is performed by one of the nitrogens of the barbiturate as also found in barbiturate-metal complexes such as the bis(5,5'-diethylbarbiturato)bispicoline complex of zinc (II) (*11*). The phenyl group could either point into the S1' pocket of the collagenase or into S2', with the hydroxyethylpiperidine conversely binding in S2' or S1'. An X-ray structure of the lead compound with MMP-8 was obtained early, confirming the zinc binding concept and showing that indeed the phenyl ring points into S1' and the hydroxyethylpiperidine extends into S2' (Fig. 7). The barbiturate C5-atom occupies approximately the same spatial position as the C-atom which is origin of the P1' residue in succinates like batimastat. Whereas many results for P1' residues are known and good residues are often quite similar, there is a wide variety of possibilities for S2'. However, most of the S2' residues are amino acids or derivatives thereof. For a quick optimization of both residues we used a two-track strategy, optimizing each residue independent of the other. Whereas one residue was optimized by classical chemistry in combination with drug design, the other residue was optimized by drug design guided parallel synthesis (Fig. 1). In the structure-based combinatorial chemistry approach used for the optimization of the P2' residue, the residues for coupling with the parent compound 5-amino-5-phenyl-barbiturate were selected by using the size information of the S2'/S3' area. The structural restraints for the P2'-P4' residues were:

1. Extension in two directions, i. e., preference was given to ring systems rather than to unbranched aliphatic chains;
2. The length of the residue should be at least three atoms and not more than the length of a typical three-membered ring system like anthracene;
3. There can be two residues on the piperidine nitrogen in 5-[4-(2-hydroxy-ethyl)]piperidino-5'-phenyl-barbiturate.

Another selection criteria was the commercial availability of the residue.

For the first compounds we have chosen the 5-amino-5-phenyl-barbiturate as a parent compound since it seemed to be easy to perform a simple amide formation for the combinatorial chemistry approach. This educt has been obtained from phenylmalonic acid diethylester, sodium methanolate and urea, followed by Br_2/HBr benzylamine and hydrogenolysis to the amine. Using the 5-amino-5'-phenyl-barbiturate we have applied combinatorial chemistry to make a simple acylation.

In a first round we have acylated the amino group mainly by using either benzoic acid derivatives (36 compounds) or by using 2-phenyl-acetic acid derivatives (17 compounds, Table 4). In addition we varied the chain length between the amide and the phenyl ring (6 compounds, Table 4). The approach turned out to be not very successful. The best 5-acylamino-5'-phenyl-barbiturate we found was

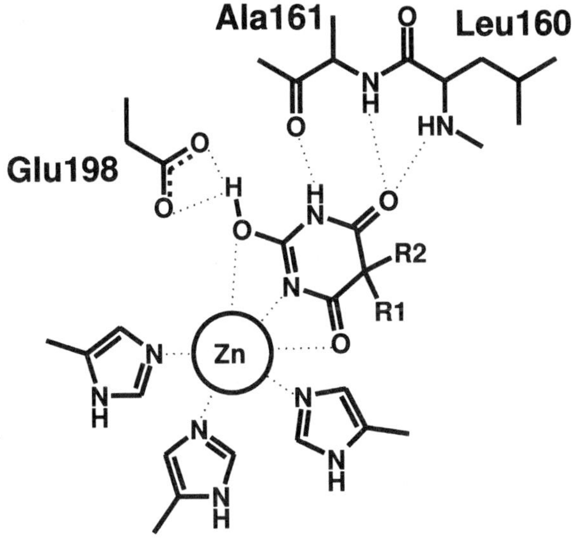

Fig. 7. Binding of barbiturates to MMP-8.

the naphthalen-2-yl derivative with 84% inhibition at 2.7 μM. The large group (annelated phenyl) in *meta*- and *para*-position seems to be favorable. In contrast the naphthalen-1-yl derivative has the same ring displaced to *ortho*- and *meta*-position. Here the inhibition is clearly worse (66%). Another relatively active compound having a large and hydrophobic residue is the 1-fluorenyl derivative. It exhibits a similar activity as the napthalene-2-yl derivative. Anyway, the large and hydrophobic residue makes it less attractive for further optimization. The 3,4-dimethylphenyl derivative as naphthalene-2-yl analogue showed only an inhibition of 42% at 2.7 μM. However, also other residues in *meta*- (*meta*-methoxyphenyl, 73%; *meta*-Cl-phenyl, 60%) or *para*-position seem to be positive (*para*-ethoxyphenyl, 63%; *para*-Br-phenyl, 56%). An exception is the basic dimethyl-aminophenyl derivative (36%), which is less favorable. A direct comparison of the substituents in *ortho*-, *meta*-, and *para*-position is possible in three cases. The methyl-, methoxy-, and chloro-residue is always best in *meta*-position. For the methyl-group the activity is similar in the *ortho*-position and worse in *para*.

Variation of the chain length between the amide bond and the phenyl ring displayed a clear preference for an even number of C-atoms in the connecting chain, a similar effect as seen with the malonic acid derivatives, although a different binding site is presumably involved. To further optimize entropic effects we tried to stabilize the 3-phenyl-propionamide skeleton by introducing a double bond, i. e., by using cinnamic acids (Table 4). However, independent of the substituent we used, the cinnamic acid derivatives could not improve the phenylpropionic acid derivative structure. All compounds were showing an approx 50% inhibition at 3 μM.

Table 4

	Number of compounds synthesized	Best hits	Inhibition of MMP8 (at concentration)
Benzoic acids	36	napthalen-2-yl 3-methoxy-phenyl	84% (2.7 μM) 73% (3.4 μM)
Phenyl acetic acids	17	m-Cl-benzyl	74% (3.4 μM)
$-(CH_2)_n-C_6H_5$	6	n = 0 2 4	54% (3.3 μM) 52% (3.3 μM) 55% (3.5 μM)
Cinnamic acids $-CH=CH-C_6H_3R1R2$	7	4-Cl-	56% (2.6 μM)

These disappointing results led us to use more of the original structure. However, since not many 4-substituted piperidines are commercially available, we decided to use the related, readily accessible piperazines, which are similarly active. For the combinatorial chemistry approach we used the 5-bromo-5-phenyl-barbiturate which was coupled with more than 100 different piperazines. The para-nitro-phenyl-piperazine derivative turned out to be the most active compound (81% inhibition of MMP-8 at 0.5 μg/ml). Reduction of the nitro-group decreased the inhibitory potency dramatically (13% inhibition at 1 μg/mL). No substituents (78% inhibition at 5 μg/mL) or different substituents at the phenyl ring, e.g., ortho-methoxy (46% at 5 μg/mL), meta-methoxy (74% at 5 μg/mL), para-methoxy (77% at 5 μg/mL), ortho-ethoxy (8% at 5 μg/mL) and para-chloro (25% at 5 μg/mL) also failed to reach this strong potency.

In parallel to the identification of the 4-(nitrophenyl)piperazine residue as an interesting P2′ residue, we have optimized the P1′ residue independently from this, keeping the 4-(2-hydroxyethyl)piperazine fixed as a P2′ residue. The optimization of this residue was done using classical chemistry and drug design. Elongation of the P1′ phenyl ring in para position with small substituents like hydroxy, methoxy, or methyl improved the potency of the lead compound 5-

Table 5^a

Compound	R	M [g/mol]	IC50 MMP 8 [nM]	IC50 MMP 2 [nM]	IC50 MMP 9 [nM]
49	(Marimastat)	331.30	12.1	14	10
50	pyrimidin-2-yl	402.50	24.8	93	17.4
51	pyrazin-2-yl	402.50	34.8	94	16.9
52	4-nitrophenyl	445.52	35.9	202	15.9
53	3,5-dichloro-pyridin-4-yl	470.40	42.5	124	7.6
54	3-trifluoromethyl-pyridin-2-yl	469.51	61.8	>1μM	11.5
55	4-trifluoromethyl-pyrimidin-2-yl	470.50	70.1	181	10.8
56	2-nitrophenyl	445.52	85.3	138	15.3
57	4-methanesulfonyl	478.61	96.1	162	10.2
58	4-difluoromethyl-pyridin-2-yl	469.51	110.8	108	14.1
59	2-fluorophenyl	418.52	129	191	16.2
60	4-hydroxyphenyl	416.52	192.8	321	18.8
61	hydroxyethyl	368.5	204	344	81

^aIC50 values from selected 5-octyl-5-piperazinyl-barbiturates against MMP-8 (catalytic domain), -2 and -9 (full length enzymes). Results were obtained using the fluorogenic substrate Dnp-Pro-Leu-Gly-Leu-Trp-Ala-D-Arg-NH$_2$.

phenyl-5′-[4-(2-hydroxyethyl)]piperazine (IC$_{50}$ for MMP-8 approx 2 μM) up to a factor of 3 (860nM, 800nM, 1500nM, respectively). Finally we found that an exchange of the substituted phenyl with an n-octyl group improved the potency to approx 200nM for MMP-8. Interestingly the same residue has also been identified for the malonic acids (*see* Subheading 2.1.).

The n-octyl as an optimized P1′ residue and the 4-(nitrophenyl)piperazine as an optimized P2′ residue have been used to generate a compound with both residues in one molecule. This was done without having further evidence from X-ray crystallography confirming that the assumed binding of the two residues is correct. However, the result of the kinetic analysis of this inhibitor confirmed our assumption with an IC_{50} of 37nM for MMP-8 and the same or even better data for the gelatinases (37 nM and 17 nM for gelatinase A and B, respectively).

For further optimization of the compound we used the octyl group as P1′ instead of the phenyl group and kept the 5-piperazinyl-group for P2′. Now we were able to identify more compounds having IC_{50}s between 10 and 100nM, which is a range useful for drug applications. One of the best compounds found (**50**) had an IC_{50} of 24.8 nM against MMP-8. Since we did not determine the K_i-values, we used marimastat (**49**) as a reference compound showing an IC_{50} of 12.1 nM in this assay. We also examined the inhibition of MMP-2 (Gelatinase-A) and MMP-9 (Gelatinase-B) with the better compounds (Table 5). Interestingly, the barbiturates proved to be excellent MMP-9 inhibitors. Nearly all of the compounds in Table 5 have IC_{50}'s below 20nM. One of them (**53**) is even better than marimastat (7.6 vs 10nM). A comparison of marimastat with the barbiturate inhibitors in a MMP-1 assay showed that our inhibitors are more specific than the succinate inhibitor. Whereas our inhibitors did not inhibit this enzyme efficiently, marimastat did (at 200 nM: marimastat: 100% inhibition, 5-[4-(2-hydroxyethyl)]piperazin-1-yl)-5-octyl-barbiturate: 14% inhibition).

3. SUMMARY AND OUTLOOK

We have described three different types of nonsubstrate-like binding inhibitors. Whereas the malonic acid hydroxamates use the classical hydroxamate function for zinc ligation, this is done by the thiol or barbiturate moiety in the other series, respectively. Due to their unusual β-turn like binding behavior also the malonic acid derivatives are very different from the well known succinate MMP inhibitors. All three series could be optimized to affinities in the nanomolar range. At least the barbiturates have inhibition constants similar to the well known succinate hydroxamate inhibitors such as batimastat or marimastat. However, they have been optimized for gelatinase specificity and indeed in contrast to marimastat they inhibit MMP-1, for example, only very weakly. Several inhibitors described in this chapter have been tested in animal models for antitumor/antimetastatic effects and some compounds show very promising results. The outcome of these experiments will be described later.

ACKNOWLEDGMENT

We thank Prof. H. Tschesche for providing the catalytic domain of MMP-8 and Prof. Hideaki Nagase for providing MMP-3.

REFERENCES

1. Grams, F., Reinemer, P., Powers, J.C., Kleine, T., Tschesche, H., Bode, W. X-ray Structures of Human Neutrophil Collagenase Complexed with Peptide Hydroxamate and Peptide Thiol Inhibitors—Implications for Substrate-Binding and Rational Drug Design. *Eur. J. Biochem.* 1995; 228:830–841.

2. Nishino, N., Powers, J. Peptide Hydroxamic Acids as Inhibitors of Thermolysin. *Biochemistry* 1978; 17:2846–2850.

3. Johnson, W.H., Roberts, N.A., Borkakoti, N. Collagenase Inhibitors: Their Design and Potential Therapeutic Use. *J. Enzyme Inhibition* 1987; 2:1–22.

4. Graf v. Roedern, E., Grams, F., Brandstetter, H., Moroder, L. Design and Synthesis of Malonic Acid-Based Inhibitors of Human Neutrophil Collagenase (MMP-8). *J. Med. Chem.* 1998; 41:339–345.

5. Brandstetter, H., Engh, R.A, Graf von Roedern, E., Moroder, L., Huber, R., Bode, W., Grams, F. Structure of Malonic-Acid-Based Inhibitors bound to Human Neutrophil Collagenase—A new binding mode explains apparently anomalous data. *Protein Science* 1998; 7:1303–1309.

6. Graf v. Roedern, E., Brandstetter, H., Engh, R.A., Bode, W., Grams, F., Moroder, L. Bis-Substituted Malonic Acid Hydroxamate Derivatives as Inhibitors of Human Neutrophil Collagenase (MMP-8). *J. Med. Chem.* 1998; 41:3041–3047.

7. Becker, J.W, Marcy, A.I, Rokosz, L.L, Axel, M.G, Burbaum, J.J, Fitzgerald, P.M, Cameron, P.M, Esser, C.K, Hagmann, W.K, Hermes, J.D, Springer, J.P. Stromelysin-1: three-dimensional structure of the inhibited catalytic domain and of the C-truncated proenzyme. *Protein Sci.* 1995; 4(10):1966–76.

8. Müller, J.C., Graf v. Rodern, E., Grams, F., Nagase, H., Moroder, L. Non-Peptidic Cysteine Derivatives as Inhibitors of Matrix Metalloproteinases. *Biol. Chem.* 1997; 378:1475–1480.

9. Michoud, C., Fotouhi, N., Visnick, M., Piettranico, S., Hanglow, A., Birktoft, J.J., Vermeulen, J., Lugo, A., Kammlott, U.R. The design and synthesis of stromelysin inhibitors. *Drug Design and Discovery* 1996; 13:156–157.

10. Foley, M.A., Hassman, A.S., Drewry, D.H., Greer, D.G., Wagner, C.D., Feldman, P.L., Berman, J., Bickett, D.M., McGeehan, G.M., Lambert, M.H., Green, M. Rapid synthesis of novel dipeptide inhibitors of human collagenase and gelatinase using solid phase chemistry. *Bioorg. Med. Chem. Lett.* 1996; 6:1905–1910.

11. Nassimbeni, L., Rodgers, A. Crystal structure of the bis(5,5′-diethylbarbiturato)bispicoline complex of zinc (II). *Acta Crystallogr.,* Sect. B, 1974; B30 (8), 1953–1961.

10 Matrix Metalloproteinase Inhibitors
Therapeutic Applications Outside of Oncology

Michael R. Niesman, *PhD*

CONTENTS

1. INTRODUCTION

The previous chapters in this volume describe the rationale for the therapeutic use of matrix metalloproteinase inhibitors (MMPI) in oncology and the experience to date with these agents. However, both experts and those new to the field will realize that matrix metalloproteinase (MMPs) are involved in other disease processes. Therefore, it is probable that inhibitors of MMPs will prove useful for the treatment of diseases other than cancer. This chapter is designed to provide a brief overview of the evidence suggesting the involvement of MMPs in other diseases and an update on preclinical experiments or clinical trials that indicate MMPI impede or alter the progression of these diseases. This article is by no means an exhaustive review of the large body of MMP work outside of oncology, but it is hoped that it will provide a useful starting point for investigators interested in applications of MMPI in disease processes other than cancer. Other more comprehensive reviews have been published *(1–5)*, as has a

From: *Cancer Drug Discovery and Development:*
Matrix Metalloproteinase Inhibitors in Cancer Therapy
Edited by: Neil J. Clendeninn and Krzysztof Appelt © Humana Press Inc., Totowa, NJ

recent volume compiling the proceedings of a recent conference dedicated to this topic *(6)*.

2. ARTHRITIS

Cartilage breakdown is a major component of the pathological process that occurs in patients with arthritis. Because MMPs are directly involved in the degradation of this component of the extracellular matrix (ECM), the use of inhibitors of MMPs is a logical approach for the treatment of the disease. Current treatments for osteoarthritis and rheumatoid arthritis reduce the inflammatory response in the joint and relieve pain, but do not halt the progression of the disease. That is, the degradation of the joint continues unabated in arthritis patients despite the best treatments currently available.

Inhibitors of MMPs have proven to be effective in the treatment of animal models of arthritis *(7,8)*. Several of the MMPs have been implicated in this process *(9,10)*, with MMP-3 (Stromolysin-1) considered a key target *(11)*. One compound in clinical trials (BAY 12-9566) is an MMPI designed to inhibit MMP-3 although sparing collagenase-1 (MMP-1). The rationale given for this MMP-3 directed, MMP-1 sparing design for BAY12-9566 was that MMP-1 is widely distributed throughout the body. On the other hand, MMP-3 seems to be up-regulated mostly within the affected joints in patients with arthritis. Furthermore, MMP-3 has the ability to degrade collagen and aggrecan and activate other MMPs *(11)*. As the field matures, it will be interesting to learn whether this approach proves successful. An alternative approach now seems possible, given the recently reported cloning of the gene for aggrecanase *(12,13)*. Aggrecanase is another degradative enzyme thought to be critical to the pathological breakdown of the joint structure in patients with arthritis.

Whereas arthritis may be an obvious disease target for MMPI, no drug is currently approved for use in patients with this disease. The first disease indication with an FDA-approved drug is periodontal disease.

3. PERIODONTAL DISEASE

Periodontitis is an inflammatory process that is initiated by the microflora of the subgingival environment. It leads to the destruction of the structures that support the teeth, including the gingiva, periodontal ligament, root cementum, and alveolar bone *(14)*. It is generally accepted that the destruction present in the disease is a result of the host response. Recent research suggests that a significant contributor to this destructive process is MMP-8 *(14,15)*. MMP-8 is produced mainly by neutrophils, which is consistent with the inflammatory nature of the disease and the hypothesis that the host response is responsible for the tissue damage present in patients with periodontitis. MMP-13, also designated bone cell collagenase or collagenase 3, may also be involved in the host response seen in this disease *(16)*.

The accessibility of the gingival area for testing has made it possible to accurately measure the amount of MMP activity at the site of disease and this allows for relatively easy monitoring of treatment. For example, one can monitor collagenase activity in gingival crevicular fluid (GCF). This has allowed the CollaGenex Corporation to test subantimicrobial doses of doxycycline (SDD) as treatment for adult periodontitis *(17)*. Doxycycline has been shown to be an MMPI at doses well below those that demonstrate antibacterial activity. In clinical trials, the administration of SDD reduced the collagenase activity in the GCF, improved the clinical attachment scores and pocket depth, and reduced the bleeding seen in response to probing in these patients *(17)*. Following successful Phase III trials, the FDA approved SDD under the trade name Periostat®. It is the only MMPI currently approved by the FDA for marketing in the US.

The successful treatment of periodontitis with an MMPI is a milestone in MMP research. This is a disease in which the pathological contribution of MMPs to the disease process was clearly established. The effectiveness of an MMPI in periodontitis lends support to the hypothesis that an MMPI with the appropriate efficacy and safety profile will be able to alter disease progression in other diseases in which MMPs contribute to the pathological process.

4. OPHTHALMOLOGY

Neovascularization (i.e., pathological angiogenesis) is a component of many of the most serious diseases involving the eye. Neovascularization is present in patients with the neovascular form of age-related macular degeneration (AMD), diabetic retinopathy, neovascular glaucoma, pathologic myopia, and retinopathy of prematurity (ROP) *(18–21)*. When considered together, neovascular diseases are the leading cause of blindness in the United States *(20)*. As the understanding of angiogenesis has grown, it has become apparent that MMPs play an important role in the process of neovascularization. This has been shown both in tumors (*see* preceding chapters) and other angiogenic processes *(21)*.

Several investigators have demonstrated that MMPI can prevent or reduce angiogenesis in animal models of retinal neovascularization. Freeman, et al. *(22)* and Penn, et al. *(23)* have both presented the result of experiments in which MMPI reduced retinal neovascularization. In recently published experiments, Das and coworkers *(24)* employed an oxygen injury model of ocular neovascularization in mice for experiments with an MMPI. They demonstrated that messenger RNA levels of MMPs 2, 9, and 14, as measured by the polymerase chain reaction (PCR), were elevated in the retinas of animals with neovascularization. When the animals were treated with a broad spectrum MMPI (batimastat, BB-

94), the neovascular response was reduced by approx 3.5-fold at 1 mg/kg and 10-fold at 15 mg/kg *(24)*. Thus, in these experiments where the drug was administered during the active phase of angiogenesis, the inhibition of an MMPI had a beneficial effect.

Recent evidence suggests that MMPs may contribute to ocular disease in humans. Steen, et. al. *(25)* recently reported evidence of the presence of MMPs in ocular lesions from patients with AMD. The authors used *in situ* hybridization to analyze surgical specimens—subfoveal fibrovascular membranes—removed from five patients with neovascular AMD. MMP-2 and MMP-9 were detected in all of the samples. Interestingly, MMP-2 appeared to be associated with a majority of the endothelial cells and MMP-9 appeared to be located at the advancing borders of the lesion. The authors suggested that this supports the hypothesis that MMP-2 and MMP-9 are involved in the formation of the choroidal neovascular membranes present in AMD patients *(25)*. Although the study needs to be viewed with some caution due to the small sample size, the hypothesis does appear sound in light of the accumulated knowledge that supports the involvement of MMP-2 and MMP-9 in the process of angiogenesis *(21)*.

The lack of optimal treatments available for patients with neovascular AMD has spurred interest in developing a treatment for the condition. One antiangiogenic agent currently in clinical trials for AMD is an MMPI. That agent is prinomastat (AG3340). The characteristics of this agent have been described previously in this volume. It has demonstrated ocular antiangiogenic activity in preclinical experiments *(22)*. It is currently in Phase II clinical trial being conducted in North America.

Other ocular conditions may be amenable to therapy with MMP inhibitors. It has been demonstrated clearly that MMPs are up-regulated in the response of the cornea seen following injury. Fini and coworkers *(26)* reported the presence of several MMPs in the cornea following injury. The levels of MMP-2, MMP-3, and MMP-9 were elevated compared to those seen in normal tissue. It appeared that MMP-9 was produced by resident cells of the cornea in response to injury. When the injured corneas were removed from the animals and examined in vitro, preservation of the basement membrane was seen in corneas cultured in the presence of an MMP inhibitor. Other evidence of MMP activity in the cornea has been reported *(27,28)*. Taken together, these studies suggest that topical application of MMPI may prove beneficial in some corneal disease conditions.

Finally, there is emerging evidence that inhibitors of MMPs might prove beneficial for the treatment of proliferative vitreoretinopathy (PVR). This disease occurs most often as a complication of retinal detachment. It is the major cause of failure of surgery to repair retinal detachments. An exact understanding of the etiology of the disease is lacking. However, in the simplest terms, the disease process can be characterized as abnormal wound healing, or "scarring" in the central nervous system (i.e., the retina). Nonneuronal cells proliferate and migrate in response to a growth factor or factors released from the cells of the injured retina following retinal detachment. It may be that MMPs also serve to liberate growth factors, such as fibroblast growth factor (FGF), which is known to be sequestered in the ECM of the retina *(29)*. A recent report has demonstrated the effectiveness of one MMPI in a subacute model of PVR *(30)*. Additional work will be required to confirm this study and gain an understanding of the mechanisms involved for the positive effect that was measured. In total, research to be completed over the next few years may demonstrate the rationale for employing MMPI in several diseases of the eye.

5. NEUROLOGICAL DISEASES

The number of investigations designed to understand the role of MMPs in the central nervous system (CNS) is rapidly expanding and these studies were the subject of recent international conference *(31)*. The information that is emerging from these studies is briefly summarized below. The discussion is organized according to the diseases in which MMPs appear to influence disease progression.

5.1. Multiple Sclerosis (MS)

Several reports have shown the presence of MMPs in this disease *(32)*, either in the preclinical animal model designed to mimic MS (experimental autoimmune encephalitis; EAE) or in the human disease itself. For example, various members of MMP family have been measured in brains of animals with EAE *(33)* as well as in patients with MS *(34,35)*. Using immunohistochemistry, MMP-7 was found to be up-regulated in perivascular macrophages and astrocytes in an animal model of EAE in rats *(33)*. MMP expression appeared to be up-regulated in astrocytes, microglia, and perivascular macrophages in the brain samples from patients with MS *(34,35)*. Several experiments in animals have demonstrated beneficial effects from the administration of inhibitors of MMPs *(36–38)*. A discussion in a recent review article suggests the beneficial effect seen in these experiments should be interpreted with caution. The reduced severity of the disease could result from the inhibition of one or more MMPs, the inhibition of TNF-α converting enzyme (TACE), a reduction in the breakdown of the blood brain barrier, or a combination of these factors. Although further investigations into animal models and human disease are needed to clearly understand the underlying pharmacology, it appears that MMP inhibitors may prove useful for patients with MS.

5.2. Alzheimer's Disease (AD)

The role of MMP in AD is controversial. In tissue culture experiments, mixed cultures of neurons and glial cells from the hippocampus increased MMP production when exposed to amyloid-β proteins (Aβ) *(39)*. One investigator has shown data suggesting that MMP-2 can cleave Aβ at the α-secretase site *(40)*, which would be beneficial for patients with AD. On the other hand, it has been reported that MMP-2 could have β-secretase activity *(41)*, which would suggest it would function to increase amyloid deposits. Others have shown evidence that tissue inhibitors of metalloproteinases (TIMPs) are components of the amyloid plaques and neurofibrillary tangles seen in AD patients. Because TIMPs are both inhibitors of MMPs and also are associated with activated MMPs, it is not clear how to interpret this association.

No clear consensus exists regarding the role of MMPs in AD. As the etiology of this condition becomes better understood, it should become more readily apparent whether or not MMPI will prove beneficial for patients with this disease.

5.3. Proteolytic Disruption of the Blood Brain Barrier (BBB)

Early experiments with bacterial collagenase demonstrated that intraventricular injection of bacteria collagenase increases capillary permeability in the rat *(42)*. A more recent study demonstrated that the injection of purified, mammalian MMP-2 opens the BBB *(43)*, which suggests the possibility that proteolytic enzymes, specifically MMPs, may be involved in the BBB breakdown seen in pathological conditions in the brain. Other reports have indicated that in the transient middle cerebral artery occlusion (MCAO) model, MMPs are involved in two phases of BBB permeability increase, with the early permeability increases associated with an increase in MMP-2 and the delayed increase related to increased levels of MMP-9 *(44)*. In a model in which lipopolysaccharide (LPS) is injected to simulate neuroinflammation, MMP-9 increases appear to be responsible for the loss of integrity of the BBB *(45)*. Thus, for patients with brain edema from neuroinflammatory conditions, stroke, or even head trauma, MMPI use may prove to be beneficial, especially considering the lack of alternative therapies.

5.4. CNS Injury and Recovery

As pointed out by Yong et al. *(32)*, the fact that MMPs appear to be up-regulated following most insults to the CNS needs to be kept in mind as testing of inhibitors is pursued. For example, might MMPs be required to clear cellular debris following neuronal injury? Might this not facilitate recovery and synaptic reconnection? This is clearly an area of great scientific interest and no clear answers to these questions have yet emerged. Future work will undoubtedly shed light on the role of MMPs in CNS pathology and thereby allow for MMP inhibitors to be used for the benefit of the patients with these diseases.

6. CARDIOVASCULAR DISEASE

In several papers presented at a recent conference, evidence was presented implicating MMPs in the etiology of plaque rupture and aneurysm expansion

(46–48). Abdominal aortic aneurysm (AAA) was the focus of one of the presentations *(46)*. MMP-9 appears to be the most prominently expressed MMP in AAA, both in organ culture and in vivo *(46,49–51)*. The authors speculate that one reason for the abundance of MMP-9 is the fact that it is the main inducible product of mononuclear phagocytes *(50)*. Recent results suggest that infiltrating mononuclear phagocytes can induce MMP-2 expression in fibroblasts and smooth muscle cells, other cellular constituents of the pathological tissue *(52,53)*.

In a pilot experiment, patients with AAA preparing to undergo elective surgery were treated with 100mg of doxycycline twice a day for seven days prior to surgery *(46)*. When tissues from the doxycycline-treated group were compared to tissues from untreated patients, there was a significant reduction (3–4-fold) in the amount of MMP-2 and MMP-9 mRNA in the treated group. This suggests that it is feasible and rational to perform a clinical study to determine if MMP inhibition will halt or slow the rate of progression of AAA. This might be extremely beneficial to patients considering that although the morbidity rate for this surgery is decreasing, it is still significant.

7. CONCLUSION

It is clear from the other chapters presented in this volume that the inhibition of MMP activity may prove extremely beneficial for patients with various forms of cancer. The data reviewed in this chapter suggest that MMPs contribute to disease processes other than cancer, including arthritis, periodontitis, and ocular, cardiovascular, and CNS disease. As our understanding of the role of MMPs in these other diseases increases, it is likely that specific inhibitors of these metalloproteinases may have a positive impact on patients with these conditions.

REFERENCES

1. Nagase H, Woessner JF Jr. MMP Matrix metalloproteinases. *J Biol Chem* 1999; 274:21491–21494.
2. Jones L, Ghaneh P, Humphreys M, Neoptolemos JP. The matrix metalloproteinases and their inhibitors in the treatment of pancreatic cancer. *Ann. N. Y. Acad. Sci.* 1999; 880:288–307.
3. Kugler A. Matrix metalloproteinases and their inhibitors. *Anticancer Res* 1999; 19:1589–1592.
4. DeClerck YA, Imren S, Montgomery AM, Mueller BM, Reisfeld RA, Laug WE. Proteases and protease inhibitors in tumor progression. *Adv. Exp. Med. Biol.* 1997; 425:89–97.
5. Beeley NR, Ansell PR, Docherty AJ. Inhibitors of matrix metalloproteinases (MMP's). *Curr. Opin. Ther. Patents* 1994; 4:7–16.
6. Greenwald RA, Zucker S, Golub LM. eds. (1999) *Inhibition of Matrix Metalloproteinases: Therapeutic Applications. Annals of the New York Academy of Sciences Volume 878.* New York Academy of Sciences, NY.
7. Chau T, Jolly G, Plym JM. Inhibition of articular cartilage degradation in dog and guinea pig models of osteoarthritis by the stromelysin inhibitor, BAY 12-9566. *Arth. Rheum.* 1998; 41(9S), S300.

8. Zernicke RF, Wohl GR, Greenwald RA, Moak SA, Leng W, Golub LM. Administration of systemic matrix metalloproteinase inhibitors maintains bone mechanical integrity in adjuvant arthritis. *J. Rheumatol.* 1997; 24:1324–1331.

9. Woessner JF Jr, Guanja-Smith Z. Role of metalloproteinases in human osteoarthritis. *J. Rheumatol. Supp.* 1991; 27: 99–101.

10. Lohmander LS, Hoerrner LA, Lark MW. Metalloproteinases, tissue inhibitor, and proteoglycan fragments in the knee synovial fluid in human osteoarthritis. *Arth. Rheum.* 1993; 36:181–189.

11. Leff RL. Osteoarthritis, Matrix Metalloproteinase inhibition, cartilage loss. Surrogate markers, and clinical implications. *Ann. N.Y. Acad. Sci.* 1999; 878:201–207.

12. Tortorella MD, Burn TC, Pratta MA, Abbaszade I, Hollis JM, Liu R, Rosenfeld SA, Copeland RA, Decicco CP, Wynn R, Rockwell A, Yang F. Duke JL, Solomon K, George H, Bruckner R, Nagase H, Itoh Y, Ellis DM, Ross H, Wiswall BH, Murphy K, Hillman MC Jr, Hollis GF, Arner EC, et al Purification and cloning of aggrecanase-1: a member of the ADAMTS family of proteins. *Science* 1999; 284:1664–1666.

13. Arner EC, Pratta MA, Trzaskos JM, Decicco CP, Tortorella MD. Generation and characterization of aggrecanase. A soluble, cartilage-derived aggrecan-degrading activity. *J. Biol. Chem.* 1999; 274:6594–6601.

14. Manson JD Eley BM. eds. *Outlines of Periodontics* Wright Publisher, Elsevier, Oxford, 1996; 1–285.

15. Ryan ME, Ramamurthy NS, Golub LM. Matrix metallopteteinases and their inhibitors in periodontal treatment. *Curr. Opin. Peridontol.* 1996; 3:85–96.

16. Sorsa T, Mäntylä P, Rönkä H, Kallio P, Lallis G-B, Lundqvist C, Kinane DF, Salo T, Golub LM, Teronen O, Tikanoja S. Scientific basis of a matrix metalloproteinase-8 specific chairside test for monitoring periodontal and peri-implant health and disease. *Ann. N.Y. Acad. Sci.* 1999; 878:130–140.

17. Ashley RA, and SDD Clinical Research Team. Clinical Trial of a matrix metalloproteinase inhibitor in human periodontal disease. *Ann. N.Y. Acad. Sci.* 1999; 878:335–346.

18. Elman MJ, Fine SL. (1989) Exudative age-related macular degeneration in Retina, S.J. Ryan (ed.) Chapter 68, pp. 1103–1141.

19. Carcia CA, Ruiz RS. Ocular complications of diabetes. *Clin. Symp.* 1992; 44:2–32.

20. Lee P, Wang CC, Adamis AP. Ocular neovascularization: an epidemiologic review. *Surv. Ophthalmol.* 1998; 43:245–269.

21. Moses MA. The regulation of neovascularization of matrix metalloproteinases and their inhibitors. *Stem Cells* 1997; 15:180–189.

22. Rivero ME, Garcia CR, Hagedorn M, Zhang KE, McDermott C, Bartsch DU, Ruoslahti E, Keefe KS, Appelt K, Freeman WR. Intraocular properties of AG3340, a selective matrix metalloproteinase inhibitor with antiangiogenic properties. *Invest. Ophthalmol. Vis. Sci.* (Suppl.) 1998; 39:S585.

23. Penn JS, Roberto KA, and Bullard LE. Inhibition of retinal neovascularization by a broad spectrum matrix metalloproteinase inhibitor in an animal model of ROP. *Invest. Ophthalmol. Vis. Sci.* (Suppl.) 1999; 40:S618.

24. Das A, McLamore A, Song W, McGuire PG. Retinal neovascularization is suppressed with a matrix metalloproteinase inhibitor. *Arch Ophthalmol.* 1999; 117:498–503.

25. Steen B, Sejersen S, Berglin L, Seregard S, Kvanta A. Martix metalloproteinases and metalloproteinase inhibitors in choroidal neovascular membranes. *Invest. Ophthalmol. Vis. Sci.* 1998; 39:2194–2200.

26. Fini ME, Parks WC, Rinehart WB, Girard MT, Matsubara M, Cook JR, West-Mays JA, Sadow PM, Burgeson RE, Jeffrey JJ, Raizman MB, Krueger RR, Zieske JD. Role of matrix metalloproteinases in failure to re-epithelialize after corneal injury. *Am. J. Pathol. Oct* 1996; 149:1287–1302.

27. Fini ME, Cook JR, Mohan R. Proteolytic mechanisms in corneal ulceration and repair. *Arch. Dermatol. Res.* 1998; 290:Suppl:S12–23.

28. Ye HQ, Azar DT. Expression of gelatinases A and B, and TIMPs 1 and 2 during corneal wound healing. *Invest. Ophthalmol. Vis. Sci.* 1998; 39:913–921.
29. Hageman GS, Kirchoff-Rempe MA, Lewis GP, Fisher SK, Anderson DH. Sequestration of basic fibroblast growth factor in the primate retinal interphotoreceptor matrix. *Proc Natl Acad Sci USA* 1991; 88:6706–6710.
30. Ozerdem U, Cheng LY, Mach-Hofacre B, Chaidawangul S, McDermott C, Appelt K, Freeman WR. The effect of AG3340 a potent inhibitor of matrix metalloproteinases on a subacute model of proliferative vitreoretinopathy. *Invest. Ophthalmol. Vis. Sci.* (suppl.) 1999; 40: S974.
31. International Conference on metalloproteinases and their inhibitors in the nervous system: physiology and disease. Banff, Alberta, Canada. Feb. 27– Mar. 3, 1999.
32. Yong VW, Krekosk CA, Forsyth PA, Bell R, Edwards DR. Martix metalloproteinases and diseases of the CNS. *Trends Neurosci.* 1998; 21:75–80.
33. Clements JM, Cossins JA, Wells GM, Corkill DJ, Helfrich K, Wood LM, Pigott R, Stabler G, Ward GA, Gearing AJ, Miller KM. Matrix metalloproteinase expression during experimental autoimmune encephalomyelitis and effects of a combined matrix metalloproteinase and tumour necrosis factor-alpha inhibitor. *J. Neuroimmunol.* 1997; 74:85–94.
34. Maeda A, Sobel RA. Matrix metalloproteinases in the normal human central nervous system, microglial nodules, and multiple sclerosis lesions. *J. Neuropathol. Exp. Neurol.* 1996; 55:300–319.
35. Cuzner ML, Gveric D, Strand C, Loughlin AJ, Paemen L, Opdenakker G, Newcombe J. The expression of tissue-type plasminogen activator, matrix metalloproteases and endogenous inhibitors in the central nervous system in multiple sclerosis: comparison of stages in lesion evolution. *J. Neuropathol. Exp. Neurol.* 1996; 55:1194–1204.
36. Gijbels K, Galardy RE, Steinman L. Reversal of experimental autoimmune encephalomyelitis with a hydroxamate inhibitor of matrix metalloproteases. *J. Clin. Invest.* 1994; 94:2177–2182.
37. Hewson AK, Smith T, Leonard JP, Cuzner ML. Suppression of experimental allergic encephalomyelitis in the Lewis rat by the matrix metalloproteinase inhibitor Ro31-9790. *Inflamm Res* 1995; 44:345–349.
38. Chandler S, Miller KM, Clements JM, Lury J, Corkill D, Anthony DC, Adams SE, Gearing AJ. Matrix metalloproteinases, tumor necrosis factor and multiple sclerosis: an overview. *J Neuroimmunol* 1997; 72:155–161.
39. Deb S, Gottschall PE. Increased production of matrix metalloproteinases in enriched astrocyte and mixed hippocampal cultures treated with beta-amyloid peptides. *J. Neurochem.* 1996; 66:1641–1647.
40. Miyazaki K, Hasegawa M, Funahashi K, Umeda M. A metalloproteinase inhibitor domain in Alzheimer amyloid protein precursor. *Nature* 1993; 362:839–841.
41. LePage RN, Fosang AJ, Fuller SJ, Murphy G, Evin G, Beyreuther K, Masters CL, Small DH. Gelatinase A possesses a beta-secretase-like activity in cleaving the amyloid protein precursor of Alzheimer's disease. *FEBS Lett.* 1995; 377:267–270.
42. Robert AM, Godeau G. Action of proteolytic and glycolytic enzymes on the permeability of the blood-brain barrier. *Biomedicine* 1974; 21:36–39.
43. Rosenberg GA, Kornfeld M, Estrada E, Kelley RO, Liotta LA, Stettler-Stevenson, WG. TIMP-2 reduces proteolytic opening of blood-brain barrier by type IV collagenase. *Brain Res.* 1992; 576:203–207.
44. Romanic AM, White RF, Arleth AJ, Ohlstein EH, Barone FC. Matrix metalloproteinase expression increases after cerebral focal ischemia in rats. Inhibition of matrix metalloproteinase-9 reduces infarct size. *Stroke* 1998; 29:1020–1030.
45. Mun-Bryce S, Rosenberg GA. Gelatinase B modulates selective opening of the blood-brain barrier during inflammation. *Am. J. Physiol.* 1998; 274: R1203–1211.
46. Thompson RW, Baxter BT. MMP inhibition in abdominal aortic aneurysms. Rationale for a prospective randomized clinical trial. *Ann. N.Y. Acad. Sci.* 1999; 878:159–178.

47. Prescott MF, Sawyer WK, Von Linden-Reed J, Jeune M, Chou M, Caplan SL, Jeng AY. Effect of matrix metalloproteinase inhibition on progression of atherosclerosis and aneurysm in LDL receptor-deficient mice overexpressing MMP-3, MMP-12, and MMP-13 and on restenosis in rats after balloon injury. *Ann. NY Acad. Sci.* 1999; 878:179–190.

48. Loftus IM, Goodall S, Crowther M, Jones L, Bell PR, Naylor AR, Thompson MM. Increased MMP-9 activity in acute carotid plaques: therapeutic avenues to prevent stroke. *Ann. N.Y. Acad. Sci.* 1999; 878:551–554.

49. Newman KM, Malon AM, Shin RD, Scholes JV, Ramey WG, Tilson MD. Matrix metalloproteinases in abdominal aortic aneurysm: characterization, purification, and their possible sources. *Connect. Tissue Res.* 1994; 30:265–276.

50. Thompson RW, Holmes DR, Mertens RA, Liao S, Botney MD, Mecham RP, Welgus HG, Parks WC. Production and localization of 92-kilodalton gelatinase in abdominal aortic aneurysms. An elastolytic metalloproteinase expressed by aneurysm-infiltrating macrophages. *J. Clin. Invest.* 1995; 96:318–326.

51. McMillan WD, Patterson BK, Keen RR, Shively VP, Cipollone M, Pearce WH. In situ localization and quantification of mRNA for 92-kD type IV collagenase and its inhibitor in aneurysmal, occlusive, and normal aorta. *Arterioscler. Thromb. Vasc. Biol.* 1995; 15: 1139–1144.

52. Lee E, Grodzinsky AJ, Libby P, Clinton SK, Lark MW, Lee RT. Human vascular smooth muscle cell-monocyte interactions and metalloproteinase secretion in culture. *Arterioscler. Thromb. Vasc. Biol.* 1995; 15: 2284–2289.

53. Davis V, Persidskaia R, Baca-Regen L, Itoh Y, Nagase H, Persidsky Y, Ghorpade A, Baxter BT. Matrix metalloproteinase-2 production and its binding to the matrix are increased in abdominal aortic aneurysms. *Arterioscler. Thromb. Vasc. Biol.* 1998; 18:1625–1633.

Index

A

AAA, see Abdominal aortic aneurysm

Abdominal aortic aneurysm (AAA), matrix metalloproteinase role, 250, 251

AG3340, *see* Prinomastat

Age-related macular degeneration (AMD), matrix metalloproteinase inhibitor therapy, 247, 248

Alzheimer's disease, matrix metalloproteinase role, 249, 250

AMD, *see* Age-related macular degeneration

4-Aminophenylmercuric acetate (APMA), effects on procollagenase activity, 56

Angiogenesis,
matrix metalloproteinase inhibitor therapy in ophthalmology, 247–249
matrix metalloproteinase roles, 93, 94, 96, 97
prinomastat inhibition, 155–157
TIMP inhibitor suppression, 76

APMA, *see* 4-Aminophenylmercuric acetate

Apoptosis,
prinomastat effects, 154, 155
TIMP modulation, 74, 75

Arthritis, matrix metalloproteinase inhibitor therapy, 246

B

Barbiturate-derived matrix metalloproteinase inhibitors,
acylation of parent compound, 238, 239

collagenase-2 binding, 238
lack of sedative effects, 237
matrix metalloproteinase specificity, 241
optimization, 239–242
screening, 225, 237
structures, 240

Batimastat (BB-94),
angiogenesis prevention in eye, 247, 248
angioplasty restenosis prevention, 130
binding to matrix metalloproteinases, 119, 120
clinical trials, 131, 132
design, 114, 115
matrix metalloproteinase specificity, 114, 119
oral bioavailability, 121–123, 131
tumor inhibition studies, 92, 93, 128, 129, 131, 132

BAY 12-9566
arthritis trials, 246
binding to matrix metalloproteinases, 178
discovery, 178
matrix metalloproteinase specificity, 178, 179
phase I trials,
anticancer efficacy, 189, 190
pharmacokinetics, 186–188
safety and tolerability, 188, 189
phase III trials, 190
preclinical studies,
angiogenesis inhibition, 180, 182
metastasis inhibition,
breast cancer model, 185